OXFORD MEDICAL PUBLICATIONS

Paediatric Anaesthesia

Published and forthcoming Oxford Specialist Handbooks

General Oxford Specialist Handbooks
A Resuscitation Room Guide (Banerjee and Hargreaves)

Oxford Specialist Handbooks in End of Life Care
Cardiology: From advanced disease to bereavement (Beattie, Connelly, and Watson eds.)
Nephrology: From advanced disease to bereavement (Brown, Chambers, and Eggeling)

Oxford Specialist Handbooks in Anaesthesia
Cardiac Anaesthesia (Barnard and Martin eds.)
Neuroanaesthesia (Nathanson and Moppett eds.)
Obstetric Anaesthesia (Clyburn, Collis, Harries, and Davies eds.)
Paediatric Anaesthesia (Doyle ed.)

Oxford Specialist Handbooks in Cardiology
Cardiac Catheterization and Coronary Angiography (Mitchell, Leeson, W, and Banning)
Pacemakers and ICDs (Timperley, Leeson, Mitchell, and Betts eds.)
Echocardiography (Leeson, Mitchell, and Becher eds.)
Heart Failure (Gardner, McDonagh, and Walker)
Nuclear Cardiology (Kelion, Loong, and Sabharwal)

Oxford Specialist Handbooks in Neurology
Epilepsy (Alarcon, Nashef, Cross, and Nightingale)
Parkinson's Disease and Other Movement Disorders (Edwards, Bhatia, and Quinn)

Oxford Specialist Handbooks in Paediatrics
Paediatric Gastroenterology, Hepatology, and Nutrition (Beattie, Dhawan, and Puntis eds.)
Paediatric Nephrology (Rees, Webb, and Brogan)
Paediatric Neurology (Forsyth and Newton eds.)
Paediatric Oncology and Haematology (Bailey and Skinner eds.)
Paediatric Radiology (Johnson, Williams, and Foster)

Oxford Specialist Handbooks in Surgery
Hand Surgery (Warwick)
Neurosurgery (Samandouras)
Otolaryngology and Head and Neck Surgery (Corbridge and Warner)
Plastic and Reconstructive Surgery (Giele and Cassell eds.)
Renal Transplantation (Talbot)
Urology (Reynard, Sullivan, Turner, Feneley, Armenakas, and Mark eds.)
Vascular Surgery (Hands, Murphy, Sharp, and Ray-Chaudhuri)

Paediatric Anaesthesia

Edited by

Edward Doyle

Consultant Paediatric Anaesthetist,
Royal Hospital for Sick Children,
Edinburgh,
Scotland, UK

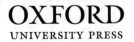
OXFORD
UNIVERSITY PRESS

OXFORD

UNIVERSITY PRESS

Great Clarendon Street, Oxford OX2 6DP

Oxford University Press is a department of the University of Oxford.
It furthers the University's objective of excellence in research, scholarship,
and education by publishing worldwide in

Oxford New York

Auckland Cape Town Dar es Salaam Hong Kong Karachi
Kuala Lumpur Madrid Melbourne Mexico City Nairobi
New Delhi Shanghai Taipei Toronto

With offices in

Argentina Austria Brazil Chile Czech Republic France Greece
Guatemala Hungary Italy Japan Poland Portugal Singapore
South Korea Switzerland Thailand Turkey Ukraine Vietnam

Oxford is a registered trade mark of Oxford University Press
in the UK and in certain other countries

Published in the United States
by Oxford University Press, Inc., New York

© Oxford University Press, 2007

British Library Cataloguing in Publication Data
Data available

Library of Congress Cataloging in Publication Data
Data available

Typeset by Newgen Imaging Systems (P) Ltd., Chennai, India
Printed in Italy
on acid-free paper by
Lego S.p.A.

ISBN 978–0–19–920279–9

10 9 8 7 6 5 4 3 2 1

Contents

Detailed contents

Section 2 Paediatric anaesthesia

4 Paediatric anaesthetic equipment   **79**
   Fiona Kelly

5 Practical procedures and postoperative care   **111**
   Francois Taljard

11 Congenital heart disease — 361

Anne Goldie

Section 6 Problems during anaesthesia, resuscitation, syndromes, and sedation

Contributors

Graham Bell
Consultant Paediatric Anaesthetist,
Royal Hospital for Sick Children,
Glasgow, UK

Alison Carlyle
Anaesthetic Department, Royal
Hospital for Sick Children,
Edinburgh, UK

Emma Dickson
Consultant Paediatric Anaesthetist,
Royal Hospital for Sick Children,
Edinburgh, UK

Pamela Eccles
Royal Hospital for Sick Children,
Edinburgh, UK

Anne Goldie
Consultant Paediatric Anaesthetist,
Royal Hospital for Sick Children,
Glasgow, UK

Fiona Kelly
Department of Anaesthesia, Royal
Hospital for Sick Children,
Edinburgh, UK

Volker Lesch
Consultant Anaesthetist,
Kantonsspital,
St. Gallen, Switzerland

Anthony Moores
Consultant Paediatric Anaesthetist,
Royal Hospital for Sick Children,
Glasgow, UK

Andrew Morrison
Fellow in Paediatric Anaesthesia,
Vancouver, British Columbia,
Canada

Manchula Navaratnam
Royal Hospital for Sick Children,
Glasgow, UK

Steve Roberts
Consultant Paediatric Anaesthetist,
Royal Liverpool Children's NHS
Trust, Liverpool, UK

Mandy Sim
Clinical Nurse Specialist, Royal
Hospital for Sick Children,
Edinburgh, UK

Carolyn Smith
Consultant Paediatric
Anaesthetist, Royal Hospital
for Sick Children,
Edinburgh, UK

Francois Taljard
Royal Hospital for Sick Children,
Edinburgh, UK

Symbols and abbreviations

♂	male
♀	female
↑	increase
↓	decrease
→	leading to
📖	cross reference
2,3 DPG	2,3-diphosphoglycerate
ACT	activated clotting time
ADH	antidiuretic hormone
ADHD	attention deficit hyperactivity disorder
AED	automated external defibrillator
AIDS	acquired immune deficiency syndrome
ALL	acute lymphoblastic leukaemia
AMC	arthrogryposis multiplex congenita
AML	acute myeloid leukaemia
APL valve	adjustable pressure limiting valve
APLS	advanced paediatric life support
ARF	acute renal failure
ASA	American Society of Anesthesiologists
ASD	atrial septal defect
ASIS	anterior superior iliac spine
ATP	adenosine triphosphate
AVSD	atrioventricular septal defect
BPD	bronchopulmonary dysplasia
BSA	body surface area
CAPD	continuous ambulatory peritoneal dialysis
CBF	cerebral blood flow
CBV	cerebral blood volume
CCPD	continuous cycling peritoneal dialysis
CHD	congenital heart disease
CMAP	compound muscle action potential
CMV	cytomegalovirus
CNS	central nervous system

CO	cardiac output
CO_2	carbon dioxide
CPAP	continuous positive airway pressure
CPB	cardiopulmonary bypass
CPK	creatinine phosphokinase
CRF	chronic renal failure
CPP	cerebral perfusion pressure
CPR	cardiopulmonary resuscitation
CSF	cerebrospinal fluid
CT	computerised tomography
CXR	chest radiograph
DA	ductus arteriosus
DDAVP	1-desamino-8-D-arginine vasopressin
DDH	developmental dysplasia of the hip
DHCA	deep hypothermic circulatory arrest
DLT	double lumen tube
DNA	deoxyribonucleic acid
DS	Down's syndrome
DV	ductus venosus
ECG	electrocardiogram
ECMO	extracorporeal membrane oxygenation
EEG	electroencephalogram
EMG	electromyogram
EMLA	eutectic mixture of local anaesthetics
ESR	erythrocyte sedimentation rate
ETT	endotracheal tube
FBC	full blood count
FG	French gauge
FFP	fresh frozen plasma
FO	foramen ovale
FRC	functional residual capacity
FVC	forced vital capacity
GFR	glomerular filtration rate
GOR	gastro-oesophageal reflux
Hb	haemoglobin
HbA	haemoglobin A
HbC	haemoglobin C
HbF	fetal haemoglobin

HbS	haemoglobin S
HDU	High Dependency Unit
HIV	human immunodeficiency virus
HVA	homovanillic acid
HME	heat and moisture exchanger
IAP	intra-abdominal pressure
ICP	intracranial pressure
ICU	Intensive care unit
IDDM	insulin dependent diabetes mellitus
IO	intraosseous
IOP	intraocular pressure
IPPV	intermittent positive pressure ventilation
ISO	International Organisation for Standardisation
IU	international units
IV	intravenous
IVC	inferior vena cava
IVH	intraventricular haemorrhage
JCA	juvenile chronic arthritis
KCl	potassium chloride
kPa	kilopascal
L	litre
LA	left atrium; local anaesthetic
LED	light emitting diode
LET	lidocaine, epinephrine and tetracaine mix
LMA	laryngeal mask airway
LV	left ventricle
LVH	left ventricular hypertrophy
MAC	minimum alveolar concentration
MAP	mean arterial pressure
mcg	microgram
MEPs	motor evoked potentials
MH	malignant hyperthermia
min	minute/s
mIBG	meta-iodo-benzyl guanidine
mL	millilitre
mmHg	millimetres of mercury
mmol	millimoles
mOsmol	milliosmoles

MPS	mucopolysaccharidosis
MRI	magnetic resonance imaging
MUA	manipulation under anaesthesia
ng	nanogram
NIPS	Neonatal/Infant Pain Scale
NSAID	non-steroidal anti-inflammatory drug
PA	pulmonary artery
PBF	pulmonary blood flow
PCA	postconceptual age
PCA	patient controlled analgesia
PCV	pressure controlled ventilation
PDA	patent ductus arteriosus
PDPH	post dural puncture headache
PEA	pulseless electrical activity
PEEP	positive end-expiratory pressure
PEFR	peak expiratory flow rate
PET	positron-emission tomography
PFC	persistent fetal circulation
PICU	paediatric intensive care unit
PNS	peripheral nerve stimulator
PONV	postoperative nausea and vomiting
PT	prothrombin time
PTT	partial thromboplastin time
PUJ	pelviureteric junction
PVR	pulmonary vascular resistance
RA	right atrium
RAE	Ring, Adair, and Elwyn endotracheal tube
RhF	rheumatoid factor
RSI	rapid sequence induction
RTI	respiratory tract infection
RV	right ventricle
sec	second/s
SCBU	special care baby unit
SPECT	single photon emission computed tomography
SSEPs	somatosensory evoked potentials
SV	stroke volume
SVC	superior vena cava
SVR	systemic vascular resistance

SVT	supraventricular tachycardia
t1/2	half life
tmax	time to maximum plasma concentration
TGA	transposition of the great arteries
TIVA	total intravenous anaesthesia
TMJ	temporomandibular joint
TT	thrombin time
U&E	urea and electrolytes
US	ultrasound
Vd	volume of distribution
VMA	vanillylmandelic acid
V-P	ventriculo-peritoneal
VSD	ventricular septal defect
vWD	von Willebrand's disease
vWF	von Willebrand factor
WCC	white cell count

Section 1

Physiology, pharmacology, and psychology

Anatomy, physiology, and psychology

Volker Lesch

Introduction

Providing safe anaesthesia for children requires a clear understanding of the anatomical, physiological, pharmacological, and psychological differences between patients in different age groups from premature neonates to adolescents. Several specific anatomical, physiological, pharmacological and psychological issues should be clearly understood when anaesthetising children.

Special consideration is needed for neonates. Neonates and infants are at much greater risk of morbidity and mortality than are older children—risk is generally inversely proportional to age.

The first two chapters of this book address aspects of anatomy, physiology, psychology, pharmacology, fluids, and electrolytes that are relevant to the practice of paediatric anaesthesia. Differences from adults are emphasized, rather than presenting material that is covered in general texts.

Upper airway

Several anatomical features of the neonatal and infant airway differ from that of adults and are important to the anaesthetist. These combine to make airway management and endotracheal intubation more difficult than in older children and adults. From about 4 years of age the anatomy is more adult and many of the airway problems associated with anaesthetizing children become less frequent.

Anatomy of the infant and neonatal airway
- Relatively large head
- Prominent occiput
- Short neck
- Relatively small mandible
- Larynx lies at the level of C3/4 rather than C5/6 seen in later life
- Relatively large tongue
- Relatively large epiglottis
- Cricoid ring is the narrowest part of the upper airway

- The size of the tongue means that there is less space in the infant airway and that they are prone to upper airway obstruction.
- The tongue may also complicate direct laryngoscopy. It may be difficult to displace anteriorly with the laryngoscope and often comes around the right hand edge of the blade unless this is introduced in the extreme right side of the mouth.
- The large head, prominent occiput, and cephalad larynx combine to produce a view of the larynx which is often described as 'anterior' but is actually cephalad compared with adults.
- The epiglottis (often described as U- or omega-shaped) may fall back over the laryngeal inlet if the tip of the laryngoscope blade is in the vallecula. A better view is usually obtained if the tip of the laryngoscope is positioned on the laryngeal surface of the epiglottis.
- The orientation of the vocal cords directs the tip of an endotracheal tube against the anterior wall of the trachea where it may hold up and can create the impression that the endotracheal tube is too wide to pass through the cricoid ring.
- Endotracheal tube diameter must be narrow enough not to exert pressure on the mucosa of the cricoid cartilage but also allow a seal adequate for IPPV with a minimal leak at a peak inflation pressure of 20 cm H_2O.
- The large tongue means that for the first few weeks of life neonates and infants preferentially breathe through the nose rather than the mouth. This imposes a resistance to ventilation that is ↑ in the presence of nasal congestion from infection or the presence of a foreign body such as a nasogastric tube, oxygen prongs, or an endotracheal tube. In the latter case, IPPV is routine in neonates because of the resistance to ventilation imposed by the endotracheal tube.

Lower airway

- The tracheal length, defined as the distance from the cricoid cartilage to the carina, may be as little as 4 cm and endobronchial intubation is a continuous hazard.
- Conversely, short endotracheal tubes are prone to unintentional displacement. 📖 See Chapter 4 for appropriate endotracheal tube sizes.
- At the carina left and right main bronchi diverge at the same angle and endobronchial intubation is as likely to be left-sided as right-sided. The alveoli are thick-walled and number only 10% of the adult total. The single terminal bronchiole opens into a single alveolus instead of a fully developed clustering.
- Horizontal alignment of the soft and pliable ribs prevents the 'bucket-handle' action of the adult thoracic cage. Weak intercostal and diaphragmatic muscles (due to a lack of type I fibres) with a more horizontal attachment and a protuberant abdomen result in less efficient ventilation than in adults. There is limited respiratory reserve and earlier onset of fatigue if the work of ventilation ↑ during anaesthesia or illness.
- Specific compliance of the respiratory system is similar in different age groups. Chest wall specific compliance, however, is higher in neonates and infants (0.06 mL/cm H_2O compared with 0.04 mL/cm H_2O) in adults because of the cartilaginous ribs and lack of chest wall muscula-ture. This explains why intercostal recession or even sternal recession occur so readily in neonates and young infants with ↑ respiratory effort and during episodes of airway obstruction.
- Upper and lower airways are susceptible to a large ↑ in airway resistance (and the work of breathing) in the event of narrowing that would be trivial in an adult.

Central nervous system

The CNS in the neonate is immature and differs from the adult and older child in several ways. These differences are relevant to general anaesthesia and regional techniques in neonates and infants.

Neonatal CNS
- Incomplete myelination of neurons
- Blood–brain barrier is not fully developed
- Lower termination of spinal cord
- ↑ volume of CSF

- At birth the brain weighs approximately 330–350 g (10–15% of body weight). Adult proportions (1200–1400 g ~ 2% of bodyweight) are reached around 12 years of age.
- The cerebral cortex is not fully developed and synaptic connections are not mature. Myelination and dendritic proliferation progress in the last 3 months of pregnancy and during the first years of life.
- The sutures are open and there is a large anterior fontanelle. Palpation of the anterior fontanelle can be used to evaluate intracranial pressure in neonates and infants. Increasing intracranial pressure is partly relieved by expansion of the fontanelles and separation of the suture lines so that head size ↑ before intracranial pressure rises.
- The blood–brain barrier is anatomically and functionally incomplete. Bilirubin, opioids, and barbiturates all cross freely into the CNS.
- In the preterm neonate cerebral vessels are at risk of rupture especially in the region of the germinal matrix close to the nucleus caudatus. The germinal matrix has a rich blood supply, scarce vascular supporting tissue, and thin vessel walls leading to a high chance of intracerebral and intraventricular hemorrhage. With increasing gestational age the germinal matrix involutes and the risk of bleeding ↓.
- The spinal cord of the fetus initially occupies the entire length of the spinal canal. Differential growth of the canal and spinal cord causes the termination of the cord to move cephalad relative to the vertebral canal. It is at the level of S1 at 28 weeks' gestation, L3 at term, L2/3 at 1 year, and the adult level of L1/L2 around the age of 8 years. The intercristal line in neonates is at the level of L5–S1 compared with L4 in adults and lumbar puncture is performed below this line. Ossification of the sacral vertebrae is not complete and sacral intervertebral epidural analgesia is feasible.
- The epidural space in the infant contains fat that is loculated with distinct spaces between individual lobules. This means that a catheter introduced into the epidural space via the sacral hiatus can often be threaded to thoracic level to provide epidural analgesia for thoracic dermatomes.
- The volume of CSF is proportionately greater than in adults (4 mL/kg compared with 2 mL/kg) and this partly explains the relatively higher dose requirements for local anaesthetic (LA) solution and shorter duration of subarachnoid analgesia. The sacral hiatus is relatively large compared with later life and is not ossified. For these reasons it provides easy access to the lower epidural space.

Respiratory physiology

The incidence of respiratory complications related to anaesthesia is much higher in neonates and infants than in older children and adults. This is largely a consequence of differences in respiratory physiology with age.

Table 1.1 Differences in respiratory parameters with age

Parameter	Neonate	Child	Adult
Respiratory rate (breaths/min)	40–60	20–30	16–24
Tidal volume (mL/kg)	7–8	7–8	7–8
Alveolar ventilation (mL/kg/min)	100–150		60
FRC (mL/kg)	30	30	30
Dead space (mL/kg)	2	2	2
Oxygen consumption (mL/kg/min)	6–9		2–3
Airway resistance (mL H_2O/L × sec)	40	20	2
Airway compliance (mL/cm H_2O)	5		100

Specific chest wall compliance, 📖 see page 6.

- Similar tidal volume in all age groups. The higher respiratory rate produces higher alveolar minute ventilation in children.
- Since a neonate's tidal volume is likely to be around 25 mL (7 mL/kg) and an adult's tidal volume is around 500 mL, the pressure required to cause this volume to flow in 1 sec is similar in both despite the higher airway resistance in neonates.
- The ratio of alveolar ventilation:FRC is 5:1 in neonates and infants (2:1 in adults). There is rapid uptake of volatile agents. Changes in the concentration of inspired gases are more rapidly reflected in alveolar and arterial values.
- Similar FRC to adults but closing volume is larger then FRC. Risk of atelectasis and tendency for V/Q mismatch with a fall in arterial oxygen tension. The small available intrapulmonary oxygen reservoir (relative to oxygen consumption) can lead to rapid desaturation in the event of airway obstruction or apnoea.
- FRC is reduced further during and for a period after anaesthesia. Physiological mechanisms to maintain FRC in neonates include partial adduction of the vocal cords during expiration (laryngeal braking), early termination of expiration (tachypnoea) and inspiratory muscle activity during expiration. All these mechanism are abolished by anaesthesia and FRC falls markedly from the value when awake. This reduces the reserve of oxygen available in the event of apnoea or airway obstruction and contributes to the rapid onset of hypoxia in infants and neonates.

- As the child grows chest wall compliance ↓ and FRC is maintained above closing volume from between 6–12 months of age.
- Continuous positive airway pressure (CPAP) improves oxygenation and reduces the work of breathing.
- Similar dead space in all age groups on a mL/kg basis. The dead space in anaesthetic equipment is more significant in relation to the small tidal volumes of neonates and infants.
- Ribs are horizontal rather than downward sloping as in adults. In adults a 'bucket handle' effect allows a significant ↑ in anteroposterior and lateral thoracic diameters when a deep breath is taken. In neonates and infants rib movement will not ↑ thoracic capacity and for this reason breathing is mainly diaphragmatic in neonates and infants.
- IPPV during anaesthesia is the norm. An ETT ↑ airway resistance much more than in adults because the wall of the ETT is proportionately much thicker and has a greater influence on airway diameter than an adult ETT.
- Immature respiratory control. The peripheral chemoreceptor response to hypoxia is weak. The central chemoreceptor response to CO_2 is blunted in premature infants. Neonates are prone to periodic breathing with apnoeic phases (2–10 sec). Longer apnoeic periods in the premature neonate, especially after anaesthesia.
- Sub-anaesthetic concentrations of anaesthetic drugs in the postoperative period alter ventilatory control.
- Insensible losses from the lungs are 15–20 mL/kg/day and heat is lost with this fluid.

Cardiovascular physiology

Fetal circulation

In the fetus (Fig. 1.1), gas exchange occurs in the placenta and there is preferential distribution of oxygenated blood to the brain and myocardium. This is achieved by the preferential streaming of oxygenated blood and the presence of intracardiac and extracardiac shunts. The fetal circulation is said to be 'shunt-dependent'.

Fetal blood flow

- Deoxygenated blood reaches the placenta in the umbilical arteries and returns to the fetus in the umbilical vein.
- pO_2 in the umbilical vein is around 4.5–5.0 kPa and fetal blood is 80–90% saturated.
- In the inferior vena cava (IVC), oxygenated blood from the placenta mixes with desaturated blood from the lower body.
- In the right atrium (RA), oxygenated blood from the IVC is directed across the foramen ovale (FO) and into the left atrium (LA). In the LA, the oxygen saturation of blood is around 65%.
- This well oxygenated blood enters the left ventricle (LV) and is ejected into the ascending aorta. The majority of the LV blood is delivered to the brain and coronary circulation.
- Desaturated blood from the IVC (lower body), SVC, and coronary sinus is directed across the tricuspid valve and into the right ventricle (RV). This blood is then pumped into the pulmonary artery (PA).
- Because of the high pulmonary vascular resistance (PVR) in utero, only about 12% of the RV output enters the pulmonary circulation. The remaining 88% passes through the ductus arteriosus (DA) into the descending aorta and the lower half of the body is supplied with relatively desaturated blood (pO_2 2.5–3.0 kPa).
- Oxygen delivery in the relatively hypoxic fetus is maximized by:
  - A high haemoglobin concentration (around 16 g/dL at term).
  - A high cardiac output (250–400 mL/kg/min at term).
  - The presence of fetal haemoglobin (HbF) that has a lower concentration of 2,3-diphosphoglycerate (2,3 DPG) than HbA and shifts the haemoglobin-oxygen dissociation curve to the left (P_{50} 3.6 kPa).

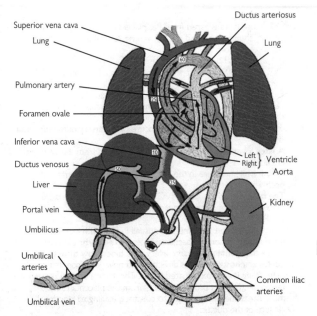

Fig. 1.1 Fetal circulation. Murphy PJ (2005). *Continuing Education in Anaesthesia, Critical Care, & Pain,* **5 (4)**, 107–12. Reproduced with permission from Oxford University Press/British Journal of Anaesthesia. Copyright: The Board of Management and Trustees of the British Journal of Anaesthesia.

Changes at birth

- Gas exchange is transferred from the placenta to the lungs, the fetal circulatory shunts close, and the left ventricular output ↑. With the onset of respiration:
  - pH and arterial oxygen tension rise.
  - PVR falls by 80% from prenatal levels within a few minutes of the start of ventilation.
  - Blood flow through the lungs and the left atrium ↑.
  - Left atrial pressure rises above right atrial pressure so closing the FO.
- With removal of the placenta and closure of the artery of the umbilical cord:
  - A large low resistance vascular bed is excluded from the systemic circulation.
  - SVR ↑ while pressure in the IVC and flow through the right atrium both ↓.
  - The fall in flow through the IVC and RA reduces RA pressure below that in the LA and contributes to functional closure of the FO.
  - The ↑ in SVR and the simultaneous fall in PVR with increasing flow in the pulmonary vascular bed lead to an aortic pressure above that in the pulmonary artery. The blood flow through the ductus arteriosus reverses direction and now goes from left to right, filling it with oxygenated blood. The ↑ local arterial oxygen tension and lack of prostaglandin E_2 from the placenta cause the muscular tissue of the ductus to constrict, leading to functional closure of the ductus.
  - Prostaglandin is used to open the ductus arteriosus in neonates with congenital heart defects where the systemic perfusion or the pulmonary blood flow depend on an open ductus e.g. coarctation of the aorta or pulmonary atresia. Conversely, the closure of the duct can be encouraged by administering prostaglandin inhibitors such as indomethacin or ibuprofen.

Transitional circulation

Under some circumstances, a normal neonatal circulation may revert to a fetal circulatory pattern (persistent fetal circulation).

- The main causes are hypoxia, hypercarbia, acidosis, and hypothermia.
- Classically associated with congenital diaphragmatic hernia, meconium aspiration, and significant respiratory distress of any cause.
- The pulmonary arterioles constrict in response to these stimuli. PVR rises and right to left flow through the functionally closed but anatomically patent FO and DA may resume. This worsens hypoxia and acidosis.

Neonatal and infant circulation

- The myocardium contains fewer contractile elements (30% versus 60% in adults) and more supporting tissue. The ventricles are less compliant when relaxed and can generate less tension during contraction. This limits the stroke volume. Therefore in neonates left ventricular end diastolic volume is relatively fixed and cardiac output is largely rate dependent.
- Reduced compliance and contractility of the ventricles lead to heart failure with increasing volume load.
- Bradycardia is not well tolerated and a neonatal heart rate below 60 beats/min does not provide adequate cardiac output. CPR should be initiated.
- Asystole is the commonest terminal rhythm. Ventricular fibrillation is very rare.
- Tachycardia is well tolerated and the neonate can cope with rates of up to 200 beats/min.
- Sinus arrhythmia is common but other irregular rhythms are abnormal.
- A term neonate has a functional autonomic and baroreceptor control mechanism; but parasympathetic tone mediated by the vagus predominates and they are prone to develop bradycardia (hypoxia, laryngoscopy).

Table 1.2 Cardiovascular parameters with age

Parameter	Neonate	Child	Adult
Heart rate (beats/min)			
Range	80–200	80–120	50–90
Average	120	100	75
Cardiac output (mL/kg/min)	200–250		80
Systolic pressure (mmHg)	50–90	95–110	95–140
Diastolic pressure (mmHg)	25–60	55–70	60–80
Estimated blood volume (mL/kg)	90	80	70

Neonatal compared with adult myocardial function

- Cardiac output: Heart-rate dependent
- Contractility: Reduced
- Starling response: Limited
- Compliance: Reduced
- Afterload compensation: Limited
- Ventricular interdependence: High

Hepatic physiology

Hepatic phase I and phase II reactions are not fully active in neonates and even less so in premature infants. Function matures rapidly after birth and from the age of about 2–3 months can be regarded as normal in healthy infants (and often exceeds that of adults).

- Phase I reactions include oxidation, reduction, and hydrolysis. These produce less active or inactive compounds that undergo phase II conjugation reactions such as glucuronidation (opioids) or sulphation (paracetamol) to produce polar compounds, which are eliminated in urine or via the gastrointestinal tract.
- Phase I reactions are catalyzed by the cytochrome P450 mixed function oxidase system which in neonates has about 28% of adult activity.
- Deficient phase I activity is also present for other systems such as alcohol dehydrogenase (chloral hydrate metabolism), plasma esterase (amino-ester LA metabolism), and N-acetyl transferase (isoniazid and hydralazine metabolism).
- The phase II reactions acetylation, glycination, and glucuronidation are very deficient at birth but sulphation is highly active. This pathway can metabolize opioids before glucuronidation matures and is also responsible for paracetamol metabolism in neonates.
- Bilirubin is produced from the breakdown of erythrocytes (80%) and from ineffective erythropoiesis (20%). The enzyme which catalyzes the transfer of glucuronic acid to bilirubin (uridine diphospho-glucuronyl transferase) to form glucuronides and allow excretion in bile has only 1% of adult values at term (this reaches adult values at 3–4 months of age).
- Physiological jaundice refers to a period from the second or third day of life lasting for about 10 days when most term and virtually all premature infants experience a period of unconjugated hyperbilirubinaemia. This is a consequence of high production (100–140 mcg /kg/day compared with 50–70 mcg/kg/day in adults) from erythrocyte breakdown (neonates are relatively polycythaemic), limited metabolism and excretion, and ↑ enterohepatic recirculation of bilirubin (due to limited capacity to form urobilinogen and urobilin).
- If this ↑ in plasma bilirubin concentration is excessive (>200 micromol/L) there may be damage to basal ganglia, cerebellum, and hippocampus comprising the syndrome known as kernicterus which results in cerebral palsy, mental handicap, and deafness (now very rare in the developed world).
- A number of factors ↑ the plasma bilirubin concentration and predispose to excessive jaundice:
  - Reduced albumin concentration.
  - The presence of drugs which are highly protein bound and displace bilirubin from plasma proteins.
  - Gestational diabetes.
  - Delayed passage of meconium.
  - Neonatal infection/sepsis.
  - Haemolysis.

- The commonest treatment to prevent this is phototherapy that converts unconjugated bilirubin to photoisomer products such as lumirubin that are excreted in bile or urine without the need for glucuronidation.
- Vitamin K-dependent clotting factors (II, VII, IX, and X) are low at term. Vitamin K is given to most neonates to prevent haemorrhagic disease of the newborn. It is important to ensure that this has been given during the preoperative assessment of a neonate.
- The ductus venosus, the connection between the inferior vena cava, portal vein, and umbilical veins, remains patent for 7–10 days after birth. This shunt bypasses the hepatic vessel bed and might ↓ the clearance of drugs metabolized in the liver. Drug metabolism and effect may be prolonged.
- Hepatic glucose storage is low and activity of the rate-limiting enzyme in gluconeogenesis (phospho-enolpyruvate carboxykinase) is around 10% of adult values. The neonate who is not feeding is prone to develop hypoglycaemia. Regular blood glucose measurements are required and a glucose infusion is usually necessary until enteral feeding is established.
- In clinical practice, the limited capacity of liver metabolism in the neonate or infant does not affect the practical conduct of anaesthesia very much. It is more relevant during the postoperative period when the metabolism and elimination of drugs—particularly opioids—may be limited and require modification of dosages, dosage intervals, or infusion rates. The perioperative care of neonates should include attention to glucose homeostasis and measurement of bilirubin so that, if necessary, phototherapy can be given.

Renal physiology

In utero the kidney is a quiescent organ and the placenta performs all necessary excretory functions. Nephrogenesis is complete in the term neonate but nephron formation continues after birth in the premature infant. Production of urine starts between 9 and 12 weeks of gestation. At term the kidneys produce approximately 20–30 mL/hour of filtrate. This constitutes a large part of the amniotic fluid.

- Glomerular filtration rate (GFR) is a function of postconceptual age and is both lower and slower to ↑ in premature than term neonates. High renal vascular resistance largely determines renal perfusion. There is a low renal blood flow at birth (6% of cardiac output increasing to 18–20% by one month) and a low GFR of 10 mL/min/1.73m^2 at birth.
- The renal blood flow and GFR approximately double during the 2nd to 4th week of life due to a fall in renal vascular resistance, loss of placental shunt and an ↑ in arterial blood pressure. The GFR is around 20–30 mL/min/1.73m^2 at 2 weeks of age. After 12 months, adult values relative to body surface area (120 mL/min/1.73m^2) are reached.
- The GFR of the neonate ↑ with fluid loading but there is limited ability to deal with a fluid load.
- Most renally filtrated drugs can be administered on a mg per kg basis after the 1st week of life.
- There is also limited tubular function despite complete nephron formation at term. Concentrating ability is limited (short loops of Henle, low urea concentration in the medullary interstitium, and limited sensitivity to anti-diuretic hormone) and the most concentrated urine which can be produced is only marginally more concentrated than plasma. Concentrating ability matures quickly and a urine osmolality of over 1000 mOsmol/L is possible by 2 months of age. The limited ability to concentrate urine is relevant if fluid administration is insufficient to handle dietary solutes and insensible water loss.
- Marked tubular immaturity leads to impairment in modifying the glomerular filtrate for conservation or excretion of solutes. There is a limited tubular capacity to absorb sodium and a relatively high renal loss of sodium, worse in the preterm. Adequate replacement in the region of 2–4 mmol/kg/day (5–10 mmol/kg/day in the preterm) is required. These losses might be ↑ by an excessive fluid intake when neonates tend to become hyponatraemic.
- Renal tubular mechanisms for acid excretion may be mature in the term child but not in the premature. This excretory capacity ↑ with gestational age. The renal threshold for bicarbonate is lower than in adults, which leads to plasma bicarbonate levels 16–20 mmol/L in preterm infants and 19–21 mmol/L in term neonates compared with 24–28 mmol/L in older children.
- Glucose reabsorption is limited in the preterm neonate and glycosuria may occur. The resulting osmotic diuresis in a patient with marked hyperglycemia may produce dehydration.

- Overall, neonates and young infants have limited renal mechanisms to maintain fluid, electrolyte and acid–base homeostasis in the face of derangements. These effects are more pronounced in the premature infant. These limitations of renal function require careful electrolyte and fluid administration in the neonatal period, frequent measurements of U&E and frequent assessments of fluid balance.

Central nervous system physiology

Cerebral metabolic rate, blood flow, oxygen requirements, and glucose (the main substrate for the CNS) consumption are all higher in small children than in older children and adults. This makes them particularly vulnerable to any interruption in perfusion of the brain during anaesthesia or at other times. The global CBF in children aged 6 months to 4 years is twice that of an adult. This is due to the accelerated cerebral development during this period. The low cerebral mass and metabolism in the preterm neonate is reflected in the low CBF.

Table 1.3 Cerebral metabolism in children and adults

Age	Cerebral blood flow	Oxygen consumption	Glucose requirement
Premature	40 mL/min/100 g		
Neonate	40–50 mL/min/100 g		
Child	100 mL/min/100 g	5.8 mL/min/100 g	6.8 mg/min/100 g
Adult	50 mL/min/100 g	3.5 mL/min/100 g	5.5 mg/min/100 g

- Cerebral perfusion pressure (CPP) equals mean arterial pressure (MAP) less central venous pressure (CVP) or intracranial pressure (ICP) (whichever is greater).

    CPP = MAP – ICP (or CVP)

- Autoregulation keeps CBF constant despite changes in CPP within an adult range of 50–150 mmHg. The thresholds of CPP autoregulation in the infant and young child are not known. Animal models suggest that the limits of autoregulation are lower than those in adults. Cerebral autoregulation might be compromised in severely ill children when blood flow becomes pressure dependent. Hypotension may induce cerebral ischemia.
- ICP in neonates and infants (2–5 mmHg) is lower than in older children and adults (8–18 mmHg). Chronic ↑ are absorbed to some extent by expansion of sutures and fontanelles. Acute ↑ cannot be compensated for in this way.
- Incomplete myelination of nerve tissue in neonates and infants allows effective blockade with low concentrations of LA solution. The concentration of lignocaine required to reduce the action potential by 50% in the myelinated A fibres of the sciatic nerve is 120 micromol/L in the newborn dog and 280 micromol/L in the adult dog. Similar values for bupivacaine are 19 and 27 micromol/L respectively. The fact that neonatal nerves and nerve roots can be blocked by very dilute solutions of LA is useful in light of the fact that pharmacokinetic factors mean that neonates are given lower doses of LA by bolus and infusion than older children (☐ Chapter 2, p.40).

- The sympathetic nervous system is likewise not fully developed and in children under the age of 6 years high sympathetic blockade from spinal or epidural anaesthesia usually causes little change in heart rate or blood pressure.
- In premature neonates the baroreceptor reflex is poorly developed and hypovolaemia results in little or no tachycardic response.

Thermal control

Temperature maintenance is particularly important during anaesthesia and surgery. Children are more prone to hypothermia than at other times and the consequences of this are important.

- Thermoregulatory mechanisms are inhibited during anaesthesia.
- There may be a reduction in metabolic heat production.
- Peripheral arteriovenous shunts open and heat is lost from the core to the periphery.
- Radiation to the environment usually accounts for 40–50% of heat loss and is proportional to the difference between body surface and ambient temperatures.
- Lower temperatures act directly on body enzymes and slow their speed of action.
- Oxygen consumption ↓ by 8% for each degree of temperature drop below 37°C.
- Hypothermia ↑ sympathetic stimulation and shivering and results in discomfort.
- It may also reduce drug metabolism, delay recovery from anaesthesia and impair coagulation.

Neonates

- Neonates are particularly sensitive to hypothermia because of proportionally ↑ heat loss, reduced ability to produce endogenous heat, and less efficient compensatory mechanisms. The range of ambient temperatures that neonates can tolerate without hypothermia is narrow. Premature infants are more at risk.
- In addition to the problems described, cold stressed infants may develop cardiovascular depression and hypoperfusion acidosis.
- They have relatively high losses of body heat (conduction, evaporation, convection, radiation) for several reasons:
  - ↑ thermal conduction to the environment because of thin skin and little or no insulating subcutaneous fat.
  - ↑ body surface area to body weight ratio (children with less than 0.5 m^2 body surface area are especially at risk of hypothermia).
  - High minute ventilation and insensible fluid loss with heat of vapourization.
- There are also relatively ineffective compensatory mechanisms:
  - Shivering is ineffective because infants have a limited muscle mass.
  - Limited vasoconstrictor response.
  - Non-shivering thermogenesis, in which triglycerides from adipose tissue in the shoulders and back known as brown fat which is rich in mitochondria is metabolised under adrenergic stimulation (via β3-adrenergic receptors). Adrenaline and noradrenaline stimulate uncoupled oxidative phosphorylation to produce heat rather than adenosine triphosphate (ATP). This is not an efficient process and ↑ oxygen consumption significantly. It compensates poorly for the lack of shivering and limited vasoconstriction compared with older children and adults.
  - Brown fat is deficient in premature neonates.

- Comparison of the neutral temperature (at which heat loss, oxygen demand and energy expenditure are minimal) and critical temperature (lowest sustained temperature compatible with survival) at different ages illustrates the difficulties for the neonate in maintaining an adequate body temperature (Table 1.4).
- Core temperature should be monitored during all procedures in neonates.
- Measures to reduce heat loss and actively warm neonates and infants are required to maintain core temperature above 36°C.

Table 1.4 Neutral and critical temperature in neonates and adults.

	Neutral temperature	Critical temperature
Preterm neonate	34°C	28°C
Neonate	32°C	23°C
Adult	28°C	1°C

Measures to maintain temperature in during anaesthesia and surgery

- Avoid unnecessary exposure. Cover neonates and infants with warm gamgee when exposed.
- Reduce the difference between patient and ambient temperature—operating theatre 20–22°C (26–28°C for neonates).
- Overhead radiant heater while neonates and infant are exposed for cannulation, intubation, and other preoperative procedures. Also used at the end of surgery when uncovered for extubation.
- Warm fluids for surgical skin preparation and irrigation.
- Warm intravenous fluids.
- Use of an active warming device—warming mattress and/or warm air blanket.
- Appropriate size disposable heat and moisture exchange filter to warm and humidify anaesthetic gases to some extent. These usually provide a relative humidity of over 50%. Passive airway humidification is more effective in children than in adults because of the higher minute ventilation per kg body weight.
- Use of a circle system.
- Active warming and humidification of inspired gases using a thermostatically controlled water reservoir and heating element in the inspiratory limb of the anaesthetic circuit.

Psychology, anxiety, and preoperative preparation

As well as purely medical preoperative considerations (☐ see Chapter 3) the anaesthetist approaching a child should be aware that considerable anxiety is often experienced by both child and parents about the proposed anaesthetic (and surgery or investigation). As well as explaining the proposed anaesthesia and analgesia, the anaesthetist may need to consider this anxiety during the preoperative assessment. The effects on children of hospitalization, anaesthesia, and surgery are not simple or predictable—significant cognitive and behavioural changes may occur after these procedures.

- Many children, particularly those operated on as day cases for relatively minor procedures with little postoperative pain, appear completely unaffected by the admission.
- On the other hand it is not uncommon to meet children and parents with vivid and distressing memories of previous anaesthetics (usually the induction) and great anxiety about the upcoming anaesthetic.
- Parental anxiety about their child undergoing anaesthesia and the risks of this is relatively common and when possible this can be allayed.
- Parents often have an exaggerated view of the risks of serious complications associated with anaesthesia for children and a simple explanation, if requested, of the true risks of cardiac arrest, brain damage, and death can give considerable reassurance.
- An assumption is often made that alleviating parental anxiety has beneficial effects for the child although there is little evidence to support this view.
- Children who undergo multiple procedures may be particularly distressed by repeated visits to theatre, although this is by no means always the case.

Developmental stages

Children have developmental stages and beliefs and fears at various ages.
- Birth–6 months:
  - The parents are usually more concerned than the child.
  - Infants tolerate separation from mother well as long as there is a surrogate mother.
  - Anxiolytic premedication is unnecessary.
- 6 months–4 years:
  - Separation anxiety (from parents) is usually prominent.
  - May be frightened by strange environment.
  - Aware that something unusual is happening but may not understand explanations.
  - Preoperative preparation is important.
  - Anxiolytic premedication is occasionally helpful.
- 4–6 years:
  - Communication and explanations are now easier.
  - Used to adults other than parents from nursery and school etc.
  - Understand some simple explanations.
  - Fear of unknown and strangers.
  - Separation anxiety remains prominent.
  - Occasional misconceptions of surgical procedure and effects of surgery on appearance.
  - Premedication may be helpful.
- 6–13 years:
  - Concerns about loss of autonomy and self-control.
  - Occasional fears about death.
  - Concerns about awareness during anaesthesia.
  - Occasional misconceptions and concerns about extent of surgery and postoperative appearance and scarring.
  - Premedication can be helpful.

These issues affect the manner in which each patient and parents are approached. To provide the child with as smooth a perioperative course as possible a multifaceted approach is needed (Chapter 3).

Preoperative preparation and parents in the anaesthetic room

There are several common methods of attempting to reduce anxiety in children and parents.

● Preoperative preparation. Explanatory leaflets or booklets sent with the appointment letter, hospital visits before the day of surgery where one or more of explanatory videos, parties with role play, guided tours of ward and anaesthetic room (when not in use), and explanations about coming into hospital are used to familiarize children and parents with the hospital environment and the processes involved in an admission for elective surgery.

● Parental presence at induction of anaesthesia. This is now very common and is routine in many UK centres even for non-elective surgery. At its best the anxiety of child and parents is relieved, the child does not suffer separation anxiety, and the parents feel that they have done all that is possible for the child during the preoperative period. At the other end of the spectrum some parents transmit their own anxieties to the child and fail to reassure them and neither child nor parents derive any benefit from their presence. The following matters are important when parents come to the anaesthetic room with a child:

  • Understanding, and acceptance by the parents of the proposed plan for induction of anaesthesia e.g. intravenous or gaseous induction, preoxygenation if indicated, and the possible need for restraint of the child during a gaseous induction.
  • Easily accessible anaesthetic rooms.
  • Continuing support by a member of staff for the parents once they have left the anaesthetic room.

● Dedicated members of staff known as play specialists often perform extensive preoperative preparation of children to explain the likely sequence of events after admission and familiarize them with relevant equipment such as face masks, oximeter probes, ECG leads, and monitoring screens. They may organize the preoperative visits, bring children and parents to the anaesthetic room from the ward, and return with the parents to the ward from the anaesthetic room.

● Use of sedatives and anxiolytics. Despite the various methods of preoperative preparation, a significant number of children remain anxious and uncooperative during the preoperative period. It is humane to offer these children a short-acting oral anxiolytic such as midazolam (0.5 mg/kg; maximum 20 mg) to reduce distress.

● There is little which can be done in the way of preoperative preparation for emergency cases other than a brief explanation to the parents about procedures in the anaesthetic room. For non-elective cases that are not true emergencies then some element of preoperative preparation is often possible as is anxiolytic premedication.

Paediatric pharmacology and fluid administration

Volker Lesch

Paediatric pharmacology

- There are important differences between adults and children in the response to drugs, including anaesthetic and analgesic agents.
- These differences are most pronounced and clinically important in neonates, premature babies, and infants up to the age of 3–6 months. After this age most differences are not clinically significant.
- Differences are pharmacokinetic, pharmacodynamic, or both.
- Relevant pharmacokinetic differences include:
  - Age-dependent body composition which influences drug distribution. A higher proportion of body weight is water in neonates (80%) and premature babies (90%) and there is a larger volume of distribution for water soluble drugs.
  - The relative size of body fluid compartments in infants and young children are different from those in adults. The extracellular fluid comprises 45% of body weight at birth and 25% at 1 year of age.
  - The large extracellular fluid compartment. Drugs that are distributed in this space may need to be given in a larger dose expressed as mg/kg to achieve a given plasma concentration e.g. digoxin, theophylline.
  - Lower total plasma protein levels and lower levels of specific proteins especially α-1-acid glycoprotein lead to less protein binding. The free fraction of many drugs in the plasma is high. Lower doses of some drugs (e.g. barbiturates) are needed.
  - Neonates have little fat or muscle tissue. Drugs that are normally rapidly redistributed to these tissues may have a high initial peak plasma concentration.
  - Immature renal and hepatic function (📖 Chapter 1).

Pharmacokinetics

- In neonates and infants, most drugs are metabolized and eliminated slowly. They tend to accumulate with repeated doses or during infusions. This is a consequence of reduced protein binding, large volumes of distribution, prolonged half-lives, and reduced clearances.
- The processes involved in pharmacokinetics are absorption, distribution, metabolism, and elimination. There are differences in all of these processes in neonates and infants compared with older children and adults.
- Volume of distribution (V_d):
  - The volume of distribution is an 'apparent' volume derived from the total amount of drug in the body divided by its concentration in plasma.
  - Increased body water results in a large V_d for water soluble drugs.
  - A drug that is lipid soluble and widely distributed will have a low plasma concentration and a large volume of distribution. Reduced protein binding results in an increased volume of distribution.
  - A large V_d implies high tissue uptake of a drug which leaves only a small fraction of the drug in the plasma where it is accessible to clearance processes.
  - The larger the V_d, the longer the elimination half-life.
- Half-life ($t_{1/2}$):
  - The time taken for the plasma concentration of a drug to decline to 50% of its original concentration is the elimination half-life.
  - To remove a drug from the circulation completely five half-lives are required.
  - For most drugs, this time is prolonged in neonates and infants compared with adults.
- Clearance:
  - Plasma clearance is the volume of plasma cleared of a drug in unit time. It is proportional to the volume of distribution.
  - Reduced in neonates and infants.

Absorption

- Inhalational and IV drugs are absorbed normally.
- Slow absorption from IM or subcutaneous depots in neonates. Regional blood flow may be reduced by cold or hypovolaemia.
- Relevant to IM injections e.g. ketamine or opioid analgesia and subcutaneous infusions e.g. opioids.
- This is one of the reasons these routes are rarely used in neonates.

Distribution

- Movement of a drug from the blood into the various body compartments.
- High cardiac output means rapid distribution.

- Protein binding limits the amount of drug able to diffuse from the blood to the extracellular fluid and act on receptors or tissues. Protein binding in neonates and young infants is reduced and free concentrations are increased.
  - There are reduced concentrations of plasma proteins.
  - Persisting fetal albumin has a reduced affinity for drugs.
  - Increased concentrations of unconjugated bilirubin compete for binding sites with acidic drugs.
  - A tendency to acidosis which results in increased concentrations of free drugs.
- Increased body water and extracellular fluid volume increase the volume of distribution of highly ionized drugs notably neuromuscular blockers.
- The blood–brain barrier is less well developed and there is a greater uptake from blood of partially ionized drugs such as morphine.

Metabolism

- The conversion of lipid soluble drugs to water soluble compounds that can be excreted.
  - Phase I reactions include oxidation, reduction, and hydrolysis.
  - Phase II reactions involve conjugation—glucuronidation, methylation, and sulphation.
- The concentrations and activities of the enzymes involved are reduced. Conjugation processes are immature in small infants and are only fully developed after about 3 months.
- Hepatocellular enzyme activity and hepatic blood flow are the main determinants of the rate of metabolism of a drug by the liver. Hepatic blood flow can be reduced in the infant by increased abdominal pressure, cardiac failure and, in the first postnatal days, a patent ductus venosus.
- These factors explain why half-lives of liver-dependent drugs in the neonate and small infant are generally longer than in the older population.
- Older infants and children demonstrate rapid elimination of some drugs due to mature enzyme activity and high hepatic blood flow.
- Non-specific esterase activity in plasma and other tissues is reduced in neonates but this does not produce a clinically significant effect.
- Hofmann degradation is independent of age.

Excretion

- Most drugs and metabolites are excreted by the kidneys.
- The relevant processes are glomerular filtration and tubular secretion.
- Glomerular filtration rate relative to surface area is reduced in neonates and increases to adult values during the first year.
- Proximal tubular secretion reaches adult values by 6 months of age.
- Excretory capacity is usually similar to older children by 6 months of age.

Intravenous anaesthetic agents

Propofol

- Used for induction, maintenance of anaesthesia, and sedation.
- Usually preferred to thiopental for induction in short cases because of the improved quality of early recovery from anaesthesia compared with thiopental
- Induction: 3–5 mg/kg in infants, 1.5–2.5 mg/kg in children (not recommended for induction under 1 month of age or for maintenance if aged <3 years).
- Causes more pronounced hypotension, respiratory depression, and suppression of pharyngeal and laryngeal reflexes than an equipotent dose of thiopental.
- Recovery is initially due to redistribution but metabolism and elimination are quicker than with thiopental.
- Advantages:
- Facilitates LMA insertion.
  - Rapid, clear headed emergence after brief procedures.
  - Anti-emetic properties.
- Drawbacks:
  - Pain on injection distresses most children and lignocaine (0.2 mg/kg) is usually added to prevent this.
  - If used for maintenance of anaesthesia there is no objective measurement of plasma concentration, unrecognized infusion pump failure, disconnection, or extravenous injection might lead to awareness.
  - Propofol infusion syndrome (metabolic acidosis, rhabdomyolysis, life-threatening cardiac failure, cardiac arrest) has been described after the use of propofol by infusion for sedation of children in ITU. Now contraindicated for this use.

Thiopental

- Short-acting agent for induction of anaesthesia, potent anticonvulsant by bolus or infusion.
- Reduced dose required in neonates.
- Induction : neonate 2–4 mg/kg, child 5–6 mg/kg.
- Plasma protein binding is reduced in neonates and the unbound fraction is twice that in older children, partly explaining the reduced dose required.
- Recovery is due to redistribution. Reduced clearance and prolonged elimination half-life of 19 hours in neonates compared with 6–12 hours in older children.
- Hypotension and respiratory depression are dose related and more pronounced in hypovolaemic patients.

Ketamine

- A phencyclidine derivative that acts as an antagonist at NMDA receptors. Produced as a racemic mixture and as the S(+)-enantiomer.
- Produces dissociative anaesthesia characterized by catalepsy, catatonia, and amnesia. The eyes may remain open and display nystagmus.
- Ketamine has potent analgesic properties.
- Can be given IV, IM, or orally.
- Induction: 1–2 mg/kg IV or 5–10 mg/kg IM (onset in 3–5 min).
- Anaesthesia after a single IV dose lasts 5–10 min (15–30 min after IM). The analgesic effect lasts longer. To prolong anaesthesia a further bolus of half the original dose can be given, an infusion started (20–40 mcg/kg/min) or a volatile agent used.
- Dose for analgesia: 0.25–0.5 mg/kg IV.
- Rapid redistribution, metabolized in liver to norketamine. Clearance depends on hepatic blood flow. Elimination half life is approximately 3 hours. Neonates have a larger apparent V_d and a lower clearance than older children.
- Advantages:
  - IM route is very useful in some situations.
  - Has sympathomimetic effects which usually prevent hypotension. Elevation of blood pressure and heart rate is mediated by the release of endogenous catecholamines. Effect is not dose-dependant.
  - Airway is maintained. Some preservation of protective airway reflexes but not guaranteed to protect against aspiration.
  - Minimal respiratory depression compared with thiopentone and propofol.
  - Has a bronchodilator effect.
- Drawbacks:
  - Increased salivation and airway secretions. An antisialogue (atropine 20 mcg/kg or glycopyrronium bromide 5–10 mcg/kg) is usually given concurrently.
  - Distressing nightmares or hallucinations on emergence (may be prevented by benzodiazepines).
  - High incidence of PONV.
  - Tolerance develops after repeated ketamine anaesthetics.
- Ketamine is also used in postoperative pain management in combination with opioids by infusion or PCA to influence opioid tolerance.
- Preservative free ketamine is often added to LA solutions for caudal epidural use (📖 Chapter 8).

Inhalational anaesthetic agents

Nitrous oxide

- As in adults, used commonly as a carrier gas for volatile anaesthetic agents. Traditionally used to reduce the percentage of volatile required to achieve an effect in younger children who are particularly susceptible to myocardial depression and bradycardia (reduced cardiac output) from volatile agent—'*The heart is sensitive, the brain is resistant*'.
- Mild cardiovascular depression in neonates.
- Faster uptake in infants and young children compared with adults.
- Also used to provide procedural analgesia as a 50% mixture with oxygen—Entonox® or Equanox®.
- Use is declining:
  - Adverse effects caused by absorption into air filled spaces causing increased pressure in non-compliant spaces e.g. middle ear and expansion of compliant spaces e.g. pneumothorax, cuff of ETT.
  - Causes PONV.
  - Potential toxicity due to effects on methionine synthetase and vitamin B_{12} during prolonged administration.
  - Relatively contraindicated for many procedures—laparoscopic surgery, bowel surgery, middle ear surgery, some ophthalmic procedures, emphysema.
  - Ready availability of piped air.

Volatile anaesthetic agents

- Indications and contraindications are similar to those in adults.
- Metabolism similar.
- Sevoflurane is the commonest agent for inhalational induction but halothane is still used especially for airway surgery or the potentially difficult airway.
- Isoflurane and desflurane are unsuitable for inhalational induction.
- All cause a degree of cardiovascular depression.
- All decrease airway resistance by direct relaxation of bronchial smooth muscle.
- MAC values of volatiles vary with age. Infants and small children need higher concentration of volatiles; premature babies and neonates need less.
- Contraindicated if previous malignant hyperthermia (MH), suspected MH, family history or risk factors for MH.

Table 2.1 MAC value and age

	Sevoflurane	Isoflurane	Desflurane	Halothane
Preterm		1.3		
Neonate	3.3	1.6	9.1	0.9
Infant	3.2	1.9	9.4	1.2
Child	2.5	1.6	8.6	0.9
Adult	2.0	1.16	6.0	0.76

Sevoflurane

- Commonest agent for inhalational induction in the UK. Its lack of pungency means that a concentration of 8% can be used from the start which speeds induction.
- Significant respiratory depression or apnoea at high concentrations. Its relatively low potency means that, in some cases, the child may be apnoeic but still too light the have the airway instrumented.
- Delirium and distress on emergence after maintenance with sevoflurane is sometimes seen in children.
- Unlike all the other volatiles it is not metabolized to trifluroacetate which stimulates formation of antibodies and immune-mediated hepatitis.

Isoflurane

- The commonest agent for maintenance.
- Little or no concern about coronary vasodilatation and 'coronary steal' in children.

Desflurane

- Useful for maintenance in prolonged anaesthesia with IPPV.
- In most children too irritant for induction or spontaneous ventilation.

Halothane

- Its potency and smoothness make halothane useful for management of a potentially difficult airway and in the provision of anaesthesia for airway endoscopy.
- When used in high concentrations for management of airway problems, dysrhythmias are much less of a problem in young children than in adults.
- As a potent bronchodilator it is very useful in severe asthma or in a child with irritable airways caused by a viral infection.

Neuromuscular blockers

- The neuromuscular junction in the neonate is immature and maximal acetylcholine release is limited (one third of that in adults).
- The volume of distribution of neuromuscular blockers is relatively large because of the large extracellular volume and the half-life is prolonged.
- A similar dose in mg/kg results in lower plasma concentrations than in adults. Despite this the response is similar because of lower acetylcholine levels. Clinically, neuromuscular blockers are given in similar doses to all age groups. The highest doses are required by small children.
- The main difference between neonates/young infants and older children/adults is that organ-dependent elimination takes longer and the duration of action is prolonged (not atracurium and mivacurium).
- Because of the respiratory physiology of the neonate—high alveolar ventilation, high closing capacity, high oxygen consumption—even a minor degree of residual paralysis can compromise oxygenation severely.

Suxamethonium

- Used mostly as part of a rapid sequence induction. Use is declining because of increasing concern about side effects and the availability of suitable alternative drugs e.g. mivacurium and techniques e.g. TIVA for rigid bronchoscopy.
- Higher are doses are needed to reach sufficient plasma levels with the high volume of distribution in small children.
- Dose 3 mg/kg in neonates, 2 mg/kg in infants, 1–1.5 mg/kg in older children; onset 60 sec; duration 4–6 min.
- Duration of action is similar in all age groups.
- Fasciculations are often not seen especially in young children.
- Side effects and contraindications are the same as in adults.

Non-depolarizers

- Indications, contraindications and side effects similar to adults.
- Onset of action often very quick in young children because of their relatively high cardiac output.
- Choice is often a matter of personal preference.

Aminosteroid compounds

- Vecuronium. Dose 0.1 mg/kg; onset 90 sec–3 min; duration 30–50 min.
- Rocuronium. Dose 0.2 mg/kg; onset 2–3 min; duration 30–45 min. For rapid sequence induction 0.9–1 mg/kg; onset 60–90 sec; duration 60 min.

Benzylisoquinolinium compounds

- Atracurium. Dose 0.5 mg/kg; onset 1.5–2 min; duration 30 min. A cutaneous reaction to histamine release is often seen but systemic reactions are very rare.
- Mivacurium. Dose 0.2 mg/kg; onset 1.5–2 min; duration 10–15 min.

Opioids

- Lower clearance and longer half-life in neonates.
- Immature liver metabolism and immature blood–brain barrier. Similar plasma level of morphine lead to higher concentrations in the CNS of neonates and young infants compared with older children and adults.

Morphine sulphate
Dose
- Intraoperative: 100–150 mcg/kg IV; 25–50 mcg/kg IV if <3 months of age.
- Postoperative: 10–40 mcg/kg/hour by infusion; 5–20 mcg/kg/hour if <3 months of age; bolus dose 20 mcg/kg for PCA; 200–300 mcg/kg oral 2–4-hourly (maximum 15 mg).

Diamorphine
- Full name 3,6-diacetylmorphine. Acts as a prodrug and is metabolized to morphine.
- Very potent and has a rapid onset because of high lipid solubility.
- Can be given by the intranasal route in children >1 year of age. May be used in the emergency department for fractures if venous access is difficult.
- Can be used as an additive to a LA solution for epidural infusion.
- More commonly used in the palliative and terminal care setting than in anaesthesia.

Dose
- Intraoperative: 50–100 mcg/kg IV.
- Intranasal: 100 mcg/kg in 0.2 ml 0.9% saline.

Codeine phosphate
- Used for mild to moderate pain. Acts as a prodrug and approximately 10% is converted to morphine after administration.
- Administered IM, orally or rectally. Not given IV.

Dose
- Intraoperative: 0.5–1 mg/kg IM; not given to neonates and young infants because it may not be absorbed completely and leave a depot.
- Postoperative: 1 mg/kg oral 4-hourly; 0.5 mg/kg oral 4-hourly aged <6 months (maximum 60 mg).

Fentanyl citrate
- Alternative to morphine sulphate for intraoperative use.
- Rarely used intravenously or orally postoperatively.
- Common additive to a LA solution for epidural infusion (📖 Chapter 6).

Dose
- Intraoperative: 2–4 mcg/kg IV; 1–2 mcg/kg IV if <3 months of age.
- Infusion: 5–10 mcg/kg/hour. Largely superseded by remifentanil for infusion.

Remifentanil
- Used by infusion intraoperatively or as a bolus to facilitate endotracheal intubation.
- Elimination by plasma and tissue esterases means that its effects will wear off rapidly and predictably even in neonates since glucuronidation is not required.

Dose
- Intraoperative: 0.25–0.5 mcg/kg/minute.
- Bolus: 0.1–1 mcg/kg (bradycardia and muscular rigidity may occur).

Non-steroidal anti-inflammatory drugs (NSAIDs)

- NSAIDs probably have a higher analgesic potency than paracetamol.
- Commonest for perioperative use in children are ibuprofen and diclofenac sodium.
- Not licensed below 5 kg or 3 months (ibuprofen) and 1 year (diclofenac) but are frequently used off licence.
- Similar indications and contraindications as in adults.
  - Absolute contraindications: gastrointestinal bleeding, peptic ulcers, allergy, coagulation disorders, renal impairment, hypovolaemia, and NSAID/aspirin sensitive asthma. Aspirin is not used in children under 12 years of age where it is associated with Reyes syndrome. Asthma is not regarded as a contraindication.
  - Relative contraindications: surgery with high risk for diffuse bleeding (tonsillectomy, adenoidectomy, cleft palate repair, neurosurgery, and craniofacial surgery). These vary from hospital to hospital.
  - Rarely used for analgesia in neonates because of the effects on renal prostaglandins and perfusion of the immature kidney.
  - Short term perioperative use in healthy children causes very few side effects.

Diclofenac sodium
Dose
- 1 mg/kg oral 8-hourly (maximum 50 mg); 1–2 mg/kg rectal (maximum 100 mg); 1 mg/kg IV. Maximum by all routes 3 mg/kg/day or 150 mg/day.

Ibuprofen
- Often given preoperatively as an analgesic premedication.

Dose
- 5–10 mg/kg oral 6-hourly. Maximum 400 mg single dose or 40 mg/kg/day.

Paracetamol

- Analgesic and anti-pyretic.
- Commonest analgesic drug in children.
- Sulphation rather than glucuronidation is the most important metabolic pathway in neonates.
- Rectal administration results in slow absorption and has very variable bioavailability depending on the patient and the preparation of paracetamol. Often associated with sub-therapeutic plasma levels even after a dose of 30 mg/kg.
- IV administration is preferable to rectal when the oral route is unavailable.

Dose
- Oral: loading dose 20 mg/kg followed by 15 mg/kg 4-hourly.
- IV: 15 mg/kg 6-hourly.
- Rectal: loading dose 40 mg/kg (20 mg/kg in neonates) followed 20 mg/kg 6-hourly.
- Maximum dose by oral and rectal routes 90 mg/kg/day above 3 months of age (4 g/day in adolescents); 60 mg/kg/day in neonates and infants up to 3 months of age. 60 mg/kg/day IV.

Local anaesthetics

- Lower levels of albumin and α-1-acid glycoprotein in neonates and young infants. Lower protein-binding and increased free or unbound fraction.
- Larger volume of distribution and longer half-life compared with adults.
- The large volume of distribution decreases peak plasma levels after a single injection but increases the risk of accumulation with multiple doses or infusion.
- Bupivacaine, levobupivacaine, and ropivacaine are given in reduced doses in neonates and infants up to 6 months of age. The 'free' fraction in plasma is higher due to lower levels of α-1-acid glycoprotein and albumin. The dose is arbitrarily reduced to 50% that used in older children.
- Prilocaine is avoided in infants <3 months of age. There is a risk of methaemoglobinaemia produced by the metabolite 4,6-hydro-xytoluidine (a potent oxidizing agent) in the presence of reduced activity of the enzyme methaemoglobin reductase (full activity is reached at about 3 months of age).

Table 2.2 Maximum doses of LA in children

Drug	Bolus mg/kg	Bolus <6 months mg/kg	Infusion mg/kg/hour	Bolus <6 months mg/kg/hour
Levobupivacaine	2.5	1.25	0.4	0.25
Ropivacaine	3.0	1.5	0.4	0.25
Bupivacaine	2.5	1.25	0.4	0.25
Lidocaine	3.0–7.0	1.5		
Prilocaine	6–10	3-5		

- In case of toxicity cerebral signs usually appear before cardiovascular collapse in patients who are not anaesthetized e.g. postoperative epidural infusion. Since most regional techniques are performed in anaesthetized children the first manifestation of toxicity is often cardiovascular. Treatment is discussed in Chapter 8.

Fluid balance and fluid administration

- Total body water content is large in neonates and infants. Comparable to adult values after the age of 1 year.
- As the amount of muscle mass rises, intracellular water content rises.
- Water turnover in the infant is more then double that of an adult. In infants approximately 40% of extracellular water is lost every day as urine, stool, sweat, and insensible losses via skin and airways and lungs. Dehydration can easily follow a reduction of intake or increased loss of fluids.

Table 2.3 Body water and blood volume with age

	Water % body weight	Extracellular volume % body weight	Blood volume ml/kg
Premature	90	60	100
Term neonate	80	40–45	90
1 year	60	25–30	80
Adult	55	18	70

- Clinical assessment of fluid balance in children is aided by recognition of situations where deficits are likely:
  - Gastrointestinal losses, vomiting, diarrhoea, pancreatitis
  - Ileus
  - Sepsis
  - Burns
  - Trauma
  - Postoperative bleeding.
- Hypovolaemia and dehydration are diagnosed clinically
  - Capillary refill time prolonged to >2 sec
  - Tachycardia (can also be caused by pain, fever, anxiety)
  - Oliguria
  - Cool peripheries
  - Increased core-peripheral temperature gap
  - Sunken fontanelle
  - Thready pulse
  - Reduced level of consciousness 'the child that is confused might not be perfused'
  - Hypotension is a late sign; often occurs only after >30% of blood volume is lost.
- Shock is the clinical state when demand is higher then delivery of oxygen and nutrition to the cells.

Preoperative fluids and fluid resuscitation

- Replace circulating volume with crystalloids (0.9% saline, Hartmann's solution) or colloids (plasma protein solution, Gelofusine or a starch solution). Blood products are given for major or ongoing losses.
- Extracellular fluid losses are replaced with isotonic crystalloid solution e.g. 0.9% saline, Hartmann's solution.
- Some situations are managed according to a local protocol e.g. burns, pyloric stenosis, diabetic ketoacidosis.
- Blood volume is estimated at 90 mL/kg in neonates, 85 mL/kg in infants and 80 mL/kg in children.
- In shock give fluid boluses of 20 mL/kg crystalloid or colloid then reassess.
- After 40, 60, and 80 mL/kg without stabilization (depends on the dynamics of the clinical situation and expected ongoing losses) consider endotracheal intubation, inotropic support, and blood products.
  - Consider blood after 15–20% of circulating volume is lost.
  - Consider fresh frozen plasma after 50% of circulating volume is lost.
  - Consider platelets after 100% of circulating volume is lost.
  - Rapid laboratory testing for specific factors and selective replacement may minimize blood product administration and the associated risks and costs.

Intraoperative fluid administration

- Required to replace a fluid deficit if any, provide maintenance requirements and replace intraoperative losses.
- Fluid deficits are rarely a problem for elective cases. Current fasting times are relatively brief and IV fluids are given to children unable to drink. Some non-elective cases may come to theatre with a fluid deficit but in most cases this is dealt with during preoperative resuscitation and preparation.
- Maintenance fluids during surgery can be given as a dextrose-containing solution or as a dextrose-free crystalloid e.g. Hartmann's solution or 0.9% saline. The latter approach is preferable.
  - Glucose containing fluids are usually unnecessary other than in premature babies, neonates, and some other at risk children e.g. those receiving parenteral nutrition.
  - Hypoglycaemia is rare in healthy children during anaesthesia and surgery. Most children show an increase in plasma glucose concentration during the perioperative period as part of the response to fasting and surgery.
  - Fluids containing 4% or 5% dextrose usually cause hyperglycaemia during surgery.
  - Glucose containing solutions are isotonic when administered but once the glucose is metabolized they become hypotonic and effectively result in the administration of free water. There is a risk of hyponatraemia if hypotonic solutions are given.
  - ADH is secreted during the perioperative period (stress, pain, hypovolaemia, drugs) and further reduces plasma sodium concentration and osmolarity.
  - Children develop hyponatraemia more readily than adults and are more susceptible to the effects on the CNS. It is now considered to be a major risk in the perioperative care of children.
- Most fluid losses during surgery are isotonic. Losses are replaced with crystalloid, colloid, or blood products depending on the clinical situation.

Maintenance fluid regimens

- **Neonatal regimens**
  - Fluid requirement during the first 5 days in the neonate:

    Day 1:   60 mL/kg/day
    Day 2:   90 mL/kg/day
    Day 3:   120 mL/kg/day
    Day 4:   150 mL/kg/day
    Day 5:   150 mL/kg/day.

  - Electrolyte requirements:

    Sodium: 2–4 mmol/kg/day (in contrast to fluid requirements
                 this is relatively stable)
    Potassium: 2–3 mmol/kg/day.

  - Dextrose requirements:
    Usually provided using a 10% solution for maintenance. A 20% is
    solution is occasionally required in septic or fluid restricted
    neonates.

- **Infants and children**
  - Several formulae may be used to calculate maintenance fluid
    requirements. These are derived from the relationship between
    body weight and metabolic rate (energy requirements). Infants
    require 100 kcal/kg/day and children 75 kcal/kg/day. 1 mL of water
    per kcal is required for metabolism.
  - A common formula is the 4–2–1 regimen:

          4 mL/kg for first 10 kg
    plus: 2 mL/kg for next 10 kg
    plus: 1 mL/kg thereafter.
    e.g. a child of 17 kg requires 40 + 14 = 54 mL/hour; a child of 24 kg
    requires 40 + 20 + 4 = 64 mL/hour.

  - Electrolyte requirements:

    Sodium   2–4 mmol/kg/day
    Potassium   2–3 mmol/kg/day

- Additional losses: depending on their nature are replaced as
  appropriate e.g.:
  - Nasogastric losses: volume for volume with Hartmann's solution or
    0.9% saline with 10 mmol KCl per 500 mL.
  - Stoma losses: 50–75% of losses as 0.9% saline with 10 mmol KCl
    per 500 mL.
- Fluids should be administered through a volumetric pump with a
  pressure limit set.
- Common solutions for maintenance are:
  - 0.45% saline/5% dextrose
  - 0.45% saline/2.5% dextrose
  - 0.225% sodium/5% glucose
  - 0.18% sodium/4% glucose
  - 10% dextrose is commonly used in premature children and
    neonates.

- Monitoring of electrolyte concentrations is required if maintenance fluids are given for more than 24–48 hours. The formulae used are only a guide and generally over estimate fluid requirements. Under these circumstances, electrolyte derangements can occur. Hyponatraemia is a particular risk and may be devastating.
- Some anaesthetists restrict maintenance fluids to 50–75% of the calculated requirement during the postoperative period to reduce the risk of these problems.

Section 2

Paediatric anaesthesia

Principles of paediatric anaesthesia

Pamela Eccles

Range of patients

Many features of paediatric anaesthesia differ somewhat from adult practice.

- The age of patients ranges from premature neonates to mature teenagers.
- Patients with weights of 600 g and 90 kg may be anaesthetized one after the other.
- There is considerable variation in anatomical, physiological, and pharmacokinetic characteristics of patients (◻ Chapters 1 and 2).
- The pattern of pathology requiring anaesthesia and surgery is different. Congenital abnormalities form a major part of the surgical workload.
- There is a much greater requirement for general anaesthesia for examinations, investigations, and imaging which are performed without general anaesthesia in adults.
- The pattern of paediatric trauma is different as is the nature of the remainder of the non-elective workload.
- The involvement of parents at every stage of the patient journey including their presence in the anaesthetic and recovery rooms.
- The requirement to communicate with the family as well as (or instead of) the child (the patient).
- Limited understanding of the hospital admission in many young children, lack of cooperation, and the issues around venous access.
- Variations in the requirements for consent to treatment depending on the age of the child.

Preoperative assessment

- The goal of the preoperative assessment is to:
  - Obtain the relevant clinical history and examination findings
  - Develop a rapport with the child and the parents or carer(s)
  - Explain the procedures involved in anaesthesia and analgesia
  - Agree a method of induction
  - If appropriate, gain verbal or written consent for invasive procedures e.g. epidural, central venous access or for administration of a suppository during anaesthesia
  - Discuss risk if appropriate.
- Avoid wearing a white coat.
- Involve the parents, but address questions to the child where possible.
- Stay at eye level with the child where possible.
- Keep information simple, clear and truthful—needles can hurt, anaesthetic gas does smell etc.

History

- Previous anaesthetic history, including any problems e.g. PONV, difficult IV access, anxiety.
- Perinatal events and any problems at delivery.
- Prematurity:
  - Gestation at birth and current postconceptual age.
  - Requirement for IPPV in SCBU, current oxygen requirements, if any, residual lung damage (bronchopulmonary dysplasia).
  - Ex-premature children have a higher risk of postoperative apnoea, especially if they are anaemic, and should be admitted to hospital overnight until >56 weeks' post conceptual age.
  - An apnoea monitor and pulse oximeter should be used for 12–24 hours postoperatively and for 12 hours after any apnoeic episodes.
  - IV access is often very difficult in ex-premature patients.
- Current medical conditions.
- Respiratory:
  - Current or recent respiratory tract infection
  - Asthma and its treatment
  - Stridor
  - Obstructive sleep apnoea.
- Cardiovascular:
  - Heart murmurs
  - Colour changes
  - Ability to keep up with peers
  - Failure to thrive.
- Infectious diseases and vaccinations (see below).
- Family history of inheritable diseases:
  - Plasma cholinesterase deficiency
  - Sickle cell disease
  - Muscular dystrophies/myotonias
  - Bleeding diathesis
  - Malignant hyperthermia
  - cystic fibrosis

- Drug history including over the counter and herbal preparations.
- Allergies:
  - Drugs
  - Latex
  - Sticking plasters and dressings
  - Food allergies may be significant (e.g. soya bean oil is used in propofol emulsion).

Examination

- Airway:
  - Mouth opening
  - Micrognathia
  - Loose teeth
  - Enlarged tonsils, drooling
  - Macroglossia
  - Some syndromes have known airway implications (e.g. Down's, Pierre Robin).
- Respiratory:
  - Cough
  - Nasal secretions
  - Wheeze
  - Spinal and chest wall deformity.
- Cardiovascular:
  - Colour
  - Cyanosis or arterial oxygen saturation
  - Peripheral perfusion
  - Murmurs and added heart sounds.
- Temperature.
- Neurological:
  - Muscle tone
  - Airway protective reflexes
  - Ability to communicate.

Investigations

Most children do not require preoperative testing.

- A full blood count is indicated:
  - In children at risk of sickle cell disease who have not already been tested. Alternatively, a Sickledex® test can be performed as a screening test for the presence of haemoglobin S in children >6 months of age.
  - In children with significant systemic disease.
  - If significant surgical blood loss is anticipated.
- Routine biochemistry is indicated if the child has:
  - A metabolic, endocrine, or renal disorder.
  - Has been receiving IV fluids.
  - Has suffered abnormal fluid losses e.g. vomiting, nasogastric aspirates.
  - Is clinically dehydrated.
- Other investigations will be dictated by the clinical state of the child.

Consent

A formal written consent procedure for anaesthesia and related procedures is not routine in the U.K., although this may change in the future. It is important to gain parental (and if appropriate the child's) agreement to the proposed measures.

- Allow time for the child and parents to ask questions.
- The type of induction can be discussed – allowing children to have a choice in the process where possible gives them some control in an unfamiliar environment.
- Consent for a suppository, regional or peripheral nerve block, if indicated, including attendant risks.
- The risks of general anaesthesia may need to be discussed.

Preoperative fasting

As in adults, the aim of preoperative fasting is to reduce the volume of gastric contents and minimize the risk of passive regurgitation and pulmonary aspiration during anaesthesia.

- Fasting is often one of the most difficult and distressing aspects of a surgical procedure for many children and parents.
- Under some circumstances, a prolonged fast may contribute to dehydration (or hypoglycaemia in neonates). More commonly it is simply unpleasant for the child.
- Formula milk has slower gastric emptying than breast milk.
- There is evidence that formula milk can be safely given to children under 3 months of age up to 4 hours prior to anaesthesia.
- Allowing clear fluids to be given up to 2 hours prior to anaesthesia reduces discomfort and may improve compliance with 'Nil by mouth' instructions.
- Many infants feed during the night and many children wake relatively early in the morning and are fed. For inpatients, fasting instructions should not be 'fast from midnight' which may in fact require a fast from 19.00–20.00 (bedtime) the evening before for some children. A fasting time related to the likely time of surgery is preferable so that fasting times are not unnecessarily prolonged.
- For day case procedures where timings are usually predictable the written fasting instructions sent to parents usually encourage clear fluids until 06.30–07.00 for children on morning lists and breakfast with clear fluids until 11.00 for those on afternoon lists.
- Every hospital has a written fasting policy and most are variations of the 2/4/6 theme:
    - Clear fluids: 2 hours before anaesthesia.
    - Breast milk: 4 hours before anaesthesia.
    - Formula milk: 6 hours before anaesthesia.
    - Food: 6 hours before anaesthesia.

Parental presence at induction

📖 See also Chapter 1.

- Most paediatric anaesthetists in the UK allow one or both parents into the anaesthetic room.
- The aim of parental presence is to ↓ a child's anxiety at induction. High anxiety is associated with emergence delirium and postoperative behavioural changes.
- It is not suitable for all patients (e.g. some emergency procedures, neonates who are induced in the operating theatre rather than the anaesthetic room) or all parents.
- Randomized control trials have not shown an improvement in distress or postoperative behavioural problems with parental presence at induction. However, most parents who have been present at induction feel their presence was of benefit to the child, and would choose to be present again.
- A calm parent will cause a child to be less anxious, while an anxious parent will often exacerbate a child's fears. Providing written and verbal information to parents regarding their role at induction and what happens to a child as they are anaesthetized (child may have involuntary movements, have noisy breathing, go limp) can be useful to ↓ parental anxiety.
- A member of staff must be designated to look after the parent(s) and escort them from the theatre once the child is anaesthetized.

Play specialists and distraction

The use of play therapists is now widespread in paediatric practice. This can be extended into the perioperative period and in many UK hospitals play therapists make an important contribution to the perioperative care of a child and in providing information and support for parents.

- Outpatient:
  - Preadmission programmes including a video or photographs of the stages the child will experience (admission to the ward, application of EMLA cream or amethocaine gel, arriving in theatre, checking procedures).
  - Visits to theatre. Parents and children may visit the preoperative reception area, anaesthetic room, operating theatre, and recovery areas.
  - Children can play with some of the equipment e.g. face masks, oximeter probe, and stethoscope.
- Preoperative:
  - Escort the patient to theatre with their parent(s).
  - Employ distraction techniques during venous cannulation or inhalational induction to ↓ child anxiety.
  - Involve parent(s) in the distraction therapy.
- Postoperative:
  - Visit the child on the ward.
  - May phone the family the next day (if a day case patient).
- Distraction techniques:
  - These aim to reduce the child's anxiety during a potentially stressful time.
  - Various techniques are used—books, music, hand-held video games.
  - Results of studies examining the effect of distraction techniques on child anxiety during induction have been mixed.
  - Most parents think these interventions are helpful.

Premedication

As in adults, indications for premedication include:
- Sedation or anxiolysis
- Analgesia
- Antisialogogue effects
- Antacid effects
- Prokinetic effects.

The route of administration should be oral. IM injections in children are avoided unless there is a strong clinical indication.

Sedative

Preoperative preparation, topical EMLA cream, or tetracaine gel, parental presence at induction of anaesthesia and the use of play therapy has ↓ the use of sedative premedication in many centres. Despite these various methods of preoperative preparation, a significant number of children remain anxious and uncooperative during the preoperative period. It is humane to offer these children a short acting oral anxiolytic to reduce distress.

- Benzodiazepines are used most commonly and are preferable to phenothiazines such as trimeprazine because of a more predictable effect and fewer side effects.
- Midazolam (0.5 mg/kg; maximum 20 mg) is commonly used.
  - Onset of effect is in 10–15 min and duration is approximately 45–60 min. Ideally it is given 30 min before induction.
  - With midazolam, the timing of administration is important since after 60 min it often starts to wear off.
  - Since there are no active metabolites, midazolam is particularly useful for day case patients who need a sedative premedication.
  - An oral formulation is available. Alternatively, the IV preparation can be used. This has a bitter taste that needs to be disguised in diluting fruit juice or something similar.
  - A minority of children are not sedated by midazolam and in some cases suffer disinhibition and become boisterous or tearful.
- If precise timing is difficult then a longer acting drug such as diazepam (0.2–0.3 mg/kg; maximum 10 mg) may be useful since this takes longer to wear off. Diazepam should be given 45–60 min before induction.
- Ketamine is used alone or in combination with midazolam.
  - It is not a first line sedative but is often used in cases where midazolam alone has proved ineffective. Consider in children with more severe behavioural problems (ADHD, autism).
  - Dose is 3–6 mg/kg.
  - May prolong recovery time and hospital stay.
  - Dysphoria and hallucinations may occur if a benzodiazepine is not given concurrently.

Analgesic

An analgesic is often given preoperatively. This practice is often termed 'pre-emptive analgesia' although there is little evidence that efficacy is improved by preoperative administration.

- Typically non-sedating analgesics such as paracetamol (20 mg/kg; maximum 1 g) or ibuprofen (10 mg/kg; maximum 400 mg) are used.
- Analgesic syrups can also be used to disguise the taste of other medicines such as midazolam or ketamine.
- Clonidine (4 mcg/kg) can be used for both its sedative and analgesic effects, especially in cases where relative hypotension is desirable (e.g. scoliosis surgery). The prolonged sedation it produces makes clonidine unsuitable for day case surgery.

Antisialogogue

- Indicated in the child with excessive secretions as sometimes seen in cerebral palsy and in the anticipated difficult airway.
- Some anaesthetists use vagolytic agents routinely in neonates and infants to prevent laryngospasm from secretions and bradycardia from stimulation of the vagal nerve during laryngoscopy.
- Atropine 40 mcg/kg oral 90 min before induction
- Glycopyrronium bromide 100 mcg/kg oral 1 hour before induction.

Antacid

Considered in children at ↑ risk of regurgitation of gastric contents. This is classically a child with severe cerebral palsy who refluxes freely and is likely to undergo fundoplication at some point.

- Particulate antacids are rarely given to children.
- H_2 receptor antagonists are more commonly used.
- Cimetidine 6 mg/kg oral 2 hours before induction or 3 mg/kg IV 1 hour before.
- Ranitidine 2 mg/kg oral 2 hours before induction or 1 mg/kg IV 1 hour before.

Prokinetic

Not common.

- Metoclopramide 100–150 mcg/kg, to allow for children <1yr, oral 2–4 hours before induction or IV 30 min before.

Venous access

- Establishing IV access can be very difficult, even for an experienced paediatric anaesthetist.
- Small gauge cannulae e.g. 24G are used in infants and neonates and 22G in children unless there is a clinical need for a wider gauge cannula.
- Common sites for insertion are the dorsum of the hands, dorsolateral aspect of the foot, long saphenous vein, the antecubital fossa, or the radial aspect of the wrist. In young children, the small veins on the palmar aspect of the wrist may be the most prominent. In infants, scalp veins can be used.
- Some staff avoid using words such as 'needle', preferring to use more neutral words, such as a 'plastic tube' or 'straw'.
- Topical local anaesthetic creams make cannulation more tolerable for patients, parents, and staff. When used in combination with distraction techniques, it is often possible to place an IV cannula without the child being aware.

Topical cutaneous anaesthesia

This is routine before venous cannulation and venepuncture. EMLA cream, tetracaine gel, and ethyl chloride spray are commonly available. Choice depends on circumstances and hospital policy.

EMLA (eutectic mixture of local anaesthetics) cream

- Consists of a eutectic mixture (a mixture of two or more substances in proportions which gives the lowest possible melting point of any combination of those substances) of 2.5% lidocaine base and 2.5% prilocaine base in an emulsifier with a thickening agent.
- The eutectic mixture forms an emulsion with a concentration of local anaesthetic in the droplets of 80%. This fact accounts for the efficacy of the preparation since the effective concentration of local anaesthetic in contact with the skin is 80% despite an overall concentration of only 5% in the cream.
- Licensed for use from 1 year of age.
- Covered with an occlusive dressing.
- Recommended application time of 1 hour.
- The mean depth of skin analgesia depends on the duration of application and after 120 min this exceeds the mean skin thickness.
- After application for 1 hour, it is effective in 65% of children. It is more effective if left in place for 90–120 min.
- Duration of action 30–60 min after removal.
- Blanching of the skin at the site of application occurs in almost all applications. This is not a side effect but a predictable pharmacological effect of the compound. Both lidocaine and prilocaine have vasoconstrictor and vasodilator effects that are dependent on concentration. Constriction or blanching occurs at lower concentrations and dilatation at higher concentrations.

- EMLA has a biphasic action on the cutaneous blood vessels with a vasoconstrictor effect that is maximal after 1.5 hours followed after 2–3 hours by vasodilatation and erythema.
- The initial vasoconstriction sometimes makes venepuncture difficult.

Side effects

- Occasional erythema at the application site caused by the late vasodilator effect.
- Conjunctivitis if there is contact with the eyes.
- Methaemoglobinaemia from the oxidative effect of prilocaine. Methaemoglobin (HbM) is formed by the oxidation of the ferrous iron in haemoglobin to the ferric state. This is not a problem in normal clinical use.

Tetracaine

- Tetracaine is available as a 4% gel. It is more lipophilic than lidocaine and prilocaine and crosses the stratum corneum barrier more easily.
- Licensed for use from 1 month of age.
- Like EMLA, it is covered by an occlusive dressing.
- Efficacy is as good as or better than EMLA.
- It has a more rapid onset time of 40 min and an ↑ duration of action of around 4 hours following removal.
- Tetracaine forms a depot in the stratum corneum from which it slowly diffuses. This helps limit its systemic uptake and accounts for its prolonged duration of action.
- Erythema at the site of application occurs in 30–40% of patients after 40 min (and more after longer application times) and is due to local vasodilatation that is a predictable pharmacological effect rather than a side effect.

Side effects

- Itch in 10% of subjects and local oedema in 5%.

Ethyl chloride

- Used to provide instantaneous skin analgesia prior to venepuncture or cannulation.
- Presented in a glass phial with a nozzle for spraying.
- On contact with skin, it vapourizes causing a transient drop in local temperature to between −10°C and −20°C that causes transient anaesthesia of the affected skin.
- Its main advantage is the instantaneous onset of effect that is particularly useful where there is no time to wait for a local anaesthetic preparation to be effective.

Inhalational induction of anaesthesia

- This is one of the core techniques in paediatric anaesthesia and it is used commonly. It may be:
  - Clinically indicated as in suspected epiglottitis or another cause of a potentially difficult airway
  - Requested by the patient (or parents), especially in patients undergoing repeat procedures.
  - The preference of the anaesthetist because of poor venous access in a chubby toddler or a child born prematurely who has had many IV cannulae previously.
- An IV cannula is sited after the induction and preferably before any airway instrumentation or surgical intervention.
- Inhalational induction is usually performed with sevoflurane in oxygen. Nitrous oxide is often included to provide a second gas effect. Many anaesthetists prefer to induce with oxygen and volatile alone so that the child is well oxygenated in the event of airway obstruction during the induction, especially if problems are anticipated.
- Halothane is used less commonly than sevoflurane but is more potent. It is frequently used in the (anticipated) potentially difficult airway.
- Most children will tolerate a gradual introduction of nitrous oxide and then volatile anaesthetic agent. The child may hold the mask, or the anaesthetist may hold the tubing in a cupped hand close to the child's face. As the child becomes more sedated, the mask can be applied to the face and a gentle chin lift performed if required.
- Sevoflurane, with its non-irritant odour, can be given in a high concentration quickly or even from the start. Halothane must be increased incrementally (0.5% every 4 breaths is one rule of thumb) in order not to distress the child.
- Many anaesthetists use scented facemasks or rub the facemask with scented lip balm to disguise the smell of volatile agent. The benefit, if any, of this is probably more in the ritual and sense of control it gives the child rather, than its efficacy in disguising the smell of anaesthetic agent.
- Patience is important. Stimulating the child when he/she is at an inadequate plane of anaesthesia may result in breath holding, coughing, or laryngospasm and airway obstruction. For this reason, avoid placing oral airways early and be gentle when applying chin lift or jaw thrust.
- It is important to reduce the inspired concentration of volatile agent once the child is adequately anaesthetized because of the depressant effects on the cardiovascular (and to a lesser extent respiratory) systems of high concentrations of volatile. In particular, 'bagging' the child with a high concentration must be avoided. This will bypass the inherent safety feature of an inhalational induction—hypoventilation with overdose—and result in cardiovascular depression.
- Inhalational induction may be inappropriate in a child with limited cardiovascular reserve as in severe hypovolaemia, cardiac failure, right to left shunts and fixed cardiac output states. Myocardial depression and vasodilatation may cause profound hypoperfusion and cardiac arrest in these patients.

- Atmospheric pollution in the anaesthetic room is a feature of inhalational induction and many anaesthetists and anaesthetic assistants report ↑ fatigue after a number of these in the same day.
- A difficult and prolonged inhalational induction if often remembered as one of their most unpleasant experiences by many children.

The child with a 'cold'

The management of a child presenting with an active or recent cold, or respiratory tract infection (RTI) is a common dilemma for anaesthetists.

- These are usually viral infections with rhinoviruses, adenoviruses, parainfluenza, respiratory syncytial virus in infants, and influenza viruses (during annual winter epidemics).
- Bacterial super infection is occasionally present.
- Often referred to as an upper RTI these are, in fact, infections of the whole respiratory tract including the lower airways and abnormalities of these are present for up to 6 weeks after a viral RTI.
- Should be distinguished from allergic rhinitis—chronic condition, may be seasonal, child is well and the parents give s clear history which distinguishes this from a RTI.

A RTI is defined as a minimum of two of:

- Sore throat
- Sneezing
- Rhinorrhoea
- Nasal congestion
- Malaise
- Cough
- Fever or laryngitis
- Confirmation by a parent

The reasons for concern are:

- Even if a child is systemically well, the incidence of respiratory complications during anaesthesia is 5–7 times above normal in children with a RTI. This may not apply to very brief procedures performed with a facemask such as insertion of grommets.
- This ↑ to approximately 10-fold if an endotracheal tube is used.
- In general, infants and toddlers are more prone to respiratory complications during anaesthesia for anatomical and physiological reasons, explored in 📖 Chapter 1.
- These complications may be relatively benign—coughing, a short period of laryngospasm, transient mild hypoxia.
- Occasionally laryngospasm may be severe and result in profound hypoxia, bradycardia, and a requirement for emergency intubation.
- A child with a viraemia may have a carditis and be at risk of dysrhythmias during anaesthesia.

Under some circumstances, the decision to defer elective surgery is clear:
- Elective surgery should usually be cancelled if the child has evidence of a lower RTI, including a productive cough, or purulent nasal secretions, fever > 38°C, constitutional symptoms (lethargy, loss of appetite, diarrhoea or vomiting).

Less clear cut factors which may lead to a decision to cancel are:
- The child is under 1 year of age
- Also has asthma
- The procedure requires endotracheal intubation.
- The parents express concern about the safety of anaesthesia in the child's current medical state.

Elective surgery is usually deferred for 4–6 weeks.

Factors that may encourage a decision to proceed include:
- A preschool child may have as many as eight colds a year and some are never free of respiratory symptoms.
- In many cases (particularly ENT), the surgical pathology is partly responsible for the respiratory symptoms and the child will never be symptom free until after surgery.
- Families often make special arrangements so the child can attend hospital. As well as the time and inconvenience involved, it may be a financial burden if the operation is cancelled.

Elective surgery often proceeds if the child:
- Has recovered from the RTI and has only residual symptoms
- Is 'as well as he/she normally is' on parental report
- If the surgery is brief
- Endotracheal intubation is not required.

With urgent procedures, there is no choice about whether to proceed.

If the surgery is to proceed, there are two approaches to management of the airway:
- When appropriate a 'minimal interference technique' with a facemask or LMA, spontaneous ventilation, and a local anaesthetic analgesic technique.
- If this is inappropriate and especially if endotracheal intubation is required then consider:
  - Preoperative administration of a bronchodilator.
  - Atropine to reduce the incidence of vagal reflex bronchoconstriction.
  - IPPV with PEEP to help to prevent atelectasis.
  - Manual ventilation to expand collapsed areas of the lungs if the patient is hypoxic (exclude other causes of hypoxia).
  - Suction of secretions via the ETT prior to extubation.
  - Extubate awake.
  - Postoperative supplementary oxygen may be necessary.
  - Postoperative physiotherapy if required.

Respiratory complications are likely in children who:
- Are exposed to second hand cigarette smoke.
- Have nasal congestion.
- Have a productive cough.
- Undergo endotracheal intubation.
- Normally have obstructive sleep apnoea.

Babies and infants have a higher risk compared with older children. It is relatively common to find a mismatch between the preoperative assessment of risk and actual complications during anaesthesia i.e. proceeding in a child who is asymptomatic and believed to over the worst and having a torrid time with hypoxia, bronchospasm, and secretions.

Heart murmurs

- Most pathological murmurs are detected in the neonatal period, but may, rarely, present as a preoperative finding.
- Parents and the general practitioner are aware of most innocent and abnormal murmurs and they are documented in the notes.
- It is common to assess a child who is known to have congenital heart disease and has often undergone treatment. The relevant information is in the notes and further investigations are not required on the day of surgery.
- The dilemma occurs when a murmur is heard for the first time during the preoperative assessment.
- Functional or flow murmurs occur in up to 50% of normal children at some time.
- Discrimination between innocent and pathological murmurs depends on salient features of the history and examination.
- With 'innocent' or physiological murmurs, the child is asymptomatic with normal growth and exercise tolerance. On auscultation, the murmur is soft, systolic, and accompanied by normal heart sounds.
- Symptoms indicating a pathological condition include failure to thrive, poor exercise tolerance, or cyanotic episodes. Signs may include diastolic or pansystolic murmurs, abnormal heart sounds, a praecordial heave, or reduced femoral pulses.
- If any of these abnormal features are present, review by a paediatric cardiologist is arranged prior to surgery. An ECG with or without an echocardiogram is required.
- If a previously unknown murmur is heard preoperatively, a decision is required on whether it is probably innocent or pathological. If pathological, surgery is deferred and the patient referred for investigation. If innocent, the options are to proceed (with antibiotic prophylaxis if surgery will cause a bacteraemia) or defer for investigation. This decision may depend on the personal preference of the anaesthetist or there may be a local policy concerning this decision. Some anaesthetists request an ECG at this stage.
- If surgery proceeds, the child is referred for investigation postoperatively to allow classification of the murmur and documentation in the medical notes.
- Prophylaxis against bacterial endocarditis is required in a child with a structural heart lesion. The regimen used will depend of the type of surgery to be performed and the local policy. A high risk patient has a prosthetic heart valve, other prosthetic material such as a modified Blalock–Taussig shunt or has had endocarditis previously.

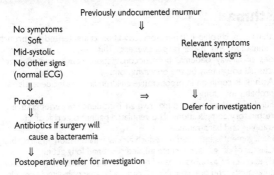

Fig. 3.1 Algorithm for management of previously undocumented heart murmour.

Asthma

Asthma is a chronic inflammatory condition characterized by bronchial inflammation and hyper-responsiveness. This results in recurrent episodes of airway oedema, bronchoconstriction, cough, and wheeze. A nocturnal cough may be the only symptom.

- Asthma is common in preoperative children and the incidence is probably increasing.
- Surgical patients with asthma have an ↑ incidence of perioperative respiratory complications. The ventilated patient is at risk of air trapping and barotrauma.
- Management is intended to reduce airway inflammation and irritability.
- Classes of drugs used include inhaled short and long-acting β_2-adrenergic agonists, inhaled corticosteroids, leukotriene-receptor antagonists, and oral steroids. Occasionally, aminophylline is used in severe cases. Sodium cromoglycate is an anti-inflammatory agent used in children with mild asthma.
- In most cases, asthma is well controlled and the usual anaesthetic technique for a given procedure does not need modification. Most of the modifications suggested would only be required in a severe asthmatic or in a symptomatic child anaesthetised for urgent surgery.

Preoperative

History

- Is the diagnosis of asthma appropriate? Children may have post-viral bronchitis, a fixed airway obstruction (associated with stridor) or gastro-oesophageal reflux causing nocturnal cough.
- Establish severity of disease and current level of control. Asthmatics who are well controlled use short-acting β_2-agonists less than 3 times a week. Nocturnal cough can be a sign of poor control.
- Exercise tolerance is an indicator of severity.
- Determine triggers for asthma attacks—RTI, cold, pollen, exercise.
- Previous admissions to hospital and admissions to ITU with asthma indicate severe disease.
- Children may be atopic and have allergies to agents including latex.
- Current medication.

Examination

- Usually no clinical signs when well.
- Children with current wheeze or an RTI may need to have surgery postponed to improve their preoperative condition.

Premedication

- Continue all regular medications.
- Sedative premedication, such as midazolam, can be given safely.
- β_2 agonists are usually give prior to anaesthesia to reduce airway irritability.

Intraoperative management

Induction
- Inhalational or IV inductions are used as appropriate.
- Propofol produces less bronchoconstriction than barbiturates in asthmatics, although idiosyncratic reactions to propofol have occurred.
- Ketamine is the induction agent of choice in patients with severe asthma, as it has a direct bronchodilator effect. An anticholinergic is often given with ketamine to reduce airway secretions.

Airway management
- Avoiding endotracheal intubation may reduce the incidence of adverse respiratory events.
- Bronchoconstriction is more likely if the patient is not at an adequate plane of anaesthesia when the airway is instrumented.
- Spraying the larynx with topical lignocaine is sometimes done to reduce airway responses to endotracheal intubation. However, this may itself provoke bronchospasm.

Maintenance
- On theoretical grounds, histamine-releasing agents are often avoided e.g. fentanyl and vecuronium are used rather than morphine and atracurium. This is not usually an important factor.
- During IPPV consider limiting airway pressures and using a long expiratory time. Pressure controlled ventilation is a good mode.
- Have a high index of suspicion for the development of complications such as bronchospasm or anaphylaxis (📖 Chapter 14).
- Patients on oral steroids may have suppression of the hypothalamo-pituitary-adrenal axis and need steroid replacement to prevent an adrenal crisis.

Emergence
- The decision to extubate 'deep' or awake will depend on the nature of the case and the experience of the anaesthetist. Deep extubation avoids mechanical stimulation from the ETT, while awake extubation ensures a secure airway immediately after extubation.
- Airway secretions are suctioned prior to extubation.

Analgesia
- For any given procedure analgesia rarely needs to be modified from that given to a child without asthma.
- Regional anaesthetic techniques are used as normal.
- NSAIDs are used unless the patient has a history of problems with these or has nasal polyps
- Opioids are given as required. Oral opioids such as codeine or morphine in the usual doses. IV infusion (or PCA) using morphine is usually trouble free.

Attention deficit hyperactivity disorder (ADHD)

- ADHD is the most common neurobehavioural disorder of childhood, with an incidence of 5% in schoolchildren.
- Characterized by inattention, poor impulse control, motor overactivity, and restlessness.
- ADHD is more common in boys and in lower socio-economic groups.
- Aetiology is multifactorial and approximately 50% of children will have other behavioural, emotional, learning, and language disorders.
- Inadequate dopamine and noradrenaline in the fronto-subcortical-cerebellar regions may cause under stimulation of inhibitory pathways. The effectiveness of stimulants in treatment supports this theory.
- Poses similar problems to anaesthetists as the autistic spectrum of disorders.
- Two main issues emerge in the care of these children—management of the perioperative period and possible interactions between current medications and anaesthetic agents.

Perioperative management

- Children tolerate poorly waiting for long periods in hospital and behaviour may become disruptive on the ward.
- Minimize waiting times where possible. Plan to do the case early in the day when the child is more cooperative (ideally, first on a morning list).
- Providing a quiet room to wait in can reduce preoperative anxiety and adverse behaviours.
- Distraction techniques may help while the child is waiting and at induction of anaesthesia.
- Sedative premedication is used frequently in this group of patients. Effects are less predictable and more variable in patients on stimulants.
- Medications modify noradrenergic and dopaminergic function in the CNS. They may reduce the seizure threshold and predispose to PONV.

Stimulants

- Methylphenidate is by far the most common drug used to treat children with ADHD or autistic spectrum disorder. Its mechanism of action is to block dopamine transport and ↑ extracellular dopamine in the corpus striatum.
- Dexamphetamines block dopamine and noradrenaline reuptake and inhibit the enzyme monoamine oxidase.
- May ↑ the MAC of anaesthetic agents.
- Pro-seizure activity and cardiovascular effects may be exacerbated by a number of drugs including tramadol, pethidine, and ephedrine.

Non-stimulants

- Atomoxetine is a highly selective inhibitor of the presynaptic noradrenaline transporter, especially in the prefrontal cortex. Use sympathomimetics with caution. Potentiates the cardiovascular effects of salbutamol.
- Bupropion is a selective inhibitor of neuronal uptake of catecholamines.
- Caution with agents that can alter the seizure threshold or have cardiovascular effects, as for stimulants.
- Clonidine has been used alone and in combination with stimulants in the treatment of ADHD.

Infectious diseases

The management of a child with an infectious disease involves protection of staff and other patients as well as the patient.

- Important concepts are the incubation and infectious periods, when surgery should be delayed (if possible), and the management of a child with an infectious disease if surgery cannot be delayed.
- Incubation period is the time between contact with a person with the disease until the onset of the disease.
- Infectious period is the time when the infected patient is able to infect others.
- Anaesthetic agents affect the immune system, and may impair the child's ability to mount an effective immune response. This may ↑ the risk of developing severe complications of the disease.
- Children with an infectious disease are often unwell and have ↑ oxygen and fluid requirements because of ↑ metabolism.
- Secondary infections and/or pneumonia may complicate these conditions e.g. measles, varicella, pertussis. In some cases, lung pathology can persist for months.
- Staphylococcus pneumonia with bullous lung disease may complicate measles.
- Myocarditis can occur in severe forms of many diseases e.g. mumps.
- Septicaemia and multi-organ failure (including thrombocytopaenia or encephalopathy) can occur.

Table 3.1 Incubation and infection periods

Disease	Incubation period (days)	Infectious period
Diphtheria	2–5	14 days after start of illness and malaise
Measles	7–18	From onset of symptoms until 5 days after appearance of rash
Mumps	12–25	Several days before and 9 days after start of parotitis
Pertussis	6–20	21 days after coughing started or six days after start of antibiotic therapy
Rubella	14–23	10 days before and days after appearance of rash
Varicella (chickenpox)	10–21	2 days before spots appear until all lesions have dried and crusted

Immunizations

Immunization aims to protect individuals and the population from the devastating consequences of a number of infectious diseases.

- There are two types of vaccine:
  - Live attenuated. These are more likely to induce an immunological response, but have a higher risk of causing a mild form of the disease or infecting non-immune people.
  - Inactivated or detoxified agents.
- Many people will develop symptoms after immunization. Most of these are mild (local redness and swelling, irritability). After inactivated vaccines, reactions are likely to have occurred within 5 days. After live vaccines, the reaction may be delayed and present as a mild form of the illness. The development of symptoms depends on the incubation period of the disease.
- Anaesthesia and surgery cause a degree of suppression of the immune system *in vitro*. This has led to concern that performing immunization and surgery around the same time may impair the ability to mount an effective immune response and ↓ the effectiveness of the vaccine. This problem has not been demonstrated in practice.
- Reactions, such as fever after anaesthesia and surgery in the recently immunized patient can cause a diagnostic dilemma.
- There has been little research in this area and considerable variation in practice. Many anaesthetists ignore the immunization history of the child. In some centres there is a policy of:
  - Discouraging opportunistic immunization during anaesthesia.
  - Avoiding immunization until 1 week after anaesthesia.
  - Avoiding anaesthesia for elective surgery which is nor clinically urgent for 7–14 days after immunization.

Paediatric anaesthetic equipment

Fiona Kelly

Paediatric face masks

- Face masks provide an interface between the child and the breathing system.
- They are used for inhalational induction, during maintenance with spontaneous ventilation, for positive pressure ventilation before intubation, and for pre-oxygenation prior to rapid sequence induction.
- For neonates and infants, face mask dead space may be significant (possibly >30% of tidal volume).
- An ideal face mask for paediatric use should:
  - Provide a good seal around the mouth and nose (to prevent leaks during positive pressure ventilation and dilution of anaesthetic gases during spontaneous ventilation).
  - Have a soft rim to minimize pressure and prevent trauma.
  - Be of the correct size to avoid pressure on the eyes.
  - Have minimum dead space.
  - Be transparent to allow observation of lip colour, vomit, other secretions, and the presence of breathing.
- Round, transparent, plastic face masks with an inflatable rim are used for neonates and infants (sizes 1 and 2) while a teardrop shape is generally used for older children (sizes 3 and 4).
- Although the round masks have a larger dead space, they are easier to position.
- Acceptability to the child can be improved by the use of scented masks.
- The Rendell–Baker face mask, although originally devised to minimize dead space, does not have an inflatable cuff and is now rarely used.
- Face masks or angle pieces can be adapted for the passage of a fibreoptic bronchoscope (📖 Chapter 5).

Oropharyngeal airways

- Used to prevent the tongue and epiglottis from occluding the upper airway.
- Not often useful for neonates (because they are obligate nasal breathers) but can be of use for the prevention of gastric distension during mask ventilation. Also of use for children with micrognathia, a large tongue (e.g. Down's) or in syndromes such as Pierre Robin, Hurler's, Hunter's, or Goldenhar.
- Oropharyngeal airways must only be inserted in adequately anaesthetized patients. Insertion during lighter planes of anaesthesia can cause laryngospasm or vomiting if the pharyngeal reflexes are not sufficiently depressed to suppress the gag reflex.
- In practice, the Guedel oropharyngeal airway is now universally used. This has a curved air channel (flattened anteroposteriorly, curved laterally) with a straight bite section made of hard plastic (to ensure the airway cannot be occluded by biting) and a flange at the oral end to prevent the airway falling into the mouth.
- The correct choice of airway size is vital. An estimate of the correct length is given by the distance between the centre of the incisors and the angle of the jaw. The distal end should lie just above the epiglottis to avoid irritating the laryngeal inlet. An incorrect choice of airway size can worsen airway obstruction and cause trauma and laryngospasm.
- In young children the adult method of insertion can cause damage, and so the oropharyngeal airway should always be inserted with the concave side down. Insertion can be aided by use of a laryngoscope to push the tongue towards the floor of the mouth or by lifting the angle of the jaw.
- Guedel airways range in size from 000 to 4 (4 to 10 cm in length). A guide to the typical choice of size is given in Table 4.1. The smallest oropharyngeal airways (sizes 000 and 00) have an exaggerated curve to fit over the relatively bulky tongue of small infants.

Table 4.1 A guide to the use of Guedel oropharyngeal airways

Age	Size	Colour
Preterm	000	White
Preterm	00	Blue
Neonate–3 months	0	Black
Infant (3–12 months)	1	White
Child (1–5 years)	2	Green
Child (>5 years)/small adult	3	Orange
Large adult	4	Red

Nasopharyngeal airways

- These provide a patent airway passage from the nostril to the nasopharynx. Not routinely used during paediatric anaesthesia.
- Better tolerated during relatively light levels of anaesthesia than oral airways.
- Can be a useful alternative for children with obstructive sleep apnoea or some congenital airway problems. It can also be used to apply CPAP.
- Paediatric sizes are commercially available, but in practice nasopharyngeal airways for children are often fashioned from tracheal tubes cut to the appropriate length and secured across the cheeks and nose.
- If an ETT is used in this way, the tube diameter in mm can be estimated from the formula (age/4) + 3.5 or from the diameter of the child's little finger. The tube length can be estimated from the distance from the tip of the nostril to the tragus of the ear. The correct length should result in the distal end lying just above the epiglottis, good air entry and no stridor.
- Nasopharyngeal airways should be well lubricated before insertion and gently pushed posteriorly along the floor of the nose to minimize bleeding and trauma to nasal mucosa or adenoidal tissue. Excess force should not be used as a false passage may be created.
- Nasopharyngeal airways are contraindicated if a fracture of the base of the skull is suspected. They should also be avoided if there is evidence of coagulopathy or nasal deformity.

Laryngeal mask airway

- The laryngeal mask airway (LMA) is now in wide and varied use in paediatric anaesthesia.
- Used instead of a face mask in a spontaneously breathing patient, an LMA:
  - Frees the anaesthetist's hands.
  - Allows the anaesthetist to stand back from the patient, surgical drapes, and operating site.
  - May provide a superior airway in some patients with a difficult airway (e.g. Hurler's syndrome).
- As an alternative to the ETT the LMA can be used:
  - For airway maintenance during spontaneous ventilation when there is no risk of aspiration.
  - For IPPV/PCV in selected cases.
  - As an aid in difficult intubation (Ⓛ Chapter 5).
  - As a method of airway maintenance following failed endotracheal intubation.
  - For resuscitation when patient position inhibits use of the laryngoscope.
  - In an emergency by staff untrained in endotracheal intubation.
- Use of the LMA is contraindicated when there is a risk of aspiration (full stomach or history of reflux) and caution is required when there is a risk the mask may be dislodged as in surgery around the head and neck.

Design and use

Normal

- The LMA is made of silicon (latex free), and can be autoclaved and used up to 40 times.
- It has an oval head surrounded by an elliptical cuff. After blind insertion into the pharynx this cuff is inflated (via a small tube with a self-sealing valve) to form a seal around the laryngeal inlet, supporting it away from the posterior pharyngeal wall. The back of the head leads to a tube, the proximal end of which has a standard 15 mm ISO male connector for connection to a breathing system. Slits at the junction between the tube and the mask head prevent the epiglottis from obscuring the tube lumen. The wide diameter of the tube offers low resistance.
- The LMA is not widely used for controlled ventilation. If used, great care must be taken not to inflate the stomach. Gastric distension is less likely if inflation pressures are kept below 20 cm H_2O and pressure controlled ventilation is used rather than volume controlled ventilation.

Reinforced

- A thinner, longer, and reinforced version of the LMA is available with a stainless steel spiral in the wall. This retains flexibility but prevents kinking and crushing.
- This version is especially useful in head and neck surgery because the breathing system can be connected away from the operating site and the end of the tube can be moved without losing the cuff seal. Throat packs can also be used.
- The narrower tube presents ↑ resistance to flow and so this type of LMA is less suitable for prolonged use.

Sizes

- Five sizes of paediatric LMA are available, suitable for patients ranging from neonates to teenagers.
- Selection is determined by patient weight (📖 see Table 4.2 which also gives the size of tracheal tube that can be passed through the mask).
- The smaller sizes often do not provide a reliable airway and the size 1 LMA is only suitable for short procedures.

Table 4.2 Suggested LMA sizes

Weight kg	Mask size	Maximum cuff volume mL	ETT mm
<5	1	4	3.5
5–10	1 1/2	7	4.0
10–20	2	10	4.5
20–30	2 1/2	14	5.0
30+	3	20	5.5

Insertion

- Pharyngeal reflexes must be adequately depressed by general anaesthesia before insertion.
- The device is checked for damage. The cuff should be fully deflated, the mask lubricated with gel and the mask advanced into position using the same technique as in adults. Correct positioning should be checked clinically.
- An alternative rotational method is occasionally used. The LMA is inserted in to the mouth with the aperture facing the hard palate i.e. 180° rotation from normal. It is then pushed cranially and backward to slide along the hard and soft palates and rotated through 180° when the cuff is in the oropharynx.
- Hyperinflation (deliberate or from nitrous oxide diffusion) of LMA cuffs carries a risk of airway morbidity by exerting pressure on laryngeal and pharyngeal structures, and cuffs should therefore be inflated only with the minimum volume of air required to form an effective seal.

Other designs

- *Intubating laryngeal mask (iLMA):* a modification designed to facilitate blind orotracheal intubation and fibreoptic intubation. Available in size 3, so potentially useful for older children.
- *LMA with oesophageal drain (LMA-ProSeal):* a second lumen is added to give access to the oesophagus and allow passage of a nasogastric tube. Recently introduced in paediatric sizes. Potentially attractive for procedures in which IPPV is desired in children and the nasogastric tube will prevent gastric distension.
- *Single use LMAs:* a variety of these are now available from several manufacturers. They are likely to replace reusable LMAs because of concerns about transmission of infection and sterilization between patients. Usually not as well made as the original version and have a higher incidence of difficulty in positioning, unsatisfactory position and airway obstruction during use particularly in younger children.

Laryngoscopes

Laryngoscopes are used to perform direct laryngoscopy and as an aid in tracheal intubation.

Anatomical factors

The main anatomical features that must be considered when performing laryngoscopy in children are:

- Small size of the mouth and airway.
- Relatively large tongue.
- Higher and more anterior (cephalad) position of the larynx (in infants, opposite C3–C4).
- Longer and narrower mobile epiglottis.

Different laryngoscope designs and laryngoscopy techniques may offer better views of the larynx in a given patient.

Design and operation

Laryngoscopes fall into two main categories—retractor-type laryngoscopes (to retract tissue to obtain a clear line of sight) and fibreoptic laryngoscopes (to allow viewing around an obstruction).

Retractor type laryngoscopes

These consist of a detachable blade (curved or straight, flanged or flat, metal or plastic, sometimes disposable), a handle containing the light source, and a bulb or fibreoptic bundle to project the light from the blade. For paediatric use:

- The light should be near the tip of the blade to ensure adequate illumination of the larynx.
- The blade should not be too bulky for a small mouth, but should prevent the large tongue from obscuring the view of the larynx.

The choice of blade design depends on patient age and on individual preference. Due to concern about transmission of prions from lymphoid tissue, disposable laryngoscope blades are now used for endotracheal intubation for tonsillectomy and/or adenoidectomy.

Curved blades

A curved Macintosh blade is usually used from the age of 3 or 4 years upwards. They can also be used in many children down to about 6 months of age if desired. Technique is the same as in adults. The laryngoscope blade is inserted to the right of the mouth, the tip is positioned in the valleculla and the blade is used to lift the base of the tongue and attached epiglottis anteriorly so exposing the larynx.

Straight blades

For infants and neonates most anaesthetists prefer a straight blade designed to pass behind the epiglottis and then lift it directly to reveal the laryngeal inlet. The classic technique involves inserting the blade to the right side of the mouth and advancing it until the tip is in the upper oesophagus. The blade is then withdrawn little by little until the tip comes out of the oesophagus and lies against the laryngeal surface of the epiglottis. In this position, the epiglottis is lifted out of the field of view and the laryngeal inlet is exposed. The little finger of the hand holding the laryngoscope can be used to apply external laryngeal pressure to help bring the vocal cords into view. The laryngeal surface of the epiglottis is innervated by the vagus nerve and, for this reason, the straight-bladed technique sometimes causes a transient slowing of heart rate. This is rarely of clinical significance. As these blades are designed to be inserted further into the pharynx and upper oesophagus, they are relatively long. Some anaesthetists prefer a flange on the medial side of the blade (Wisconsin type) to keep the tongue out of the way, while others prefer a flatter blade (Robertshaw type). The risk of trauma to the epiglottis is higher with straight blades. A straight blade is used for the retromolar technique of laryngoscopy.

A wide range of straight and curved laryngoscope blades is available for paediatric use.
- Curved blades:
  - *Macintosh*: most commonly used blade in the UK. Available in sizes 1–5. Size 1 is of very little use as straight blades are usually preferred in neonates and infants. Left handed and Polio (wide handle-blade angle) versions are available.
- Straight blades:
  - *Miller*: curved tip and flat flange requiring little mouth opening. Cross section C-shaped.
  - *Wisconsin*: similar to Miller.
  - *Robertshaw*: gently curving tip, small flange does not complete a C-shape cross section. Flat profile does not need much mouth opening to use.
  - *Oxford*: C-shaped in cross section. Curve attenuated distally.
  - *Cardiff*: straight blade but designed to be used in the same way as a Macintosh. Can be used in patients ranging from neonate to teenager. 10 cm long. The proximal 6 cm is straight so that no part of the blade can obscure the line of sight. This offers a view of the larynx with the minimum of mouth opening. The distal 4 cm of the blade is curved, displacing the tip approximately 1 cm forward of the main axis. Proximally, the blade has a reverse Z cross section, the flat blade plate being 16 mm across with a 10 mm web and a 2.5 mm flange. The web and flange are attenuated distally so that the terminal 15 mm continues as a curved spatula, narrowing to 8 mm at the tip. It terminates with a thickened, transverse bead to minimize mucosal damage. Tip is placed in the vallecula to elevate the epiglottis using the same mechanism as a Macintosh.
  - *Seward*: similar design to Cardiff with reverse Z cross section.

Fibreoptic laryngoscopes

- The flexible fibreoptic laryngoscope is now widely regarded as the instrument of choice for the management of difficult endotracheal intubation. Its flexibility allows it to follow virtually any anatomical space to return an image to the anaesthetist.
- The insertion tube typically contains two fibreoptic light bundles (feeding light from an external light source), one image bundle (from the objective lens to the eyepiece or camera), one working channel for the intended task, and two angulation wires for control of the flexible tip.
- The image from the device is best viewed with a video monitor to facilitate ease of viewing, teaching, and assistance.
- The main drawbacks of these devices are that blood and secretions easily obscure the small objective lens and the fibres are easily damaged.
- Standard flexible fibreoptic laryngoscopes are available with insertion tubes as small as 2.5 mm (external diameter) for use in infants, although this smallest size usually has no suction/working channel. A 2.2 mm diameter bronchoscope can also be used to aid intubation in children.
- Rigid fibreoptic laryngoscopes are also available (*Bullard laryngoscope* and *Upsherscope*) but are little used in the UK.

Endotracheal tubes

Endotracheal intubation is used to provide:
- A patent airway.
- Airway protection from aspiration.
- Positive pressure ventilation with ability to apply PEEP.
- Bronchial lavage and suction.

Anatomical factors

The narrowest part of the paediatric trachea is at the cricoid ring (rather than the vocal cords). After puberty with the growth of the trachea the cricoid ring ceases to be the narrowest part of the larynx. Too large a tracheal tube can compress the tracheal epithelium leading to tracheal oedema and possibly permanent subglottic stenosis.

Design

The standard tracheal tube is:
- Curved, with a left-facing bevel at the distal end, and often a hole (Murphy eye) opposite the bevel (in case the distal end is obstructed).
- Made with as thin a wall as possible to minimize resistance while avoiding kinking and fitted with an ISO 15 mm or 8.5 mm connector.
- Fitted with a radio-opaque line to aid detection of tube position on a chest X-ray.
- Marked with internal diameter (in mm) on the side of the tube.
- Marked with distance from tip of tube (in cm) at intervals along the length of the tube.

Modern ETTs are disposable, and made of plastic (PVC or polyurethane) which can be reliably sterilized during manufacture. These materials soften at body temperature, helping the tube to mould to the airway. When used for nasotracheal intubation, they can be softened before use in warm water to minimize trauma.

Uncuffed ETTs

Uncuffed tubes are generally used for children younger than 8 years old. This allows the internal diameter of the tube to be maximized (minimizing air resistance) while allowing an audible leak (minimizing the risk of tracheal damage). Potential disadvantages of uncuffed tubes include aspiration, atmospheric pollution from leakage of anaesthetic gases, inadequate ventilation because of a large leak, and the possible need for reintubation.

Cuffed ETTs

Some anaesthetists prefer to use cuffed endotracheal tubes, with low pressure, high volume cuffs even in small infants. Cuffed tubes reduce the risk of aspiration, avoid the potential requirement for reintubation and may reduce trauma. However, the cuff reduces the available lumen and is a potential cause of laryngeal trauma.

Size of ETT
- Choice of tube diameter and length is determined by patient age and weight (🕮 Table 4.3). Most ETTs are made longer than necessary giving the anaesthetist the choice of cutting before insertion, or leaving the tube uncut allowing flexibility so that the connector need not be located next to the mouth. This may reduce the risk of accidental extubation due to head movement but may ↑ the risk of kinking.
- For children younger than 4 years old, Table 4.3 provides a guide to the appropriate choice of tube internal diameter. For older children the formula size = (age/4) + 4.5 mm is often used, but pre-existing medical conditions may influence size (in Down's syndrome internal diameter is typically 1–2 mm smaller than predicted). In practice, with uncuffed tubes, it is advisable to have tubes of smaller and larger internal diameter available prior to intubation and to check the diameter by confirming that a small audible leak can be heard at an inspiratory pressure = 20 cm H_2O.
- For tube length, the formulae length = (age/2) + 12 cm (oral) or (age/2) + 14 cm (nasal) provide a rough estimate but tube length should be confirmed clinically by checking for equal bilateral chest movement and breath sounds.
- An alternative method of ensuring correct length is to look at the length of ETT through the vocal cords. In normal children without anatomical abnormalities of the airway, this should be 3 cm for ETTs of internal diameter 3.0 mm and 3.5 mm; 4 cm for those of 4.0 mm and 4.5 mm; and 5 cm for those of 5.0 mm and 5.5 mm.

Table 4.3 Suggested ETT sizes

Age	Weight kg	ETT internal diameter mm
Premature	<2	2.5–3.0
Term	3–4	3.0–3.5
0–6 months	3–5	3.5
6–12 months	5–10	4.0
1–2 years	10–14	4.5
2–4 years	12–16	5.0

Problems

The potential problems of intubation in children are similar to those encountered with adults (but with a greater risk of occurrence, especially with smaller tubes), and include:
- Kinking.
- Occlusion by secretions, foreign bodies, or the bevel lying against tracheal wall.
- Oesophageal intubation.
- Bronchial intubation.

- Inadvertent extubation.
- Trauma and injury to the airway.
- Risk of adenoidal bleeding in nasal intubation.
- N_2O diffusion into cuffs.

Varieties of paediatric endotracheal tubes

- *RAE preformed tubes:* these have a preformed bend as the tube emerges so that breathing system connections are at the chin (south facing) or forehead (north facing) and do not interfere with surgical access. They can be temporarily straightened for insertion of a stylette or suction catheter.
- *Reinforced tubes:* these are made kink resistant by a steel or nylon spiral embedded in the tube wall. They remain flexible but they cannot be cut and the thicker wall means a larger external diameter than a normal ETT of the same internal diameter (it may be necessary to drop 0.5 mm below the size predicted from age particularly in small children).
- *Microcuff™ tubes:* have a high-volume, low pressure cuff made of a microthin polyurethane material. It does not form folds during inflation, provides an effective seal at a lower cuff pressure (8–15 cm H_2O) than conventional cuffed ETTs, and potentially reduces the risk of mucosal damage. They are available in infant and neonatal sizes and allow a cuffed ETT to be used in all age groups if desired.
- *Microlaryngeal tubes:* this has a small diameter and a large cuff to improve exposure and surgical access to the larynx.
- *Laser surgery tubes:* these are made from metal or have a laser-proof coating to avoid the risk of fire or tube damage during laser surgery.
- *Endobronchial tubes* and *tracheostomy tubes* are also available.

Breathing systems

The design and choice of paediatric breathing systems is determined by the child's age and weight, and by the need for spontaneous or controlled ventilation.

Anatomical and physiological factors

The key differences between children and adults of relevance to breathing systems are:

- Smaller lung volume, and hence ↑ apparatus dead space relative to the child's dead space. This can be partially compensated for by intubation and controlled ventilation.
- Chest wall is more compliant, and the diaphragm more easily fatigued. Alveolar ventilation is therefore more dependent on respiratory rate.
- Work of breathing is greater and so apparatus resistance is particularly important when small infants are breathing spontaneously.
- Closing capacity may exceed and overlap functional residual capacity.

The ideal paediatric breathing system

Accordingly, an ideal system for use with small (<20 kg) children should:

- Have minimal functional and apparatus dead space.
- Have small internal gas volumes.
- Produce minimal resistance to flow and gas turbulence.
- Be either without valves or have very low resistance valves.
- Permit spontaneous, manual, and controlled ventilation.
- Offer the ability to provide CPAP or PEEP.
- Provide heating, humidification, and filtration.
- Be lightweight, and have universal connections.

Common paediatric breathing systems

Mapleson F

The circuit in most common use for paediatric anaesthesia is the Jackson–Rees modification to the Ayre's T-piece (📖 Fig 4.1). This system is simple and lightweight, has an open-ended 500 mL bag, no valve, and has low resistance and low dead space. It can be used for spontaneous, assisted and controlled ventilation in children of all ages, but is less efficient for children >20 kg. The bag allows assessment of tidal volume and a qualitative assessment of lung compliance (because of the low compression volume of the system). The bag must be large enough not to restrict tidal volume, but not so large that its value as a visual monitor is lost. By partially occluding the bag opening between the little finger and the palm, the anaesthetist can apply CPAP and PEEP. This system can also be used with a ventilator (e.g. Penlon Nuffield Series 200).

Fresh gas flow

The fresh gas flow required to prevent rebreathing is high—up to three times the predicted minute volume for spontaneous ventilation, with a minimum flow of 4 L/min. For controlled ventilation, a guide to fresh gas flow is given by the formula FGF = 1000 mL + 200 mL/kg. However, in practice fresh gas flow is determined by continuous monitoring of end-tidal CO_2. Pollution is a disadvantage of this system and while scavenging is possible, it makes the system less simple.

Mapleson D

The Mapleson D circuit, including the Bain co-axial version (with longer and lighter tubing), can be used for spontaneous or controlled ventilation in older (>20 kg) children. It is an efficient system for controlled ventilation. The valve is located at the proximal end of the circuit, which can be long because fresh gas is always delivered at the patient end. This makes the system especially useful when access is limited (e.g. a length of 540 cm can be used for MR scanning), and scavenging is also easy.

Fresh gas flow

Suggested values are 150–250 mL/kg/minute for spontaneous ventilation and 70–100 mL/kg/minute for controlled ventilation.

Mapleson A

The Mapleson A (Magill) system is efficient for spontaneous ventilation, but not for controlled ventilation because of preferential elimination of CO_2 in spontaneous mode. It should not be used for controlled ventilation in children. Even for spontaneous ventilation, this circuit is not suitable for use with small children <20 kg, as the expiratory valve adds resistance, and its location (next to patient) gives a large apparatus dead space. Moreover, the weight of the valve, especially if connected to scavenging apparatus, places drag on connections at the patient end.

Humphrey ADE

The Humphrey ADE system is a versatile hybrid system that can perform functionally as a Mapleson A, D, or E circuit. The mode of operation is selected by switching a single lever (□ Fig 4.2). With the lever up, the system functions in its Mapleson A mode for spontaneous ventilation. With the lever down, it functions in Mapleson E mode for mechanical ventilation. Scavenging is straightforward and a carbon dioxide absorption canister can be easily incorporated. The system is suitable for paediatric use because:

- It has narrow 15 mm tubing that gives a low internal volume.
- The tubing is smooth, giving no significant ↑ in resistance over 22 mm corrugated tubing.
- The APL valve in the system offers no significant extra resistance, but is designed to provide a small amount of PEEP (1 cm H_2O).
- A ventilator can be connected, e.g. Penlon Nuffield 200.

Fresh gas flow

This system can be used efficiently for spontaneous and controlled ventilation. In both modes an initial fresh gas flow of 3 L/min is recommended for children <25 kg.

Circle systems

The circle system, incorporating soda lime or baralyme for CO_2 absorption is now widely used in paediatric anaesthesia. Paediatric circuits use:

- Narrow 15 mm diameter tubing, reducing compression volume.
- Smaller distal connections to minimize dead space.
- A ventilator capable of ventilating small children.
- Out of circuit vapourizers.

Advantages
- Low fresh gas flow—economic as less volatile agent is used.
- Easy scavenging and reduced atmospheric pollution.
- Conservation of heat and water vapour (i.e. humidification).

Disadvantages
- Unidirectional valves can offer resistance, and valves can stick—not ideal for small infants (<5 kg) breathing spontaneously
- Loss of feel during hand ventilation due to large compression volume, and hence high system compliance.

Fresh gas flow

A high initial gas flow (several L/min) is required for 5–10 min to wash nitrogen from both the circle system and the patient's functional residual capacity. This can later be reduced to 0.5–1 L/min, although in paediatric anaesthesia the leak around uncuffed ETTs limits the extent to which fresh gas flow can be minimized.

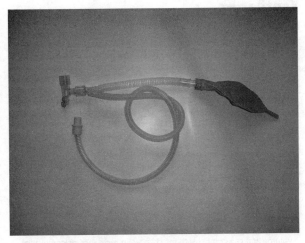

Fig. 4.1 Mapleson F (T-piece) breathing system.

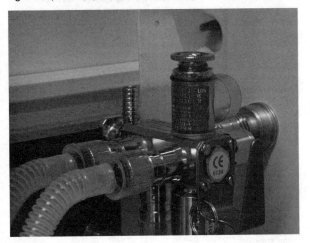

Fig. 4.2 The Humphrey ADE block with the lever in the up position for spontaneous ventilation.

Ventilators

Positive pressure ventilators are widely used during paediatric anaesthesia and in ITU.

Anatomical and physiological factors

The key differences between children and adults of relevance to ventilation are:
- Smaller tidal volumes.
- ↑ lung compliance.
- ↑ risk of barotrauma.
- Higher respiratory rates.
- Closing capacity may exceed or overlap functional residual capacity.

Most children can be adequately ventilated with inspiratory pressures of ~18–20 cm H_2O and a respiratory rate in the range 16–24 breaths/min. In practice, the precise ventilator settings are determined clinically, with the rate being adjusted to achieve normocapnia.

Design of paediatric ventilators

Ventilators can be classified as:
- Flow generators. These provide a predetermined inspiratory tidal volume and can compensate for changes in resistance or compliance.
- Pressure generators. These provide a predetermined inspiratory pressure. They do not compensate for changes in resistance or compliance, but can compensate for leaks in the circuit, changes in compression volume and changes in fresh gas flow.
- Pressure controlled ventilators are generally used in children because:
  - Of the leak generally present around uncuffed ETTs.
  - Lower risk of barotrauma.
  - Reduced compliance is not generally an issue in children.
- Other features of a ventilator designed for use with children include:
  - Ability to deliver small tidal volumes at high respiratory rates.
  - Provision for PEEP.
  - A variable I:E ratio.
  - Simplicity, including the ability to change from controlled to manual ventilation without changing circuits.
  - Compatibility with a circle system.
  - Built in alarms for pressure, expired tidal and minute volume, oxygen concentration, and disconnection.

Examples of ventilators for paediatric anaesthesia

- Many modern multi-purpose ventilators, such as the Penlon AV900, are sufficiently sophisticated that they can be set to act as time-cycled pressure generators with appropriate rates and tidal volumes for paediatric use.
- An example of a relatively simple ventilator still commonly used for paediatric ventilation in the UK is the Penlon Nuffield 200. This time-cycled flow generator can be used in paediatric anaesthesia in two different modes.

- For children >20 kg, it can be used in its normal, flow-generating mode, attached to a Bain, Humphrey ADE, T-piece or circle system. In the Bain and circle the reservoir bag is replaced by the tubing carrying the driving gas from the ventilator. The breathing system APL valve must be fully closed. Inspiratory and expiratory times are set by selecting the required I:E ratio and tidal volumes set by adjusting inspiratory time and flow rate. In this mode, the ventilator delivers a minimal tidal volume of 50 mL.
- For children <20 kg, it can be converted to a time-cycled pressure generator by connecting it to the breathing system via a Newton (paediatric) valve. In this mode, the ventilator is capable of delivering tidal volumes between 10 mL and 300 mL at frequencies between 10 and 85 breaths/min. This makes it suitable for the ventilation of premature babies and neonates. With the Newton valve connected the flow rate set on the ventilator is *not* the flow delivered to the patient. The valve is basically a simple (3.5 mm diameter) orifice that, by restricting the gas flow from the outlet, produces pressure at the end of the expiratory limb of the breathing system (which should have a minimum volume of 350 mL to prevent driving gas from diluting the inspired gas). The effect of ↑ the driving gas flow into the Newton valve can be summarized as:
  - At low flows the pressure in the valve only partially opposes the flow from the breathing system outlet, and so acts as a partial thumb occluder. The child receives a small tidal volume at a rate dependent on, but less than, the fresh gas flow into the T-piece.
  - As flow ↑, a point is reached where the valve acts as complete thumb occluder, and tidal volume equals fresh gas flow.
  - At higher flows, and hence higher pressures in the valve, some driving gas moves up the expiratory limb, and acts as a piston. Tidal volumes exceed fresh gas flow, and are determined by the ventilator settings.

Problems
- The ventilator continues to cycle even if the breathing system becomes disconnected and a disconnect (pressure) monitor is therefore essential.
- The Penlon Nuffield 200 is a gas powered ventilator, and requires high flows of driving gas (usually oxygen at ~400 kPa).

Pulse oximetry

- Pulse oximetry provides the best, non-invasive, continuous method of measuring the arterial oxygen saturation of haemoglobin (SpO_2). It can:
  - Provide an early indication of hypoxia.
  - Guard against hyperoxia, especially in premature infants at risk of retrolental fibroplasia (oxygen saturation in premature infants should be maintained in the range 90–95%).
- Fetal haemoglobin has no effect on measured SpO_2 as it has the same light absorbance properties as adult haemoglobin in the red/infrared range.
- Pulse oximeter measurements are also unaffected by jaundice, as bilirubin does not absorb light significantly in this wavelength range.
- Thus the same basic method of pulse oximetry used in adults can provide accurate SpO_2 values in all ages of children. Paediatric modifications have generally been confined to the design of dedicated probes.
- Oxygenated and deoxygenated haemoglobin have different light absorption spectra.
- The standard pulse oximeter has a photodetector and two light-emitting diodes (LEDs). One LED emits red light, at 660 nm, where the absorption of reduced haemoglobin exceeds that of oxygenated haemoglobin. The other LED emits in the infrared, at 940 nm, where oxygenated haemoglobin is the stronger absorber.
- To allow detection of the pulsatile component of absorption, the LEDs are cycled on and off at a frequency of 400 Hz. This cycle includes a phase in which both diodes are off (to allow measurement of the background level of ambient light).
- The measurements are averaged over a period of 10–20 sec. They are then converted by the microprocessor into oxygen saturation levels (SpO_2), using conversion factors derived from multi-wavelength co-oximeter measurements of healthy subjects.
- Because it is unethical to render volunteers hypoxic to a significant degree, this calibration is only accurate down to an SpO_2 ~75% (± 2%). This may be important (e.g. in cyanotic heart disease), but is not normally a serious limitation as values of SpO_2 <90% are acted upon.
- The oximeter signal is displayed as a continuous trace, showing signal quality and measured SpO_2.
- Alarm limits can be set for low saturation values and for both high and low pulse rates.

Paediatric sensors

- Standard oximeter probes are often less accurate in paediatric use because the path length of the light at the two wavelengths differs significantly in small digits (the 'penumbra' effect).
- Paediatric sensors have been developed to overcome this problem, and soft, secure sensors are now available which can be wrapped around a finger, a toe, the palm of a hand or a foot (🕮 Fig 4.3).

Problems and limitations

Inaccurate measurements can result from:
- Incorrect sensor positioning or movement.
- Interference from fluorescent lighting.
- Venous pulsation (e.g. with high airway pressure).
- Nail polish.
- The presence of dyes into the bloodstream (e.g. methylene blue).

Errors in the inferred level of oxygen saturation can arise from:
- Hypoperfusion.
- Peripheral vasoconstriction.
- Drugs which produce methaemoglobinaemia—methaemoglobin mimics the effect of additional reduced haemoglobin, and hence results in an under estimate of S_pO_2.
- Carboxyhaemoglobin, which produces an over estimate of S_pO_2.
- Slow device response time, which results in a delay in the detection of acute desaturation.
- Severe anaemia and polycythaemia.

Oximeter probes can cause pressure sores with continuous use on the same site. Burns have been reported in children following the prolonged use of finger probes.

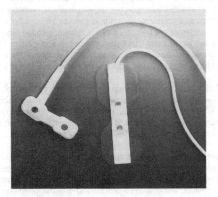

Fig. 4.3 Examples of wrap-around infant pulse oximeter probes for use on digits, palm or foot. A reusable sensor is shown on the left, a disposable sensor on the right (with adhesive fastening tape).

Blood pressure measurement

Blood pressure is lower in children than in adults, and lower still in infants and neonates. Table 4.4 gives the normal range of systolic, diastolic and mean blood pressure in children of different ages.

Table 4.4 Normal range of blood pressure (mm Hg) in children of different ages

Age	Systolic	Diastolic	Mean
Neonate (<1 kg)	40–60	15–35	25–45
Neonate (3 kg)	50–70	25–45	35–55
Newborn (4 days)	60–90	20–60	35–70
Infant (6 months)	85–105	55–65	65–80
Child (2 years)	95–105	55–65	65–80
Child (7 years)	100–110	55–70	70–85
Adolescent	110–130	65–80	80–95

- The measurement of blood pressure during anaesthesia is normally done using monitors based on the technique of oscillometry. A single cuff, controlled by a microprocessor, is used to both compress the limb, and to detect the pulsations of the returning blood flow as the cuff pressure is reduced. These devices can be used for the accurate measurement of blood pressure even in small premature infants.
- The middle of the cuff bladder should be placed over the brachial artery.
- The inflation/deflation sequence is set on the microprocessor. The cuff is inflated rapidly (to avoid venous congestion) to above (previously-measured) systolic pressure. It is then deflated gradually. The returning pulse is sensed as rapid pressure oscillations in the cuff, which are converted to electrical signals by a transducer accurate to ± 2%.
- The rapid onset of oscillations corresponds to systolic pressure, maximum amplitude corresponds to mean arterial blood pressure, and the subsequent rapid decline corresponds to diastolic pressure. In some devices, the measured systolic and diastolic pressures are also compared to the values calculated mathematically from the mean value (where the measurement technique is most accurate).
- All three pressures, as well as measured pulse rate, are displayed on the monitor and alarm limits can be set for both high and low values. Some monitors can be used to apply venous stasis to facilitate IV cannulation.

Problems

- Oscillometry becomes less accurate at extreme values of blood pressure. Systolic pressure is over estimated at low systolic pressures (<60 mmHg), and under estimated at high pressures.
- The accuracy of the blood pressure measurement can also be affected by atrial fibrillation and other dysrhythmias, arm position and external pressure on the cuff. Of particular importance in children, however, is use of the correct cuff size.
- An excessively small (or too stiff) cuff produces an over estimate of blood pressure, while an excessively large cuff produces an under estimate (although the systematic error is smaller with too large a cuff).
- The commercial labelling of blood pressure cuffs as infant, paediatric, small adult, adult and large adult can be misleading. The standard recommendations for cuff size are that:
  - The cuff should cover at least 2/3 of the upper arm length.
  - The width of the cuff bladder should be 40% of the mid-circumference of the upper arm.
- Confusingly however, especially for small children, these two alternative recipes can lead to a different choice of cuff size. If in doubt, it is better to choose a larger cuff to minimize error.

Temperature monitoring

Core temperature monitoring is important for the prevention of both hypothermia and hyperthermia.

- Hypothermia occurs most frequently in infants, in patients who receive large volume infusions of cold fluid and where it has been deliberately induced.
- Hyperthermia is uncommon during anaesthesia. However, it may occur when infants are over heated, in malignant hyperthermia, or with infection. It sometimes occurs in patients with osteogenesis imperfecta.

Skin temperature monitoring is used to measure peripheral temperature, which provides:

- An indication of peripheral perfusion, from the core-peripheral temperature gradient.
- A useful indication of the effectiveness of cooling and re-warming techniques during cardiac surgery.

A skin sensor should be used whenever an infrared heating device is used on an infant.

Measurement sites for core temperature

Pulmonary artery temperature is regarded as the 'true' core temperature but is unsuitable for routine clinical use. Core temperature is usually monitored at sites where temperature closely reflects core temperature.

- Nasopharyngeal: provides good estimate of brain temperature unless excessive cooling is caused by a large leak around the ETT.
- Oesophageal: the lower third of the oesophagus is normally used as the proximal oesophagus may be cooled by anaesthetic gases.
- Rectal: less frequently used due to a prolonged lag time (up to several hours) resulting from insulation provided by faeces.
- Tympanic membrane: provides an accurate estimate of hypothalamic temperature with minimal lag time, but the use of a thermistor probe carries a risk of perforation of the tympanic membrane.
- Bladder: accuracy varies with urine flow rate.
- The axilla is the best site for the measurement of muscle temperature, making it the best site for the early detection of malignant hyperthermia.

Temperature probes

- Temperature probes are either electrical or non-electrical.
- Electrical devices include:
  - Thermocouples: based on the Seebeck effect, in which a temperature-dependent voltage is produce at the junction of two metals with different specific heat capacities.
  - Platinum-wire thermometers: the electrical resistance of metals ↑ linearly with temperature.
  - Thermistors: the electrical resistance of semiconductors ↓ non-linearly with temperature.
  - infrared thermometers: a thermopile is used to measure the intensity of heat radiation from a surface, and the temperature of the equivalent black-body radiator derived.

- Non-electrical devices are based on:
  - The expansion of liquids/gases: e.g. the mercury thermometer.
  - The bending of bimetallic strips made of two metals with different expansion co-efficients.
  - Chemical techniques: e.g. liquid crystals that change colour with temperature.
- Continuous, intraoperative monitoring is usually performed with thermistors or thermocouples. Most modern medical temperature sensors use semi-conductor thermistors because they are compact, robust, and easy to manufacture. Thermistors produce a non-linear relationship between temperature and resistance, but this is not an issue with the calibration power of modern microprocessors.
- Flexible and durable reusable and disposable temperature probes are available. Paediatric nasopharyngeal/oesophageal/rectal probes consist of a small (3–4 mm diameter) thermistor sensor at the end of a semi-flexible nylon or vinyl tube.
- A typical skin sensor consists of a sensor disc with a stainless steel surface attached to a rigid steel handle or a flexible vinyl wire. Heat shields are available for paediatric skin probes used to reduce the risk of burns from overhead infrared heaters.
- Liquid crystal technology is used in some skin probes. Infrared thermometry is utilized in probes that can be used for the intermittent measurement of temperature from the tympanic membrane without risk of trauma.

Warming devices

All patients lose heat during anaesthesia, but children, and in particular neonates have poorly developed physiological mechanisms for maintaining body heat. Heat loss occurs primarily through radiation, but also through convection, evaporation, and conduction. Prevention of heat loss is important because of the adverse effects of hypothermia (📖 Chapter 1):
- ↑ postoperative O_2 consumption caused by shivering.
- Prolonged duration of action of neuromuscular blocking drugs.
- Delayed drug excretion.

Physiological factors

During anaesthesia the normal regulatory responses of peripheral vaso-constriction and ↑ heat production are abolished and infants cool very quickly as heat is redistributed to the periphery and then lost to the environment. Neonates are especially prone to hypothermia if placed in a cool environment because of their:
- High surface-area/volume ratio.
- Relatively large head.
- Minimal subcutaneous fat.
- Poor insulation.
- Limited vasoconstrictor response.
- Inability to shiver—non-shivering heat production occurs via metabolism of brown fat, but this is deficient in premature infants.

The neutral thermal environment, the temperature at which no meta-bolic response is required to stay warm, depends on age, maturity, and weight (34°C for a premature baby, 32°C for a neonate, 28°C for an adult).

Environment

Operating theatre

The operating theatre should be maintained at high relative humidity (around 50%) and at a high temperature. For older children an ambient temperature of 20–22°C is adequate. Infants and neonates may ideally require an ambient temperature around 32°C, but in practice a comp-romise has to be adopted to allow a tolerable working temperature of 26–28°C.

Patient covering

Exposed areas, especially the head (a major source of heat loss in infants), can be wrapped in *Mediwrap*® (laminated heat-reflective material), bubble plastic or cotton gamgee. This reduces radiation heat loss and also convective heat loss, and is important both during the operation and during transfer to and from theatre. Neonates should be transferred in an incubator.

Active warming devices

Heating blankets and mattresses

Warming blankets can be very effective in reducing radiation losses and ↑ total body heat. Mattresses and blankets can be heated by electricity, warm water, or forced warm air. In the *Bair Hugger*® for example, warm air is pumped into the blanket from a heater. The warm air then passes through the gortex cover of the mattress to surround the patient, providing heat by convection and conduction. Clear plastic drapes over (but not under) the patient can help to create a warm air microclimate.

Overhead infrared heaters

Radiant heaters are very useful in the anaesthetic room and when infants are uncovered during induction and immediately after surgery. They are very effective, and portable models are available. These must always be used with a skin temperature probe to guard against over heating.

Gases and fluids

Heat and moisture exchanging (HME) filters

Use of an HME, partial rebreathing with an Ayre's T piece, and use of a circle breathing system can all contribute to passive warming and humidification of inspired gases, reducing heat loss from the respiratory tract. A range of simple HMEs is available and they are used routinely. They usually have a transparent plastic housing (allowing obstructions and secretions to be easily seen), and contain a layer of paper or foam coated with a hygroscopic salt. On expiration the gas cools as it passes through the layer, the water condenses, and is absorbed by the salt. The water molecules are then released back into the low-humidity inspired gas. Some HMEs have an added layer of filter material. These HMEFs are designed to prevent microbes entering the breathing system from the patient, whilst conserving heat and humidity.

HMEs ↑ apparatus dead space, and so HMEs with volumes as low as 7.8 mL are available for paediatric circuits. Filters for paediatric use are tested at gas flows of 15 litres/minute rather than 30 litres/minute for adult filters.

Blood and fluid warmers

These reduce conductive heat loss associated with the administration of cold fluid. The aim is to deliver fluids to the child at a temperature of 37°C. Any of the countercurrent heat exchange, dry heat warmer, or fluid heated coil systems are suitable. The warmed fluids should be delivered as near to the IV cannula as possible to minimize heat loss to atmosphere between the warmer and the patient.

Continuous temperature monitoring is required when an active warming device is used.

Peripheral venous cannulae

- As in adults, at least one peripheral venous cannula is placed in all children undergoing anaesthesia.
- If the child undergoes an inhalational induction, a cannula is placed as soon as practical.
- Placement is often difficult and frustrating.
- Common sites are the dorsum of a hand, antecubital fossa, feet, the long saphenous vein, and the cephalic vein in the forearm. The external jugular vein is useful in chubby toddlers. Scalp veins can also be used in neonates and young infants but are less secure and reliable than other sites. Veins on the flexor aspect of the wrist should be avoided if possible. In the event of extravasation, adjacent nerves and tendons will be exposed to the extravasated fluids and drugs.
- The technique of insertion is the same as in adults. The time from penetrating the vein wall to seeing a flashback in the needle hub may be longer than in adults if a small gauge needle is used. Many people find manipulation of fine cannulae difficult initially.
- The size chosen depends on the size of the child, the anticipated fluid requirements and the venous anatomy.
- Very small cannulae are used for peripheral access in neonates and infants. Plastic cannulae are available for paediatric use in sizes as small as 26 G. Typically, 24 G cannulae are suitable for use with neonates, while 24 or 22 G cannulae are appropriate for infants and older children.
- Maximum flow rate is proportional to the fourth power of the radius of the cannula. Because of their narrow bore, the maximum flow rates through paediatric cannulae are much lower than in adult apparatus. Table 4.5 gives flow-rates for different sizes of IV cannulae. Flow rates are measured under standardized conditions (using distilled water, at 22° C, under a pressure of 10 kPa, connected to the cannula by 110 cm of tubing with an internal diameter of 4 mm). In practice, maximum flow rates are seldom required and ease of placement is often a more important consideration when choosing the size of cannula.

Table 4.5 Flow rates through different sizes of IV cannulae

Catheter size (G)	Diameter (mm)	Colour-code	Flow rate (mL/min)
26	0.46	Black	13–15
24	0.56	Yellow	36
22	0.71	Blue	56
20	0.90	Pink	40–80
18	1.27	Green	75–120

Practical procedures and postoperative care

Francois Taljard

Basic airway management

Much of the morbidity associated with anaesthesia is due to airway problems. The same basic principles as in adults apply when managing the airway in children.

- Positioning
- Oxygen
- Recognizing airway obstruction
- Simple manoeuvres
- Airway adjuncts.

Positioning

- The airway of neonates and infants obstructs easily because of the large head, short neck, large tongue, and lack of space in the airway.
- Anatomical changes with age require different positioning in different age groups. In neonates and infants the relatively large head and prominent occiput (autoflexion) avoids the requirement for a pillow to flex the neck.
- For infants and children, a neutral position with the eye in line with the ear canal is required. Further extension of the neck may obstruct the airway.
- As the child gets older, positioning changes more towards the adult 'sniffing the air position'. A pillow is often useful in teenagers.

Oxygen supplementation

- Oxygen consumption in the neonate approximates 7 mL/kg/min decreasing gradually during childhood to the adult value of 3.5 mL/kg/min.
- There is rapid onset of hypoxia in the event of airway obstruction or apnoea.
- Effective preoxygenation is often distressing to children and is usually omitted, but it is essential that oxygen (preferably 100%) be given as soon as possible after induction.

Recognizing airway obstruction

- It is easy to occlude the airway unintentionally if the fingers compress the floor of the mouth and force the tongue upwards or if the neck is over extended, which results in hyperlordosis of the cervical spine and compression of the oropharynx.
- Quiet breathing is an indicator of airway patency. Any noisy breathing i.e. stridor, wheeze, grunting noise may indicate obstruction.
- Bilateral chest expansion on inspiration is assessed. Paradoxical abdominal movement is an indicator of airway obstruction.

Simple manoeuvres

- Correct positioning and clearing the airway is frequently all that is required. Continual assessment of airway patency is required and repeated adjustment may be necessary. Some infants may require CPAP. The positive pressure aids alveolar recruitment and prevents airway collapse due to tracheomalacia.

- The triple manoeuvre—mouth opening, jaw thrust, and neck extension—can be performed. The most useful of these is mouth opening, which separates the tongue from the palate and causes some forward movement of the mandible. Neck extension should not be much beyond neutral. It is easy to provoke laryngospasm with these manoeuvres at a light level of anaesthesia.
- If positive pressure ventilation is required, low inflation pressures are used to prevent gastric distension and splinting of the diaphragm. If CPAP or IPPV is required insertion of an orogastric or nasogastric tube to decompress the stomach should be considered. Consider this early if there is abdominal distension and splinting, even in a spontaneously breathing child. Distressed children tend to swallow air when crying.
- If necessary, remove secretions with nasal or oral suctioning. Use flexible rather than rigid suction catheters in neonates and infants.

Airway adjuncts

- Insertion of an oropharyngeal airway may help. They can stimulate the gag reflex or provoke laryngospasm if placed when the child too is light. They do not always improve the airway, possibly because of down folding of the epiglottis if too large or distortion of the base of the tongue if too small.
- Nasopharyngeal airways are used less often but are useful if there is limited mouth opening. There is a risk of causing adenoidal haemorrhage.
- An LMA can be used with the same considerations about adequate depth of anaesthesia.

Advanced airway management

Insertion of the laryngeal mask airway (LMA)

- Indications for an LMA include:
  - Airway maintenance during spontaneous ventilation.
  - Airway maintenance during IPPV (some anaesthetists ventilate through an LMA, some do not).
  - Conduit for fibreoptic endotracheal intubation.
- Contraindications are mostly relative and include:
  - Patients at risk of regurgitation and aspiration (absolute unless used to deal with severe airway obstruction).
  - Limited mouth opening.
  - Long procedures.
  - IPPV.
  - Neonates.
  - Infants other than for brief procedures.
  - Many head and neck procedures.
- An appropriately sized LMA is selected.

Table 5.1 Suggested LMA sizes

Patient weight (kg)	Mask size	Maximum cuff volume (mL)	ETT (mm) that will pass through LMA
< 5	1	4	3.5
5–10	1 1/2	7	4.0
10–20	2	10	4.5
20–30	2 1/2	14	5.0
30+	3	20	5.5

- Preoxygenation prior to insertion is essential. Many anaesthetists maintain the child with volatile agent in 100% oxygen for a period before insertion so that in the event of an episode of airway obstruction caused by attempted insertion there is a reserve of oxygen to provide time for remedial measures.
- Adequate depth of anaesthesia is required to prevent laryngospasm on insertion. A useful indicator is lack of movement or other response to jaw thrust. Jaw thrust in an inadequately anaesthetized child can itself initiate laryngospasm.
- Head is positioned in sniffing position; mouth open with an assistant supplying jaw thrust improves the chances of successful insertion.
- The technique of insertion is the same as for adult patients. The laryngeal aperture faces the tongue and the LMA is pushed along the palate with a smooth motion. A characteristic stop is felt when in position.

- An alternative rotational method is occasionally used. The LMA is inserted in to the mouth with the aperture facing the hard palate i.e. 180° rotation from normal. It is then pushed cranially and backward to slide along the hard and soft palates and rotated through 180° when the cuff is in the oropharynx.
- The cuff is inflated.
- Position is assessed using the pattern of breathing, evidence of partial or complete obstruction, noisy breathing, and the ability to ventilate through the LMA.
- If the position is unsatisfactory, the LMA is removed and a period of spontaneous ventilation with volatile agent in 100% oxygen is required before further attempts at insertion.
- There is an inverse correlation between age and the incidence of problems and unsatisfactory positioning of the LMA. Partial or complete airway obstruction, change in position after insertion, hypoxia and hypercarbia are all more common in younger children. For this reason, LMAs are rarely used for airway maintenance in children aged less than six months where endotracheal intubation and IPPV are usually preferred even for brief procedures.
- Removal of the LMA is carried out either with the patient anaesthetised ('*deep*') or on emergence from anaesthesia ('*awake*'). There is little to choose between the techniques and personal preference is usually the deciding factor. In 'deep' removal, the LMA is removed at the end of surgery as anaesthetic agents are discontinued. The airway is then maintained with a facemask until emergence from anaesthesia. In 'awake' removal, the LMA is left in place until the child starts to swallow on it and in most cases expels it themselves. Some people position a bite block for 'awake' removal to prevent the child biting on the tube risking damage to teeth and making it difficult to remove. Laryngospasm is a risk with both techniques especially in younger children It is important not to stimulate the child's airway during emergence to reduce the chances of laryngospasm.

Endotracheal intubation

- Decide which route—oral or nasal and which type of ETT is indicated—cuffed or uncuffed, North or South facing, cut or uncut, armoured. *Microcuff pediatric* endotracheal tubes with ultra thin high volume—low pressure polyurethane cuff are now available and can be used as long as the pressure in the cuff is checked regularly.
- For children younger than 4 years old, Table 5.2 provides a guide to the appropriate choice of ETT internal diameter. For older children the formula size = (age/4) + 4.5 mm is often used, but pre-existing medical conditions may influence size. With uncuffed tubes, it is advisable to have an ETT 0.5 mm larger and smaller than the initial choice.

Table 5.2 Suggested ETT sizes

Age	Weight (kg)	ETT internal diameter (mm)
Premature	< 2	2.5–3.0
Term	3–4	3.0–3.5
0–6 months	3–5	3.5
6–12 months	5–10	4.0
1–2 years	10–14	4.5
2–4 years	12–16	5.0

- Anatomical differences require different approaches at various ages.
  - Relatively large tongue in infants.
  - Cephalad larynx (adult position C4–5 in infants C2–3).
  - Anterior larynx compared to adults.
  - Epiglottis shape and position (long, narrow, floppy, and angled over the larynx at 45°).
  - Cricoid ring narrowest part of upper airway as opposed to vocal cords in adults.
- Ensure all equipment is at hand and functional prior to proceeding and perform preoxygenation. Patients are usually paralysed but intubation can be done under deep inhalational anaesthesia or with a bolus of opioid such as alfentanil 15 mcg/kg or remifentanil (1–2 mcg/kg).

Oral endotracheal intubation

- Straight bladed laryngoscopes are preferred in infants, with curved blades used for toddlers and older children.
- Straight blades can be used in the same way as a Macintosh with the tip placed in the vallecula and used to elevate the base of the tongue and attached epiglottis.
- The classic technique of straight bladed laryngoscopy involves advancing the blade until the tip is in the upper oesophagus. The blade is then withdrawn little by little until the tip comes out of the oesophagus and lies against the laryngeal surface of the epiglottis. In this position,

the epiglottis is lifted out of the field of view and the laryngeal inlet is exposed. The little finger of the left hand holding the laryngoscope can be used to apply external laryngeal pressure to help bring the vocal cords into view.

- The laryngeal surface of the epiglottis is innervated by the vagus nerve and the straight bladed technique sometimes causes a transient slowing of heart rate. This is rarely of clinical significance.
- The vocal cords are identified and the ETT inserted under direct vision to an appropriate length.
- Check diameter by confirming that a small audible leak can be heard at an inspiratory pressure of 20 cm H_2O. It is essential to ensure that there is a small leak around the tube prior to securing, in order to prevent excess tracheal mucosal pressure and subsequent tracheal stenosis.
- For tube length, the formula length = (age/2) + 12 cm provides a rough estimate, but tube length should be confirmed clinically by observing the length of the tube through the vocal cords, and checking for equal bilateral chest movement and breath sounds.
- Many ETTs have a solid black mark at the distal end to provide an indication of the length of ETT that should be passed through the cords.
- An alternative method of ensuring correct length is to look at the length of ETT through the vocal cords. In normal children without anatomical abnormalities of the airway, this should be 3 cm for ETTs of internal diameter 3.0 mm and 3.5 mm; 4 cm for those of 4.0 mm and 4.5 mm; and 5 cm for those of 5.0 mm and 5.5 mm.
- Secure fixation is essential as minor movement may lead to the tube slipping out or endobronchial migration.

Nasal endotracheal intubation

- Usually more difficult than the oral route.
- Preferred for long-term intubation (ITU) since it allows more secure fixation and facilitates oral hygiene.
- Consider whether the situation warrants securing the airway by oral intubation followed by nasal intubation.
- Pass the ETT through the preferred nostril until the tip is lying in the posterior pharynx.
- Visualize the vocal cords as described for oral intubation and pass the ETT through the cords under direct vision with the help of Magill forceps. This can be difficult due to the acute angle and limited space available. Once the tip of the tube has passed through the cords, it often impinges anteriorly at the cricoid ring because the angle of approach from the nasopharynx to the plane of the trachea is acute. Use the Magill forceps to push the tip of the tube down towards the floor and away from the anaesthetist as the plane of the trachea runs down and away. An alternative is to spin or rotate the tube through 180° so that the curvature follows the plane of the trachea. Pressure on the cricoid ring may help to pass the tube.
- Confirm correct diameter and length as above (length = age/2 + 14 cm).
- Secure fixation is again extremely important.

Difficult airway management

Definitions

The problem presented by a child with a difficult airway may comprise one or more of difficult mask ventilation, difficult laryngoscopy, or difficult tracheal intubation. The definitions produced by the American Society of Anesthesiologists (ASA) are useful for clarifying discussion. Different approaches may be indicated for difficult airway and difficult intubation.

- A difficult airway is defined as '*the clinical situation in which a conventionally trained anesthesiologist experiences difficulty with mask ventilation, difficulty with tracheal intubation or both*'.
- Difficult mask ventilation occurs when '*it is not possible for the unassisted anesthesiologist to maintain the S_pO_2 > 90% using 100% oxygen and positive pressure mask ventilation in a patient whose S_pO_2 was > 90% before intervention*' or '*it is not possible for the unassisted anesthesiologist to prevent or reverse signs of inadequate ventilation during positive pressure mask ventilation*'.
- Difficult laryngoscopy occurs when '*it is not possible to visualize any portion of the vocal cords with conventional laryngoscopy*'.
- Difficult intubation occurs when 'proper insertion of the tracheal tube with conventional laryngoscopy requires more than three attempts' or 'proper insertion of the tracheal tube with conventional laryngoscopy requires more than 10 min'.

Predicting the difficult airway or endotracheal intubation

- The incidences of difficult mask ventilation and difficult or impossible conventional endotracheal intubation in children are unknown. Probably less common than in adults. There is a higher incidence in sub-specialties such as maxillofacial surgery.
- A large number of congenital syndromes and acquired conditions are associated with a potentially difficult airway but in the majority of these individual patients are often straightforward to ventilate by facemask and to intubate.
- The child is assessed for dysmorphic features e.g. macroglossia, micrognathia, abnormal ear position, wide webbed or short neck, and also limited mouth opening. These features may provide indicators of difficulty but as with formal predictive tests are insensitive and lack specificity.
- The fundamental causes of difficulties are the same as in adults—a small mandibular space, a large tongue, restricted extension at the atlanto-occipital joint, and an inability to introduce a laryngoscope into the mouth.
- The various predictive tests that have been used in adults such as the thyromental distance, Wilson score and the Mallampati test have never been assessed or validated in children.
- There is also the problem of lack of cooperation with assessment in a significant number of children.
- There is no information on the predictive value of investigations such as radiographs or magnetic resonance imaging in predicting difficult intubation in children.

- Information from previous anaesthetic records or from parents is frequently the best indicator of the degree of difficulty or otherwise experienced during previous anaesthetics, although this may not always be completely predictive of the current situation.
- In many cases, the degree of difficulty changes with age and some children become easier to manage while others become more difficult. The latter is a problem in some types of mucopolysaccharidosis (MPS). In these, airway management and endotracheal intubation usually become more difficult with age and there is a very high incidence of difficulties with airway management and endotracheal intubation.

Options for management of the difficult airway

Consider:
- Avoiding general anaesthesia—is there a place for sedation, a regional block, or a combination of these without general anaesthesia?
- Avoiding endotracheal intubation. Is a facemask or LMA technique appropriate?
- Avoiding neuromuscular blockade.
- Primary and secondary methods of achieving endotracheal intubation.
- Place of tracheostomy.
- Management of the 'can't intubate, can't ventilate' scenario.

Anticipated difficult airway or endotracheal intubation

- The use of regional anaesthetic techniques alone in children is limited to relatively minor and superficial procedures.
- Painful or invasive procedures in children often require a degree of sedation that is indistinguishable from general anaesthesia in which case any advantages of sedation are lost. In most cases, general anaesthesia is usually more appropriate than sedation.
  - Often children who are impossible to intubate conventionally have an easy airway to maintain with a facemask or LMA. In these cases, many surgical procedures are performed without endotracheal intubation. This situation might apply in temporomandibular joint ankylosis or hemifacial microsomia i.e. 'easy airway, difficult intubation' cases.
  - In children who present a difficult facemask anaesthetic ('difficult airway, difficult intubation') the LMA is often an option for maintenance of anaesthesia during surgery. This is particularly common in MPS.
- For children who require endotracheal intubation and are known or suspected to be difficult to intubate, a general anaesthetic technique that preserves spontaneous ventilation is employed.
  - If appropriate equipment and expertise are available, a fibreoptic technique can be used (□ p.123).
  - If the fibreoptic option is unavailable, a traditional approach to this problem is to perform an inhalational induction and then to attempt conventional endotracheal intubation.
  - Sedative premedication requires careful consideration. This may be helpful in an easy airway, difficult intubation scenario but contraindicated in a difficult airway situation. Antisialogogue premedication may be useful to dry secretions (atropine 40 mcg/kg

oral 90 min before induction or glycopyrrolate 100 mcg/kg oral 60 min before induction).

- The assistance of a second anaesthetist is useful. A full complement of basic airway adjuncts (different sized face masks, oropharyngeal airways, LMAs) and laryngoscope blades (straight and curved) as well as specialized difficult airway equipment such as the McCoy laryngoscope should be available. Equipment for emergency cricothyroidotomy should be available. Preparations for a surgical tracheostomy may be indicated.

- As with all difficult airway scenarios, the maintenance of spontaneous ventilation is vital. Inhalational induction with sevoflurane or halothane in 100% oxygen is the norm. The desired level of anaesthesia is that which will allow laryngoscopy. If the airway becomes obstructed, adjuncts should be used. Positioning with the head turned to the side, the lateral position or even semi-prone may improve airway patency.
  —If apnoea occurs, assisted ventilation is avoided if possible as this can lead to laryngospasm and/or gastric distension. Maintain CPAP until spontaneous ventilation resumes. Once an adequate level of anaesthesia is attained, insertion of an LMA may help in further deepening the level of anaesthesia.
  —If an adequate depth level of anaesthesia cannot be attained, the patient should be woken up.

- Once the patient is deep enough, laryngoscopy is performed. A variety of laryngoscopes are available including the common straight bladed Robertshaw, Miller, and Wisconsin types as well as levering tip types such as the McCoy and each of these may make a difference in some cases.

- Variations in the technique of laryngoscopy may also be helpful particularly the paraglossal or retromolar technique in the case of a relatively large tongue or small mandible. In this technique, the laryngoscope displaces the tongue to the left rather than anteriorly and it is useful in the case of limited anterior space for displacement of the tongue.

- Changes in the application of cricoid pressure may improve the view, as may the BURP manoeuvre that comprises backward, upward, and rightward pressure otherwise known as optimal external laryngeal manipulation (OELM) of the larynx.

- A blind approach to intubation through the nose or via an LMA is possible but requires experience in the technique and exposes the child to the risk of trauma to the airway. Rarely used in the UK.

- Light wands or illuminating stylettes are available in paediatric sizes.

- The technique of retrograde endotracheal intubation where a wire is passed through the cricothyroid membrane, retrieved through the mouth or nose, and then used to railroad an ETT has been used in children.

- Repeated attempts to intubate the trachea may cause trauma, hypoxia, and postoperative morbidity. Trauma during attempted intubation may result in postoperative oedema and swelling with critical narrowing of the airways. It is important to have a predetermined end point for the initial technique. A change to a fibreoptic technique should be made before the situation deteriorates.
- A tracheostomy may be required as either a short or long-term measure. Some children present needing a series of procedures over time and while on an individual occasion they are managed by fibreoptic intubation it is likely that at some point there will be a serious airway problem. In these cases, a temporary tracheostomy may also be the safest option.

Unexpected difficult airway or endotracheal intubation

Unexpected problems are often potentially more serious:

- The patient may have been paralysed before intubation is attempted, often as part of a rapid sequence induction.
- There may be a trainee anaesthetist or non-specialist anaesthetist.
- There may be a regurgitation/aspiration risk in non-elective cases.
- Many will occur out-of-hours when help is difficult to obtain.

The most likely scenarios are:

- A paralysed patient (not a regurgitation risk) who proves to be difficult to intubate.
  - It may be possible to continue the case using an LMA without endotracheal intubation.
  - The various manoeuvres described above may be used.
  - It is important to limit attempts at intubation to avoid trauma and the risk of problems following extubation.
  - In most elective and non-emergency cases, there is the option of abandoning the case and rescheduling when the patient is treated as an anticipated problem airway with appropriate personnel, equipment and planning in place.
- An elective patient induced but not paralysed who then proves to be a difficult facemask anaesthetic despite use of the triple manoeuvre, an oropharyngeal or nasopharyngeal airway, and two people attempting to maintain the airway.
  - Under these circumstances, the insertion of an LMA may transform the airway but the patient must be at an adequate depth of anaesthesia. Airway interventions at a light depth of anaesthesia may worsen the situation.
  - If early control of the situation is not obtained then abandonment is the best option.
  - This situation can easily degenerate into the 'can't intubate; can't ventilate' scenario.
- A rapid sequence induction performed in a patient at risk of regurgitation and aspiration.
  - In the event of difficulty with intubation during a rapid sequence induction, the failed intubation drill is followed, the patient allowed to recover from anaesthesia and senior help enlisted.

Can't intubate, can't ventilate

This is a particular danger in the 'difficult airway, difficult intubation' scenario especially if neuromuscular blockers are used before the airway is secured.

- The only objective is to oxygenate the child.
- An LMA should be used if it has not been tried already.
- A cricothyroidotomy may be performed.
  - There are commercial kits (mini-tracheostomy type and cannula type) available and these should be immediately at hand wherever children are anaesthetized.
  - Mini-tracheostomy types are connected to the anaesthetic circuit to ventilate the child.
  - Cannulae have both 15 mm and Luer lock connectors.
  - It is impossible to ventilate a patient with an anaesthetic circuit or self-inflating bag via a cannula cricothyroidotomy. The maximum pressure generated is insufficient to drive gas through the cannula.
  - The cannula is connected via the Luer lock connector and a Y-connector to the oxygen flow meter. The flow rate in L/min is set at the child's age in years. For inflation the open end of the Y-connector is occluded with a thumb for 1 sec. Chest movement is verified. If the chest does not rise, the flow rate is ↑ by increments of 1 L/min. Allow passive exhalation by taking the thumb off the connector for 4 secs.
  - Expiration of gases is not possible through the cannula. Expiration must occur through the upper airway, even when the airway is partially obstructed. It is important that the upper airway should be maintained in an optimal position during this procedure.
  - If total airway obstruction occurs the oxygen flow rate is reduced to 1–2 L/min. This will allow a degree of oxygenation but no ventilation. Insufflation will buy a little time for insertion of a surgical airway.
  - The chance of success, especially in infants, is low. The risk of life threatening complications is high. Complications are more likely in younger children and include:
    —bleeding
    —pneumothorax
    —pneumomediastinum
    —subcutaneous (surgical) emphysema
    —oesophageal placement
    —creation of a tracheo-oesophageal fistula
    —catheter dislodgement and failure of ventilation
    —haematoma
    —infection.

See also 📖 Chapter 14.

Fibreoptic endotracheal intubation

General points

- Some patients are poor candidates for fibreoptic endotracheal intubation. These include those with copious secretions, bleeding, or soiling in the upper airway where it is may be difficult to obtain adequate views through a fibreoptic instrument.
- It is often difficult to perform a fibreoptic intubation if there have been multiple attempts at conventional intubation resulting in trauma or laryngospasm.
- Fibreoptic equipment available in the UK comprises an adult fibreoptic laryngoscope (usually the LF2 model with an outside diameter of 4.1 mm) and a paediatric fibrescope the LF-P with an external diameter of 2.2 mm. There are also paediatric bronchoscopes with an external diameter of 2.8–3.5 mm. The adult instrument is suitable for teenagers. It has the disadvantage that the smallest ETT suitable for passing over the fibrescope is 5.0 mm internal diameter which too large for many patients. The fibrescope tends to obstruct the airway of smaller children during the procedure.
- The LF-P is suitable for endotracheal tubes of over 3 mm internal diameter. It has a number of disadvantages. There is no working channel to clear secretions, administer drugs or pass a guide wire to aid placement of an ETT. The instrument is very flexible and difficult to manipulate.

Routes for fibreoptic endotracheal intubation

- The oral route is preferred in most cases because it avoids the risk of adenoidal haemorrhage and allows use of an LMA for airway management and to guide the fibrescope to the larynx.
- The nasal route is used in cases with limited mouth opening or if there is a surgical indication for a nasal ETT.

Maintenance of anaesthesia during the procedure

- Usually with a volatile agent in 100% oxygen.
- Ideally using an LMA or alternatively through a facemask fitted with a bronchoscopic angle piece or by means of a nasal airway connected to the anaesthetic circuit.

Place of the LMA in fibreoptic endotracheal intubation

If the mouth can be opened enough to allow placement of an LMA this will:

- Provide a clear airway.
- Provide a route for spontaneous ventilation, oxygenation, and maintenance of anaesthesia.
- Guide the fibrescope to the laryngeal inlet.
- Allow CPAP and, if required, IPPV during the procedure.

ETT placement

- 'Railroading' over fibrescope. An ETT is threaded on to the fibrescope before use and slid off once the fibrescope is in the trachea. This may cause several problems. Too small a tube will not fit over the fibre-scope or may not slide off it into the trachea. Too big a tube will fail to enter the larynx and the procedure will need to be repeated with a smaller ETT. If an LMA is used, it can be difficult to pass the ETT through the LMA into the trachea and there is a risk of dislodging the ETT when removing the LMA.

- Using a guide wire with an airway exchange catheter. A 150 cm flexible J-tipped guide wire is passed under direct vision through the working channel of the fibrescope into the trachea and the bronchoscope removed. The bronchoscope need not pass through the larynx for this. An ETT may then be railroaded along the wire into the trachea. More commonly, an airway exchange catheter is passed over the wire to stiffen it, prevent it coiling in the airway and reduce the chances of the wire flicking out of the trachea as the ETT is passed. Position of the airway exchange catheter in the trachea is verified using capnography. The ETT is then railroaded over the airway exchange catheter. Advantages of using a wire technique include its suitability for children of all ages, availability of suction via the working channel of the fibrescope, less obstruction of the airway by fibrescope and/or combined fibrescope and ETT and the facility to change the ETT if the diameter is unsuitable without needing to repeat the whole endoscopy.

Technique

Successful fibreoptic intubation may take a long time and the anaesthetic technique must allow adequate oxygenation, ventilation, and the maintenance of an adequate depth of anaesthesia.

Oral endotracheal intubation

- The most commonly used technique involves an LMA.
- An antisialogogue is administered preoperatively. A sedative premedication may be administered, depending on the patient, if this is unlikely to cause respiratory depression or airway obstruction.
- Induction is usually inhalational with sevoflurane or halothane in oxygen. Monitors are applied, venous access is secured, the LMA positioned, and the patient observed by a second anaesthetist.
- During spontaneous ventilation through the LMA the fibrescope is introduced through an angle piece modified for bronchoscopy and advanced until the larynx is identified.
- The larynx is sprayed with 2–4 mL of 1% lignocaine though the working channel of the fibrescope.
- A guide wire is advanced along the working channel into the trachea and the fibrescope removed leaving the wire in place.
- An airway exchange catheter is passed over the wire.
- The position of the airway exchange catheter in the trachea is verified by capnography.
- The LMA is removed over the airway exchange catheter.
- An ETT is passed over the airway exchange catheter and into the trachea.
- This is checked for length and a leak. It is changed over the airway exchange catheter if required to obtain an ideal length with an adequate leak.

Variations

- An ETT may be loaded on the fibrescope and introduced directly into the trachea without using a wire technique. This leaves a laryngeal mask airway in place with an ETT passing through it.
- An oral ETT may be passed with the aid of an intubating oropharyngeal airway. The Ovassapian and Berman types are suitable for use in older children over 30 kg while the while the VBM™ model is available in smaller sizes.
- During the procedure, the airway may be maintained with a naso-pharyngeal airway or an airway endoscopy facemask.

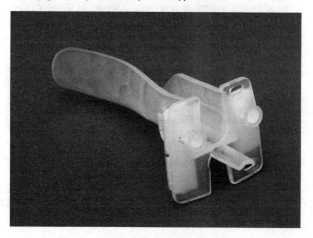

Fig. 5.1 Ovassapian oropharyngeal airway for fibreoptic endotracheal intubation

Nasal fibreoptic endotracheal intubation
- An antisialogogue and a nasal vasoconstrictor (*xylometazoline*) are given preoperatively (and sedation if indicated).
- An inhalational induction of anaesthesia is usually performed. Monitoring is applied, and venous access secured.
- Anaesthesia is usually maintained with a volatile agent in oxygen and spontaneous ventilation preserved.
- The airway is usually maintained by a second anaesthetist using an airway endoscopy mask connected to the anaesthesia circuit. The second anaesthetist monitors the patient and warns of problems.
- The fibrescope is inserted through a nostril and passed along the floor of the nose into the nasopharynx. It is gently advanced and manoeuvred to identify the larynx.
- The larynx is sprayed with lidocaine. A wire is passed along the suction channel and through the vocal cords into the trachea. The fibrescope is then removed.
- An airway exchange catheter is passed over the wire.
- The wire is removed.
- The position of the airway exchange catheter in the trachea is verified by capnography and then an ETT railroaded over it.
- The length and diameter of the chosen ETT are checked. It may be changed over the airway exchange catheter as required.

Variations
- Alternative methods of airway management include an oropharyngeal airway ('chimney airway') with a 15 mm connector to allow connection to an anaesthetic circuit or a nasopharyngeal airway.
- In older children, the ETT may be placed on the fibrescope and railroaded directly in the same way as in adults.

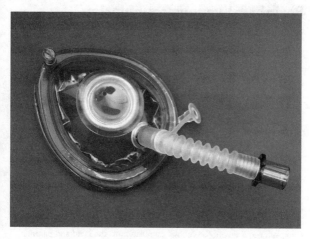

Fig. 5.2 Endoscopy face mask with removable membrane containing port for fibrescope

Peripheral venous cannulation

- Often difficult:
  - Difficulty finding veins e.g. chubby 1-year-old, neonates where scalp veins might be the best option.
  - Uncooperative child.
  - Limited number of chances to cannulate before the situation becomes very distressing for child, parents, and staff.
  - Vasoconstriction as in hypovolaemia.
- If the child is critically unwell and requires immediate access, try only a maximum of two attempts for peripheral cannulation before proceeding to intraosseus needle insertion (📖 p.134).
- Paediatric cannulae are usually narrow (22 G or 24 G) and backflow of blood may be slow. A cannula might be in the vein and mistakenly removed due to lack of backflow of blood. Sometimes necessary to check with a flush of normal saline to confirm correct placement in these cases if the insertion is felt to have been a success.

Elective or emergency anaesthesia and surgery

- Insertion after inhalational induction may be appropriate.
- Explain requirement for venous cannulation to the child and parents during the preoperative visit.
- Assess for the most promising veins during preoperative assessment.
- EMLA (1–2 hours before) or Ametop (30–40 min before) over the most promising veins is useful.
- Two or more sites should receive topical cutaneous analgesia in case of failure of the first attempt.
- Keep the needle out of sight of the child.
- Ensure child is distracted during insertion. Parents and/or play specialists can be very helpful in this situation.
- Remove the LA cream and get assistant to immobilize the limb and provide venous congestion.
  - Identify the intended vein and cannulate as in adults.
  - Rapid securing of the cannula before the child moves their hand or arm.
  - Test patency with saline flush to avoid subcutaneous injection of induction agent.
  - Anaesthetic drugs should be close at hand and can be administered as soon as the cannula is sited.
  - Ensure you have access to head and airway despite the presence of parents and play specialist as the child will desaturate rapidly once anaesthetized.

External jugular vein cannulation

- The external jugular vein is an easily identifiable and consistent landmark in the neck.
- It is formed by the junction of the posterior division of the posterior facial with the posterior auricular vein. It commences in the substance of the parotid gland, on a level with the angle of the mandible, and runs perpendicularly down the neck, in the direction of a line drawn from the angle of the mandible to the middle of the clavicle at the posterior border of the sternocleidomastoid. In its course it crosses the sternocleidomastoid obliquely, and in the subclavian triangle perforates the deep fascia, and ends in the subclavian vein, lateral to, or in front of, the scalenus anterior. It is separated from the sternocleidomastoid by the deep cervical fascia, and is covered by the platysma, the superficial fascia, and the skin. It crosses the cutaneous cervical nerve, and its upper half runs parallel with the great auricular nerve. The external jugular vein varies in size.
- After unsuccessful attempts at venous access at other sites cannulation of this vein may be very useful. An aseptic procedure is required as this vessel is a central vein.

Technique

- The patient is positioned slightly head down with the head turned to the contralateral side and arms by the sides. A small roll or bolster is placed under the shoulders to extend the neck. The vein can be made more prominent if an assistant occludes it by laying a finger across it just above the clavicle.
- Cannulation is performed with a cannula over needle as in peripheral venous cannulation. The approach is in the line of the vessel, aiming caudal and posterior. If a flashback of blood is seen as the vein is punctured, the cannula is advanced in to the vein and secured *in situ*. More often, the vessel is transfixed and the cannula is withdrawn slowly until blood is seen and then it is advanced in to the vein.
- This route can sometimes be used to insert central venous catheters over a guide wire passed down the cannula and in to the superior vena cava. Its usefulness is limited by the fact that passage is often obstructed at the point where the vein perforates the deep fascia.

Internal jugular vein cannulation

- Less frequently used in children than adults. Difficult technique in children less than 1 year of age due to the short neck and difficulty in cannulating the vein.
- Requires general anaesthesia with or without muscle relaxation. Placement is made easier by the use of muscle relaxants to prevent movement and risk of damage to other structures.
- The process of insertion is identical to adult techniques although shorter needles and shorter catheters are used.
- The internal jugular vein lies deep to the sternocleidomastoid muscle, and follows a course from just anterior to the mastoid process to behind the sternoclavicular joint.
- Lines available for use vary in diameter from 4 FG to adult sized catheters and single, double and triple lumen lines are available. Lengths vary from 6 cm to 30 cm.

Technique

- Similar to that in adults.
- The right side is preferred when possible. The internal jugular vein, superior vena cava and right atrium are in line on the right and correct placement of the tip is almost guaranteed. On the left side the catheter tip frequently ends up in a suboptimal position and the thoracic duct is at risk.
- Options are a low approach near the clavicle (high success rate but a risk of pneumothorax and haemothorax) or higher approach at the apex of the triangle formed by the two heads of sternocleidomastoid at the level of the cricoid cartilage (less risk of pneumothorax, may ↑ risk of carotid artery puncture).
- The child is positioned head down with the head turned to the contralateral side with a roll or bolster under the shoulders.
- The carotid artery is identified and the needle inserted just lateral to it at an angle of 30° to the skin surface and directed towards the ipsilateral nipple while aspirating gently.
- The end point is aspiration of venous blood in to the syringe. The needle should not be advanced more than 2.5 cm. The needle frequently transfixes and kinks the vein without aspiration and blood is only aspirated during withdrawal of the needle.
- The syringe is disconnected and, if venous blood flows freely from the needle, the vein is cannulated or a guide wire is passed and a standard Seldinger technique used to place the definitive catheter.
- Care is required to avoid air embolism as minimal amounts can cause dysrhythmias, cardiac arrest or cerebral embolism. The lumen(s) of the catheter are flushed prior to use with saline or heparinized saline.

Ultrasound
- Ultrasound guided insertion of central lines is now very common. The ultrasound device e.g. SonoSite® (SonoSite Inc., Bothell, USA) is used either to identify the vein before needle insertion or to provide real time imaging during insertion of the needle.
- Ultrasound guidance is recommended by the National Institute for Health and Clinical Excellence (NICE) as the preferred method of internal jugular vein cannulation for elective procedures. It should also be considered in the emergency situation. However, proficiency in landmark guided insertion should be maintained.
- Advantages include being able to define the anatomy before attempting the procedure, confirm that a patent vein is present, observe the position of the artery and its relationship to the vein, guide the needle during insertion and observe penetration of the vein by the needle.
- In adults, ultrasound guided central line insertion is associated with higher success rates and fewer complications than landmark guided insertion and with time this is likely to be demonstrated in children as well.

Placement
Correct placement has two aspects:
- Venous rather than arterial location is verified by transducing a venous trace and pressure from the distal lumen and by free aspiration of venous blood from all lumens.
- Catheter tip positioned at or near the junction of superior vena cava and right atrium is verified by a chest X-ray (CXR) that also excludes a pneumothorax.

Complications
Complications of internal jugular cannulation are general as for all central lines and particular to the route of insertion.
- General:
  - Air embolus
  - Haematoma
  - Thrombosis
  - Sepsis
  - Long term damage to the vein.
- Particular to the internal jugular route:
  - Carotid artery puncture
  - Pneumothorax
  - Haemothorax
  - Damage to neural structures i.e. brachial plexus, phrenic nerve, Horner's syndrome (usually transitory)
  - Damage to the thoracic duct on the left side.

Femoral vein cannulation

- This is a popular method of central venous access in children especially neonates and infants.
  - It is often easier to perform than internal jugular, subclavian or external jugular cannulation in these age groups.
  - There is less risk of serious complications and damage to vital structures.
- Femoral venous lines do not provide accurate cardiac filling pressures and have limited use in cardiac surgery.
- They are less popular for long-term use than neck lines because of concerns about infection, kinking of the catheter with leg movements and displacement during nappy changes and perineal cleaning.
- The femoral vein accompanies the femoral artery in the femoral triangle, and lies medial to the artery at the inguinal ligament where it becomes the external iliac vein.

Technique

- General anaesthesia is required to prevent movement during insertion.
- The patient is positioned supine with a small roll or bolster under the hips to bring the hips forward. Slight abduction and external rotation of the hip.
- The femoral artery is palpated 1–2 cm below the midpoint of the inguinal ligament halfway between anterior superior iliac spine and symphysis pubis.
- The needle inserted just medial to the artery and advanced at an angle of 45° to the coronal plane while aspirating gently.
- The end point is aspiration of venous blood in to the syringe. The needle should not be advanced more than 2.5 cm (risk of perforation of a viscus or penetration of the hip joint). The needle frequently transfixes the vein without aspiration and blood is only aspirated during withdrawal of the needle.
- The syringe is disconnected and, if venous blood flows freely from the needle, the vein is cannulated or a guide wire is passed and a standard Seldinger technique used to place the definitive catheter.
- Care is required to avoid air embolism as minimal amounts can cause dysrhythmias, cardiac arrest, or cerebral embolism. The lumen(s) of the catheter are flushed prior to use with saline or heparinized saline.

Placement

- Correct placement is with the catheter tip in the inferior vena cava. The catheter tip sometimes ends up in a minor tributary such as an epidural vein where erosion is a danger. This risk is minimized by transducing a venous trace and pressure from the distal lumen and by free aspiration of venous blood from all lumens. This also excludes arterial placement.
- Ultrasound is helpful in confirming the anatomy and identifying aberrant features especially when the vein is almost posterior to rather than medial to the artery.

Complications

General for all central venous lines and particular to the femoral approach:

- Femoral artery puncture (common)
- Penetration of hip joint (rare)
- Bowel perforation (rare).

Intraosseous cannulation

- This technique is used to gain rapid venous access when peripheral or central approaches are unsuccessful.
- Used for drug administration, fluid (volume) resuscitation, obtaining laboratory samples (remember to label these samples as bone marrow).
- Marrow cavities in long bones contain a mesh of non-collapsible venous sinusoids which drain into a central venous canal. The central venous canal leaves the bone through nutrient veins (with arteries) or sometimes emissary veins that pierce the shaft elsewhere. These sinusoids are effectively an approach to the venous system.
- The marrow spaces of infants contain very vascular red marrow which gets replaced by less vascular yellow marrow after 5 years of age. Although intraosseus cannulation is recommended for children less than 6 years of age, it can be used throughout childhood and even in adults.
- Specifically designed intraosseous needles are available (18 G and 20 G) and these should be available in all sites where children are anaesthetized and on resuscitation trolleys.

Indications

- During resuscitation of babies or children under 6 years of age.
- In any emergency when venous access cannot be gained rapidly after two failed attempts.
- As a temporary measure during induction of anaesthesia in a child with difficult venous access until peripheral or central venous access can be gained.

It is a temporary measure and should be replaced by conventional IV access within 24 hours if possible.

Advantages

- Easily identifiable landmarks.
- Rapid access.
- Requires no special training or expertise.
- High success rate.
- Safe with infrequent complications.
- Can be used to inject variety of drugs and fluids.

Sites

- The anterior surface of the proximal tibia, 2 cm distal to the tibial tuberosity is the most common site.
- The iliac crest may be used in older children.
- Sternal insertion is no longer recommended due to the risk of mediastinal penetration.

Technique

- Aseptic technique.
- Landmarks as described above.
- 90° to bony surface.
- Exert constant axial pressure.

- Use a boring, screwing rotational movement.
- Stop at loss of resistance.
- Unscrew cap.
- Aspirate to confirm placement and obtain marrow samples for investigation.
- Inject 10 mL 0.9% saline to confirm correct placement.

Signs suggesting correct placement
- Sudden loss of resistance (not with screw tipped needles).
- Aspiration of bone marrow (not always possible despite correct placement).
- Needle maintains an upright position unsupported.
- Fluid can be injected easily without evidence of extravasation (e.g. increasing limb circumference, localized swelling or tissue firmness).

Complications
- Transfixion of the tibia.
- Compartment syndrome of the calf.
- Osteomyelitis.
- Haemorrhage.
- Damage to the tibial growth plate.

Radial artery cannulation

- The radial artery is the commonest site for arterial cannulation in children followed by the femoral.
- As in adults used for continuous monitoring of blood pressure, arterial blood gas analysis, and frequent blood sampling.
- Complications of arterial cannulation are higher in children than in adults, especially in those less than 5 years of age. The risks and benefits of cannulation should be assessed carefully.
- The radial artery is a terminal branch of brachial artery. It arises in the antecubital fossa level with the radial neck and passes distally on the tendons and muscles attached to the radius. It lies deep to brachioradialis in the upper forearm but is subcutaneous in the lower forearm. It runs deep to abductor pollicis longus and extensor pollicis brevis tendons at the radial styloid. It enters the palm between the first and second metacarpals.
- The radial artery is preferred to the brachial for cannulation because there is less potential for forearm ischaemia. Allen's test for ulnar artery patency is often performed but is of dubious value.

Technique

- General anaesthesia or sedation and local anaesthesia are required.
- Positioned with small roll or bolster under wrist, the wrist extended (dorsiflexed) and secured with tape.
- Aseptic technique.
- Arterial pulsation identified by palpation.
- Needle inserted at 45–60° to coronal plane and advanced until the artery is punctured.
- Pulsatile flow from the needle is confirmed.
- Guide wire advanced down the needle.
- Cannula advanced over guide wire following removal of needle.
- Cannula secured with sutures and/or tape.
- It is easy to transfix the vessel during the attempt, so if cannulation appears unsuccessful the needle should be withdrawn slowly and observed for a flashback of blood.
- As well as a Seldinger technique, a catheter over the needle technique using a 22 G or 24 G cannula can be useful especially in neonates and infants.

Complications

- Haematoma.
- Haemorrhage.
- Arterial thrombosis.
- Distal hand ischaemia.
- Damage to surrounding tissues.
- Introduction of peripheral air emboli.
- Compartment syndrome of the forearm.
- Infection.
- Disconnection and haemorrhage.

Femoral artery cannulation

- The femoral artery is a much more common site for arterial cannulation than in adults.
- Especially useful in neonates and infants where the success rate is higher than for radial artery cannulation.
- A specific indication is in repair of aortic coarctation.
- The femoral artery is a continuation of the external iliac artery. It enters the thigh below the inguinal ligament midway between the anterior superior iliac spine and the symphysis pubis. Lies between the femoral vein medially and the femoral nerve laterally. Descends through the femoral triangle and enters the subsartorial canal.

Technique

- General anaesthesia is required to prevent movement during insertion.
- The patient is positioned supine with a small roll or bolster under the hips to bring the hips forward. Slight abduction and external rotation of the hip.
- The femoral artery is palpated 1–2 cm below the midpoint of the inguinal ligament halfway between anterior superior iliac spine and symphysis pubis.
- The needle inserted gently.
- The end point is aspiration of arterial blood in to the syringe. The needle should not be advanced more than 2.5 cm (risk of perforation of a viscus or penetration of the hip joint). The needle frequently transfixes the artery without aspiration and blood is only aspirated during withdrawal of the needle.
- In infants a non-aspiration technique is usually more successful as high negative pressures can occlude the artery.
- The syringe is disconnected and, if arterial blood pulsates from the needle, a guide wire is passed and a standard Seldinger technique used to place the catheter.

Complications

- Haemorrhage and haematoma if the artery is punctured but the guide wire and/or catheter will not thread.
- Venous puncture.
- Thrombosis and distal limb ischaemia.
- Perforation of hip or bowel (rare).

Recovery area (post anaesthetic care unit)

An area reserved for immediate postoperative care first described by Florence Nightingale in 1863, but only implemented in the US in 1923.

Requirements

- Requirements similar to adult units:
  - Adjacent to the operating suite and ICU.
  - Open floor area allowing good observation of patients.
  - Two bays or bed spaces for each operating theatre.
  - Monitoring equipment—ECG, NIBP, S_pO_2, temperature, invasive blood pressure and CVP monitoring capability.
  - High flow high volume suction.
  - Piped oxygen and air.
  - Electrical outlets.
- Full supply of airway equipment, IV equipment, fluids.
- Resuscitation equipment, ventilator and drugs readily available with a dedicated emergency call system.
- Adequate ventilation or scavenging to extract exhaled anaesthetic gases.
- Emergency and anaesthetic drugs readily available.
- Specific to paediatric recovery areas:
  - Child friendly with bright colours and decorations.
  - Toys available to distract and entertain.
  - Cots and beds with padded side rails essential to prevent injuries during recovery period.
  - Chairs for parents.

Use

- Takes patients recovering from anaesthesia and surgery until:
  - Awake.
  - Able to maintain airway unaided.
  - Adequate ventilatory effort to sustain oxygenation and avoid hypoventilation with CO_2 accumulation.
  - Adequate circulation and organ perfusion.
  - Pain free.
  - Normothermic.
- Time spent in the recovery varies from 15 min for healthy children after a brief procedure or examination to many hours depending on preoperative condition, extent of surgery, temperature, fluid requirements, and analgesic requirements.
- Occasionally used for postoperative IPPV until extubation or transfer to ICU.

Staffing

- Nurse to patient ratio should be >1:1 with at least one nurse to each patient and 'runners' to help with patients immediately after admission, complex patients, those who have undergone major or prolonged surgery and those suffering complications such as laryngospasm.
- Paediatric recovery nurses should be:
  - Specifically trained for this specialist work.
  - Expert at basic airway skills and manoeuvres.
  - Competent in the use of a T-piece circuit and the administration of CPAP to treat laryngospasm.
- They should have immediate access to the anaesthetist responsible for the child or a nominated deputy.

Procedures

- Procedure for thorough handover between theatre staff, surgeon, and anaesthetist to recovery nurse.
- Assessment of airway patency, vital signs, and level of consciousness are the first priorities upon admission. Other checks are also made:
  - Surgical site and dressings.
  - Patency of drainage tubes/drains.
  - Body temperature.
  - Patency of cannula and rate of IV fluids.
  - Circulation and sensation in extremities after orthopaedic surgery or regional anaesthesia.
  - Pain score.
  - Nausea and vomiting.
- Procedure for thorough handover from recovery to ward staff.
- Early contact with a parent(s) reassures most children and makes managing distressed and disorientated children easier.
- If the physical layout is appropriate, parents should come to the recovery room with a ward nurse to collect the child and return to the ward.
- It is also helpful for parent(s) to be with a child during a longer stay in recovery room.
- Protocol for administration of analgesia e.g. IV bolus of morphine sulphate, epidural 'top up'.

Discharge

Discharge to the ward when:
- Fully awake or responding to verbal stimuli.
- Airway patent.
- Ventilation adequate.
- Protective airway reflexes intact.
- Cardiovascularly stable.
- Normothermic.
- Pain free.

High Dependency Unit (HDU)

- An area where a level of care intermediate between that of a general ward and intensive care is provided.
- Greater monitoring and a higher nurse to patient ratio than a general ward are available but it does not provide facilities for IPPV.
- Usually used as step-up or step-down care area between general wards and ICU. Ideally, situated adjacent to ICU.
- Should be used to care for patients with or likely to develop, single organ failure. Should not be used to manage patients with multi-organ failure but can provide monitoring and support for patients at risk of doing so.
- Can be used to care for postoperative surgical as well as medical patients.
- Admission criteria should be less strict than in adult HDU setting but care should be taken not to overwhelm the unit with patients who can be sent to a normal ward.
- Nurse:patient ratio should not be less than 1:2 and medical staff should be readily available.
- Likely patient groups:
  - Following major surgery.
  - Receiving spinal opioid infusions.
  - Step-down patients from ICU not yet ready for ward level care.
  - Acutely ill medical patients at risk of organ failure.
- Referral and communication with senior nurse in HDU.
- Medical staff responsible for the patients should be clearly identified including joint care where different staff may be responsible for elements of care e.g. analgesia—anaesthetic, fluid balance—surgical.
- Consultant responsible for ICU should be aware of any potential multi-organ failure patients being treated in HDU especially those with potential airway compromise.

Intensive Care Unit (ICU)

- Area where level of care of the highest possible level is provided. Invasive monitoring, IPPV, and a higher nurse to patient ratio than HDU are available (higher than 1:1).
- Used to care for patients with or likely to develop multiple organ failure. Can be used to care for postoperative surgical as well as medical patients.
- Different patient population from adult ICU:
  - Diseases are skewed to infective and congenital problems—viral laryngotracheobronchitis, meningococcal sepsis, postoperative congenital anomalies, and metabolic diseases.
  - Fewer intercurrent chronic medical problems.
  - Lower mortality rates in paediatric units compared with adult units (by as much as a factor of ten).
  - Usually greater physiological reserve in children although decompensation from pathological insults is rapid and severe once the physiological reserve is exhausted.
- Likely patient groups:
  - Acutely ill medical patients with or at risk of organ failure.
  - Postoperative requiring IPPV and/or invasive monitoring e.g. faecal peritonitis after laparotomy.
  - Planned postoperative IPPV e.g. correction of oesophageal atresia, neonatal cardiac surgery.
  - Patients requiring preoperative optimization for major surgery.
- Referral and communication:
  - Referral to consultant in ICU.
  - Joint care between ICU and referring clinicians. Often multiple specialties involved. Medical staff responsible for the various aspects of the patients care should be clearly identified. Care coordinated by ICU staff.
  - Consultant responsible for ICU retains overall responsibility for patient management until the patient is ready for discharge from ICU.
- Dealing with parents can be fraught and care should be taken to be informative and realistic about the patient's condition, prognosis, and progress. Accurate communication and the documentation are essential to preclude later misunderstandings. A specific member of staff can be tasked with communication with relatives. This helps to avoid misunderstandings and ensures consistency of approach. This communicator should be a senior member of staff, able to relate to the relatives or carers but still be able to give objective information.
- Parents are usually resident and present most of the time on the ward. Access to temporary accommodation on site is required.

Section 3

Intraoperative and postoperative analgesia

Acute pain and postoperative analgesia

Mandy Sim

Principles of analgesia in children

- The same working definition is used as in adults. 'Pain is defined as an unpleasant sensory and emotional experience associated with actual or potential tissue damage or which is described in terms of such damage' (International Association for the Study of Pain).
- Pain management in children presents additional challenges not seen with adults.
- The neural pathways and neurotransmitters responsible for the perception of pain and its modulation are present in the neonate and the evoked hormonal, metabolic, and behavioural responses are similar to those seen in older children and adults.
- The requirement to provide analgesia encompasses all age ranges from premature neonates to adolescents.
- As in adults, optimum pain management requires a multidisciplinary team involving, but not limited to, anaesthetists, nurses, and pharmacists.
- Guidelines and protocols agreed between the interested professional groups should be available in every clinical area to encourage effective, safe, and consistent practice in pain management. Protocols vary between hospitals but can be summarized as the 'rights':
  - Right drug
  - Right dose
  - Right route
  - Right time
  - Right treatment for side effects
  - Right approach to child and family.
- Care should be family-centred with involvement from parents, carers, and siblings.
- Anticipation of the need for analgesia and pre-emptive treatment should be the norm.
- A multimodal approach using appropriate doses of non-steroidal drugs, opioids, and LA is used along with non-drug methods.
- As in adults, an individual child's pain can be influenced by a number of factors including:
  - Cognitive development
  - Personality
  - Previous pain experience
  - Gender
  - Family
  - Culture and religion
  - Fear or anxiety.

Pain assessment

- Pain is regarded as one of the vital signs in many hospitals and assessed regularly like temperature, pulse, and respiration.
- Treatment should be informed by valid assessments to ensure, as far as possible, efficacy without the occurrence of unnecessary side effects. A pain assessment tool should be able to detect the presence of pain, to estimate its severity and to determine the effectiveness of analgesic interventions.
- Assessing pain in children can be difficult. To ensure effective analgesia, pain should be assessed using a reliable and valid tool on a regular basis. Parental opinion should be noted.
- Given the subjective nature of pain, a child's self-report of pain is sought when possible.
- In children who are old enough to communicate, self-report numerical or visual analogue scales fulfil these requirements.
- In babies, infants, and handicapped children subjective assessments are not possible and pain assessment is based on indirect indicators. Pain assessment tools used in these groups are based on behavioural or physiological indicators. Facial expression has been coded for neonates and an objective pain score based on observed behaviour has been validated in toddlers. Of the physiological parameters, changes in heart rate and blood pressure and a reduction in respiratory sinus arrhythmia have been used in neonates and infants.
- To achieve optimum assessment the following are considered:
  - Chronological age.
  - Development of the child.
  - Type of pain that is being experienced.
  - Clinical state.
- Following assessment of pain and administration of analgesia re-assessment is essential.
- The QUESTT tool encompasses many of the important principles of pain assessment.
  - **Q**uestion the child.
  - **U**se a valid pain rating.
  - **E**valuate behaviour and physiological changes.
  - **S**ecure parents' involvement.
  - **T**ake the cause of the pain into account.
  - **T**ake action and evaluate the results.

Neonates

- Despite a variety of pain assessment tools being developed assessment of neonatal pain remains inconsistent. This may be because:
  - Assessment depends on using physiological and behavioural indicators some of which are subjective.
  - Many of the available tools are complicated and confusing with many categories or rely on blood pressure measurements that may disturb neonates.
  - The pain assessment tools do not discriminate between pain and other causes of distress such as hunger, anxiety, or cold.
- When assessing pain in neonates several physiological and behavioural markers are noted and used to inform the assessment. Most formal scoring systems use some or all of these features and give a numerical value to them in order to come up with a 'score'.
  - Facial expression—furrowed brow, open mouth, eyes shut tight.
  - Body and limb movements—clenched fingers/toes, squirming, back arching.
  - Cry—high pitched or silent.
  - Sleeplessness—constantly awake.
  - Cardiovascular—blood pressure, heart rate, palmar sweating, skin colour.
  - Respiratory—rate, oxygen saturations.
- Pain assessment tools that are available for this group include:
  - CRIES. This scale gives a score from 0–2 to the child's cry, oxygen requirement, vital signs, facial expression, and time spent asleep. The maximum possible score is 10 and a score of 4 or over is regarded as indicative of pain that requires treatment.
  - The Neonatal and Infant Pain Scale (NIPS). This scores facial expression, cry, breathing pattern, tension or rigidity in the limbs, and arousal. The maximum score is 7 and a score of 3 is regarded as indicating pain that requires treatment.
  - Comfort scale (has nine categories—alertness, calmness, respiratory distress, crying, physical movement, muscle tone, facial tension, blood pressure, heart rate).
  - The Liverpool Infant Distress Scale (LIDS) gives a score from 0–5 to eight behavioural and physiological features – body movements, excitability, finger and toe flexion, tone, facial expression, crying (quantity and quality) and sleep.
  - Neonatal Pain, Agitation and Sedation Score (N-PASS). This assesses and scores crying, behaviour, facial expression, tone in the extremities, heart rate, blood pressure, respiratory rate, and arterial oxygen saturation.
  - Premature Infant Pain Profile (PIPP). Uses facial expression, heart rate, arterial oxygen saturation, gestational age and sleep state.

Infants

- Many of the problems that exist in neonatal pain assessment also apply to infants and toddlers. For patients younger than 3 or 4 years, various pain assessment tools have been developed based primarily on observation rather than patient report.
- These scoring systems integrate behavioural observations, physiological changes, or a combination of these measurements but are dependent on the child and the context of the pain.
- A number of pain behaviours have been identified, facial expression being one of the most specific. Other behaviour includes:
  - Irritability
  - Unusual posture
  - Screaming, sobbing, or whimpering
  - Reluctance to move
  - ↑ clinginess
  - Loss of appetite, restlessness
  - Disturbed sleep pattern.
- Pain scoring systems suitable for use in this group include:
  - The Face, Legs, Activity, Cry, and Consolability (FLACC) scale. The FLACC scale is a behavioural pain assessment scale for use in non-verbal patients unable to provide reports of pain. A score from 0–2 is given to facial expression, position of the legs, activity or posture, crying, and degree of contentment or consolability. Score 0 indicates pain free; score 1–3 indicates mild pain; score 4–7 indicates moderate pain; and score 8–10 indicates severe pain.
  - The Children's Hospital of Eastern Ontario Pain Scale (CHEOPS). The CHEOPS is a behavioural scale for evaluating postoperative pain in young children from 1–7 years of age. It can be used to monitor the effectiveness of interventions for reducing the pain and discomfort.
  - The Objective Pain Score (OPS) uses five criteria—crying, agitation, movement, posture, and localization of pain. Each criterion scores from 0–2 to give a total score of 0–10.
  - The Toddler–Preschooler Postoperative Pain Scale (TPPPS) looks at facial expression, verbal expressions of pain, and motor behaviour to give a score from 0–7.

Pre-school children

- Self-report is the most reliable method of assessing pain, but only children who have achieved a certain degree of cognitive ability are able to provide information in this way.
- Several self-report tools have been developed to assist pre-school children to describe pain and indicate it severity.
- These include:
  - Faces (Fig 6.1). Face-based scales employ a smiling face to represent no pain and a crying face to represent the worst pain ever. Ensure that the child understands the scale represents pain and not happiness and sadness.
  - Colour scales (where increasing degrees of redness usually indicate increasing pain)
  - Poker chip tool (1–4 'pieces of hurt').

Wong–Baker FACES Pain Rating Scale

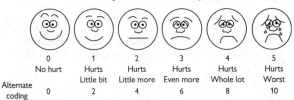

0	1	2	3	4	5
No hurt	Hurts Little bit	Hurts Little more	Hurts Even more	Hurts Whole lot	Hurts Worst

Alternate coding

0	2	4	6	8	10

Fig. 6.1 Faces Pain Assessment Tool. Reproduced with permission from Hockenberry MJ, Wilson D, Winkelstein, ML (2005). *Wong's Essentials of Pediatric Nursing,* 7th edn, St Louis. Copyright Mosby.

School children

- School-age children can usually communicate accurately about pain, its location, and severity.
- Children of this age group understand the concept of number and order and can therefore use a numeric rating scale or word graphic rating scale.
- Tools available for this group include:
  - Faces
  - Numerical rating scale
  - Colour based scales
  - Visual analogue scale.

Adolescents

- Adolescents are able to describe pain clearly because they understand words and concepts.
- Adolescents are able to characterize and accurately describe pain, intensity, and location.
- They are concerned about maintaining a degree of self-control and exhibit a high degree of control in response to their pain.
- It is important to elicit trust from adolescents to obtain an accurate report of their pain.
- Tools available for this group include:
  - Visual analogue scale
  - Eland colour scale
  - Numerical rating scale
  - Pain thermometer.
- On a practical day-to-day level children who are able to communicate should be asked to score pain using a simple four point self-report scale during a movement such as a deep breath or cough (which is a more sensitive discriminator than assessments performed at rest): 0 = no pain; 1 = mild pain; 2 = moderate pain; 3 = severe pain.

Drugs

- Multimodal therapy is the mainstay of acute pain management:
  - Paracetamol
  - NSAIDs
  - Opioids
  - LA.
- Severe pain should never go untreated. Safe protocols have been developed for the use of opioid analgesia and experience with analgesic use in children is now extensive.
- Predictable side effects should be treated pre-emptively especially nausea and vomiting.
- The use of IM injections in children is usually avoided.
- The WHO analgesic ladder was originally described for cancer pain but is useful to give general guidance on analgesic strategy in acute postoperative pain (Fig 6.2).
- Non-pharmacological measures are vital in children:
  - Parental presence
  - Play
  - Distraction

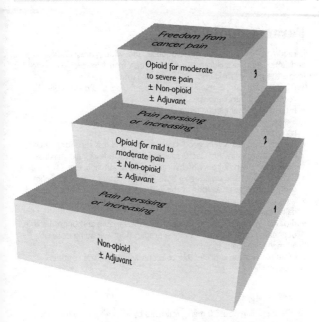

Fig. 6.2 WHO pain ladder. Reproduced with kind permission from the World Health organization (http://who.int/cancer/palliative/painladder/en/). Level 1 requires paracetamol and/or NSAID.Level 2 requires paracetamol, NSAID and codeine. Level 3 requires paracetamol, NSAID and morphine

Paracetamol

Paracetamol remains the most popular and widely prescribed analgesic and antipyretic in children. As can be seen from the analgesic ladder it forms the mainstay of almost all analgesic regimens.

- Paracetamol can be given orally (syrups, tablets and dispersible), rectally, and intravenously.
- It has a high therapeutic index with a ceiling effect.
- Side effects are rare but rashes and thrombocytopenia have been reported occasionally.
- Paracetamol has a very good safety record and it is rare for a child to suffer any toxicity. Risk factors for toxicity include regular maximal dosing for over 72 hours, dehydration and organ failure.
- Dose is calculated on a mg/kg basis. A high loading dose (20 mg/kg oral) is often given as long as the 24-hour maximum is not exceeded.
- Due to their immature metabolic pathways (□ Chapter 2), the total daily dose is reduced in neonates.
- Bioavailability after rectal administration is variable and unpredictable, depending on the patient and the preparation. A loading dose of 40 mg/kg is usually given.
- IV administration is preferable to rectal when the oral route is unavailable.

Dose:

- Oral: loading dose 20 mg/kg followed by 15 mg/kg 4-hourly.
- IV: 15 mg/kg 6-hourly.
- Rectal: loading dose 40 mg/kg (20 mg/kg in neonates) followed 20 mg/kg 6-hourly.

- Maximum dose by oral and rectal routes 90 mg/kg/day above 3 months of age (4 g/day in adolescents); 60 mg/kg/day in neonates and infants up to 3 months of age. 60 mg/kg/day IV.

Non-steroidal anti-inflammatory drugs

Ibuprofen and diclofenac are the two most commonly prescribed agents in children. They are used for mild-to-moderate pain or in conjunction with opioids for severe pain.

- Diclofenac can be given orally (tablets and dispersible) and rectally while ibuprofen is only available in oral preparations (syrups, tablets, and melts).
- NSAIDs are more potent than paracetamol but also have a ceiling effect.
- Onset time about 30 min.
- Given in conjunction with opioids they have a very useful 'opioid sparing effect' in the region of 25–30%.
- Dose is calculated on a mg/kg basis (ibuprofen 5–10 mg/kg 6-hourly, maximum 400 mg; diclofenac 1 mg/kg 8-hourly, maximum 50 mg).
- Side effects vary in severity and frequency. Gastrointestinal discomfort, nausea, diarrhoea, and occasionally bleeding and ulceration may occur.
- Consideration of the risks and benefits is required before prescribing NSAIDs for children with asthma, renal impairment, and coagulo-pathies.

Opioids

Opioids play a major role in the management of moderate and severe pain in children.

- Codeine phosphate and morphine sulphate are the two most commonly used in the paediatric ward setting.
- Codeine is available in both oral and rectal preparations and should be prescribed with paracetamol and a NSAID for moderate pain.
- Morphine can be given orally, as an IV bolus, by IV infusion, as patient controlled analgesia (PCA), or as a nurse controlled infusion.
- Onset of action is almost immediate after an IV bolus and takes about 30 min after oral administration.
- Duration of effect is commonly 3–4 hours.
- Unlike codeine, morphine does not have a ceiling effect.
- Dosing is on a mg/kg basis.
- Codeine phosphate 1 mg/kg oral 4-hourly; 0.5 mg/kg oral 4-hourly if <6 months. Maximum 60 mg. Morphine sulphate <1 month 80 mcg/kg oral 4-hourly; 1–3 months 100 mcg/kg oral 4-hourly; 3–12 months 200 mcg/kg oral 4-hourly; >1 year 300 mcg/kg oral 2–4-hourly. Maximum 15 mg.
- Side effects include nausea, vomiting, constipation, urinary retention, pruritis and drowsiness. Larger doses produce respiratory depression.
- Oral administration does not usually require enhanced monitoring but may do under some circumstances.
- IV infusions of morphine or PCA require some form of enhanced monitoring according to an agreed local protocol.
- Neonates have immature ventilatory control and are particularly prone to opioid-induced respiratory depression. They also metabolize opioids more slowly than older children and there is a risk of accumulation with repeated doses or an infusion (📖 Chapters 1 and 2).

Local anaesthetics

LA are a very important component of acute pain management for children, particularly after surgery. Local anaesthesia can provide excellent analgesia without the need of systemic analgesics and their side effects. This can facilitate the discharge of a pain free, alert child after day surgery.

- LA are ideal agents to produce analgesia as they work locally on nerves, are generally safe, and produce long-lasting, complete analgesia in the affected parts of the body.
- They can be applied topically as creams and gels, infiltrated, infused, or injected to block individual nerves or nerve plexuses.
- The agents used commonly are bupivacaine, levobupivacaine and ropivacaine. For doses see 📖 Chapters 7 and 8.
- Levobupivacaine and ropivacaine are marginally safer than bupivacaine.
- LA blocks minimize the need for opioids and are therefore ideally suited for patients sensitive to opioids.
- Children are not more resistant to local anaesthestic toxicity than adults.
- Particular care is required in neonates with infusions or repeated bolus injections since they have a reduced capacity to metabolize and eliminate LA. Doses are reduced to prevent accumulation and toxicity.

Antiemetics

- Moderate or severe postoperative nausea and vomiting (PONV) impairs the quality of recovery and ↓ patient and parent satisfaction with care. Occasionally dehydration or electrolyte derangements are caused by PONV. Risk factors include:
  - A past history of PONV.
  - Opioid use.
  - Inhalational anaesthesia.
  - Type of surgery and duration of anaesthesia.
  - Duration of preoperative fasting.
  - Level of anxiety.
- Antiemetics are given during anaesthesia to high risk patients:
  - Opioid administration.
  - Previous PONV.
  - Ophthalmic surgery.
  - Tonsillectomy or adenoidectomy.
  - Gastrointestinal surgery.
- When possible, opioid sparing techniques e.g. NSAID administration, regional technique are used along with antiemetics.
- Frequently prescribed on a regular rather than as required basis for high risk patients e.g. teenage girls using PCA.
- Various classes of antiemetic agent are available. Ondansetron is the most commonly used. Others are used if PONV persists or for some high risk procedures where two or more antiemetics with different mechanisms of action may be given e.g. strabismus surgery (📖 Chapter 10). IV administration is preferred. Oral or rectal if necessary. IM is rarely used.
- *Serotonin receptor antagonists*
  - Block the 5-HT3 receptors associated with the central connections of the vagus nerve in the brainstem in close proximity to the chemoreceptor trigger zone (CTZ).
  - Ondansetron is the commonest.
  - Can be given IV or orally.
- Anti-histamine/anti-muscarinic agents
  - Block the action of histamine on its receptors.
  - Cyclizine is an example.
  - Can be given orally, IV, or rectally
- *Dopamine receptor antagonists*
  - Block dopamine receptors and inhibit dopaminergic stimulation of the CTZ.
  - Prochlorperazine is a common example.
  - Can be given orally, rectally, or IM.
  - Metoclopramide ↑ gastric tone and dilates the duodenum causing stomach to empty more quickly. Can be given orally, IV, or IM.
- *Dexamethasone*

Table 6.1 Antiemetics used in children

Ondansetron

<2 years	2–12 years	12–18 years
Not licensed	100 mcg/kg IV (maximum 4 mg)	4 mg IV

Cyclizine

IV or oral

1 month–6 years		6–18 years
0.5–1 mg/kg up to 8-hourly (maximum single dose 25 mg)		0.5–1 mg/kg up to 8-hourly (maximum single dose 50 mg)

Rectal

2–6 years	6–12 years	12–18 years
12.5 mg up to 3 times a day	25 mg up to 3 times a day	50 mg up to 3 times a day

Prochlorperazinee

1–5 years (if over 10 kg)	5–12 years	12–18 years

Oral

1.25–2.5 mg up to 8-hourly	2.5–5 mg up to 8-hourly	5–10 mg up to 8-hourly

Rectal

2.5 mg up to 8-hourly	5–10 mg up to 8-hourly	12.5–25 mg up to 8-hourly

Metoclopramide

1 month–1 year (up to 10 kg)	1–3 years (10–14 kg)	3–5 years (15–19 kg)	5–9 years (20–29 kg)	9–18 years (30–60 kg)	15–18 years (over 60 kg)
IV or oral	IV or oral	IV or oral	IV or oral	IV or oral	IV or oral
100 mcg/kg (maximum 1 mg) twice daily	1 mg eight to twelve hourly	2 mg eight to twelve hourly	2.5 mg eight hourly	5 mg eight hourly	10 mg eight hourly

Dexamethasone: 150–200 mcg/kg IV

Acute severe pain

- Acute severe pain e.g. trauma, burns require IV opioid analgesia.
- Morphine sulphate is the most commonly used drug.
- Initial dose is determined by age and weight of child.
- Further boluses may be required to titrate the child to comfort while maintaining a balance between adequate analgesia and excessive sedation.

Preparation

Add 1 ml of morphine sulphate 10 mg/ml to 9 ml of 0.9% saline (concentration is now 1 mg/ml).

Age	Dose	Volume
3–6 months	100 mcg/kg	0.1 mL/kg
>6 months	200 mcg/kg	0.2 mL/kg

If child weighs <10 kg transfer 1 ml (1 mg morphine) of the diluted solution to a 10 ml syringe and further dilute with 9 ml 0.9% saline (concentration is now 100 mcg/ml).

Age	Dose	Volume
0–1 months	25 mcg/kg	0.25 mL/kg
1–3 months	50 mcg/kg	0.5 mL/kg

- Inject initial bolus slowly over 2–3 minutes.
- Observe for effect and side effects for 10 minutes.
- Administer a further bolus 50% of initial bolus if required after 10 minutes.

Protocols and monitoring

- As for adults, the prescription and management of common postoperative analgesic techniques is standardized and day-to-day management is usually devolved to members of the Acute Pain Service.
- Protocols for management of children receiving opioid and epidural analgesia ensure efficacy and safety. The majority of patients have an uncomplicated postoperative course when managed according to standard protocols. Occasionally, children require prescriptions outside these protocols for adequate analgesia.
- Nursing staff require competency based training usually delivered by the Acute Pain Service. Nurse:patient ratio should be 1:3 patients for opioid infusions and 1:2 for epidural infusions.
- Patients are nursed in a physical setting that allows close observation. Equipment for bag and mask ventilation and oropharyngeal suction is on hand.
- Doses are calculated using the patient's body weight.
- Anti-syphon valves are used when morphine is infused through a dedicated cannula and anti-syphon/anti-reflux valves when morphine and maintenance fluids are infused through the same cannula.
- Infusion or PCA pumps should be mounted on a drip stand at the same level as the child.
- Dedicated epidural pumps must be used for epidural infusions rather than IV infusion pumps.

Intravenous opioid infusion

- Used in young children and those where the use of PCA would be inappropriate (physical handicap or developmental delay).
- Usually prescribed as a range of infusion rates. Infusion rate is then ↑ and reduced by nursing staff within the limits of the prescription.
- Two nurses check and document all changes of infusion rate.
  - Dilution: 1 mg/kg morphine sulphate diluted in 50 mL 0.9% saline (20 mcg/kg/mL).
  - Infusion rate: 0.5–2 mL/hour (10–40 mcg/kg/hour).
  - For children >50 kg, 50 mg is diluted in 50 mL 0.9% saline and infused at 0.5–2 mL/hour.
  - Some children require higher infusion rates.
- Antiemetics are not usually added to the syringe in children.
- For exacerbations of pain there is a delay between ↑ the infusion rate and effect. If necessary a bolus of 50–100 mcg/kg is given at the same time as the infusion rate is ↑.
- When possible, combined with regular NSAID plus paracetamol to reduce opioid requirements.
- An antiemetic should be prescribed on a regular or as required basis depending on circumstances.

Monitoring and observations

- Continuous pulse oximetry while breathing air (acts an indirect marker of hypoventilation in children without other causes of hypoxia). Most children do not require postoperative oxygen and this should not be prescribed as a routine since it prevents the use of oximetry to detect hypoventilation.
- Observations of heart rate, respiratory rate and arterial oxygen saturation are documented half hourly.
- Hourly recordings:
  - Pain assessment (unless child is asleep).
  - Sedation score.
  - Syringe plunger movement.
  - Volume reading from the infusion pump.
  - Infusion site.
  - Presence and severity of PONV.
- A single sheet similar to Fig 6.3 is usually used for the prescription and recording of observations related to the infusion to aid patient assessment and ongoing audit.

Pain Management Service

OPIOID INFUSION CHART

SURNAME:
FORENAMES:
ADDRESS:
UNIT NO:
DOB:

SURGEON:
ANAESTHETIST:
WARD:
OPERATION:
DATE:
WEIGHT:

CHECKLIST PRIOR TO LEAVING RECOVERY
LINES UNCLAMPED
PUMP SETTINGS WITHIN PRESCRIBED LIMITS
SYRINGE LEVEL AT HANDOVER .... ml
RECOVERY NURSE INITIAL   ....
WARD/HDU NURSE INITIAL

MORPHINE   mgs in 50ml (1mg/kg Max 50mg)
CYCLIZINE   mgs in 50ml (1mg/kg Max 50mg)

Concentration: .... micrograms/ml

Infusion Rate: From ...... mls/hr = ... mcg/kg/hr
           To ...... mls/hr = ... mcg/kg/hr

Date	Time	Batch no. med.	Batch no. dil.	Pump No	Prepared by	Checked by	Signature				Print Name	Date/time
												Date	Time
1.							Syringe No. 1				Signed	
							Total drug given	ml			Witnessed	
							Total drug discarded	ml				
2.							Syringe No.2				Signed	
							Total drug given	ml			Witnessed	
							Total drug discarded	ml				
3.							Syringe No.3				Signed	
							Total drug given	ml			Witnessed	
							Total drug discarded	ml				

Call Doctor if severe pain (score 6), patient unrousable (sedation score 3), S_aO_2 <90%, respiratory rate <10 (over 5 year) or <20 (under 5 years), excessive nausea or vomiting, drip blocked/tissue or pump alarming.

Any problems bleep Pain Nurse Specialist or duty Anaesthetist

OBSERVATIONS CARRIED OUT HOURLY

Sedation Score
Eyes open:
0 = spontaneously
1 = to speech
2 = to shake
3 = unrousable

Pain Assess.
Tool Score
Please tick:
FLACC......
Faces......
Linear......
A = Asleep

Nausea Score
0 = None
1 = nausea only
2 = vomiting × 1 in last hour
3 = vomiting >1 in last hour

Time	S_aO_2	Resp. rate	Sedation Score	Pain Assess. Tool Score	Nausea Score	Infusion rate ml/hr	Volume (ml) Remaining in syringe Visual check	Volume infused since last check (from visual check)	Total volume infused (from visual check)	Total volume infused Pump reading	IV site check	Initials
0800												
0900												
1000												
1100												
1200												

Fig 6.3 Example of IV morphine infusion chart

Patient controlled analgesia

- Patient controlled analgesia (PCA) is suitable for children able to understand the concept and physically operate the demand button.
- PCA has been shown to be safe and effective in children as young as 5 years but each child should be assessed individually prior to surgery. In practice, it is rarely used below the age of 8 years.
- Patients may derive psychological benefit from having a degree of control over their analgesia.
  - Dilution: 1 mg/kg morphine sulphate in 50 mL 0.9% saline (20 mcg/kg/mL).
  - Bolus dose: 1 mL (20 mcg/kg).
  - Lockout interval: 5 min
  - A background infusion is sometimes added at 0.2–0.5 mL/hour (4–10 mcg/kg/hour).
  - Children weighing >50 kg receive 50 mg morphine sulphate in 50 mL 0.9% saline with a bolus dose of 1 mg and a 5 min lockout period.
- Additional NSAID, paracetamol and an antiemetic are prescribed.
- The same monitoring and observations are performed as for IV infusion with the addition of the numbers of demands made for analgesia and the number of successful demands i.e. those not made within a lockout period.

Nurse controlled analgesia

- Used to provide some of the flexibility and responsiveness of PCA in children who are unable to manage PCA.
- The child receives an IV infusion of morphine sulphate from a PCA pump and additional boluses are administered by nursing staff in response to pain.
  - Dilution - 1 mg/kg morphine sulphate diluted in 50 mL 0.9% saline (20 mcg/mL/kg).
  - Infusion: 0.5–1 mL/hour (10–20 mcg/kg/hour)
  - Bolus doses: 1 mL (20 mcg/kg) given following assessment of pain and sedation.
  - Lockout interval: 30 min.
- Monitoring and observation requirements are the same as those for IV infusions and PCA.

Epidural infusion analgesia

- Used to provide analgesia after thoracic, abdominal or major lower body surgery. Particularly useful in children with severe cerebral palsy after orthopaedic surgery to prevent painful muscle spasms. See also 🕮 Chapter 8.
- Epidural catheters are usually positioned in anaesthetized patients.
- For postoperative infusions bupivacaine, levobupivacaine, or ropivacaine are used
  - 0.1% or 0.125% bupivacaine or levobupivacaine is widely used.
  - Maximum infusion rates of bupivacaine (and levobupivacaine) are 0.25 mg/kg/hour below 6 months of age and 0.4 mg/kg/hour in older children.
  - Ropivacaine is usually infused as 0.2 mL/kg/hour of 0.2% solution (0.4 mg/kg/hour).
  - Opioids are commonly added to the LA for epidural infusion e.g. morphine 1–5 mcg/kg/hour, fentanyl 0.1–0.5 mcg/kg/hour, or diamorphine 5–25 mcg/kg/hour.
- Hypotension due to sympathetic block is unusual in children below about 8 years of age. If it does occur, in the absence of surgical bleeding, consider a subarachnoid or subdural catheter position.
- Patients with an epidural infusion are often nursed in an HDU. They can also be nursed on surgical wards with observations and management carried out in accordance with an agreed protocol by nurses with appropriate training and skills in the supervision of paediatric epidural infusions.

Monitoring and observations

- Include:
  - Continuous pulse oximetry
  - Observations of heart rate, respiratory rate and oxygen saturation are documented half hourly
  - Hourly observations
  - Pain assessment
  - Sedation score
  - Blood pressure
  - PONV score
  - Epidural catheter insertion site for inflammation or leakage
  - Dermatomal level of block
  - Accurate fluid balance
- Patient position should be changed 2-hourly to avoid damage to pressure areas.
- If 'top-up' boluses are given pulse, respiration, blood pressure, and oxygen saturation should be recorded every 5 min for 20 min, then on the half hour and the hour. The anaesthetist remains in the ward area for 20 min following a 'top-up'.
- Appropriate analgesia should be prescribed and given prior to stopping the epidural infusion.

- Side effects of epidural infusions include:
  - Nausea and vomiting, although this is usually less than that seen during IV infusions of morphine sulphate.
  - Itching.
  - Urinary retention—ideally a urethral catheter should be insertion as part of the surgical procedure.
  - Respiratory depression.
- A monitoring protocol must be in place.
- Children receiving epidural infusions must have observation and monitoring by appropriately educated staff.

Regional anaesthetic techniques: peripheral blocks

Steve Roberts

Overview and safety

- Regional anaesthesia is increasingly popular in children. The advantages of excellent intra- and postoperative analgesia, and opioid sparing effects should make the use of a LA technique mandatory unless there are specific contraindications.
- In the UK, virtually all blocks in children are performed under general anaesthesia. The principle concern with this is the masking of signs and symptoms of intravascular and intraneural injection.
- Compared to central blocks, peripheral blocks can provide more profound and targeted analgesia, greater suppression of the stress response, a safer profile, and are generally more acceptable to patients and parents.
- The main complication is a failed block. It is, therefore, prudent to take a balanced approach to analgesia provision by concurrent administration of paracetamol and/or a NSAID.
- Preoperatively, a history should be taken to elicit contraindications to LA techniques. If possible the area where the block is to be sited should be examined. Note the patient's weight to calculate the maximum safe dose of LA.
- Absolute contraindications:
  - Patient or parent refusal.
  - Local infection.
  - Allergy to LA.
- Relative contraindications:
  - Anticoagulation.
  - Neuromuscular disease.
  - Risk of masking a compartment syndrome (discuss with surgeon).
- An attempt to explain the postoperative sensation to the child should be made e.g. 'pins and needles', as they can find paraesthesiae upsetting.
- When obtaining consent a 'plan B' should be discussed in case the block fails.
- Safe nerve blockade requires a sound knowledge of anatomy, sensible block selection, IV access, standard monitoring, appropriate equipment, and aseptic precautions (this is assumed for all the blocks described subsequently).
- Short-bevelled needles should be used. It is helpful to first nick the skin to avoid missing the feel of the underlying fascia during the puncture.
- A LA with a prolonged duration of action is preferred e.g. levobupivacaine. Adequate postoperative analgesia is usually achieved with a concentration of 0.25%.
- The safe practice of incremental slow injection with repeated aspiration is mandatory for all blocks.
- The calculated maximum LA dose should never be exceeded.
- Landmark techniques for mixed nerve location can be aided by use of a peripheral nerve stimulator (PNS) as in adults.
- More recently ultrasound (US) has been used as an imaging modality; allowing real-time needle guidance, improved success rates and ↓ doses of LA. US imaging in children is of high quality as nerves are more superficial than in adults allowing the use of higher frequency probes.

- Continuous catheter techniques are particularly useful for prolonged blockade. The problem of dislodgement can largely be overcome by subcutaneous tunnelling.
- A failed block should be readily recognized intraoperatively and supplemented by LA infiltration or IV analgesia.
- In the recovery area, it can be difficult to differentiate between pain and agitation. If in doubt the former should be assumed and dealt with promptly.

Infiltration and field block

Indications
• All surgery where a specific nerve or plexus block is not possible.

Contraindications
• General.

Anatomy
• LA should be injected subcutaneously or intradermally.

Technique
• Infiltration involves the injection of a LA subcutaneously into the wound edges.
• A field block involves the injection of LA into the skin around the surgical site.
• After initial aspiration of the syringe, the needle is kept moving as LA is injected thus minimizing the risk of intravascular injection.
• It can be performed preoperatively with the benefit of allowing a lighter plane of general anaesthesia. However, this may distort the wound e.g. the vermillion border of the lip or the tissue planes e.g. herniotomy.
• Alternatively, LA is injected or instilled into the incision prior to closure. If this technique is used, a gradual emergence from general anaesthesia is preferred as it allows the infiltration to take effect.
• In the awake patient injection can be painful. This is minimized by distraction techniques, application of a topical LA e.g. EMLA or LET (lidocaine, epinephrine (adrenaline) and tetracaine mix), warmed LA, use of a 27 G needle and slow injection.

Complications
• Intravascular injection.
• LA toxicity.
• Haematoma.

Ilioinguinal/Iliohypogastric block

Indications
- Herniotomy.
- Orchidopexy (if a low scrotal incision is made, supplement with infiltration or pudendal nerve block).
- Varicocele ligation.
- Hydrocele.

Contraindications
- General.
- Relative—obstructed hernia.

Anatomy
- Both nerves originate from the primary ventral ramus of L1. The iliohypogastric runs superior to the ilioinguinal nerve.
- The nerves lie between the internal oblique and transversus abdominis muscles at the level of the anterior superior iliac spine (ASIS).
- At the level of the ASIS or more ventral the iliohypogastric nerve pierces the internal oblique muscle to lie beneath the external oblique muscle.
- Distance between the ASIS and the nerves is not related to age or weight. Both cadaver and US studies have shown the nerves to be closer to the ASIS than most traditional techniques assume.

Technique
- The numerous methods described and the 10–25% failure rate suggest that this is not a simple block to perform successfully. This may partly be due to anatomical variation between patients.
- Patient supine.
- The needle is inserted perpendicular to the skin. The needle is inserted 5–10 mm medial and just inferior to the ASIS.
- Alternatively, the needle is inserted at a point 2.5 mm medial along a line between the ASIS and the umbilicus.
- When performed blind a single fascial click technique is advised (50% of patients have only two muscles at the level of the ASIS, Fig. 7.1). This ↓ the risk of intraperitoneal injection (the average nerve–peritoneum distance is 3.3 mm).
- 0.25% levobupivacaine 0.3–0.5 mL/kg is injected slowly. US allows smaller volumes to be used, possibly ↓ LA plasma levels and the risk of femoral nerve block.
- A deep plane of general anaesthesia is maintained until peritoneal, spermatic cord, or testicular manipulation is complete since the stimulation from these manoeuvres will not be prevented by the block.

Complications
- Femoral nerve block is described in up to 11% of patients. This should be tested for before discharge
- Intraperitoneal injection
  - Bowel perforation

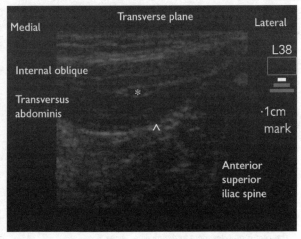

Fig. 7.1 Cross sectional ultrasound image of the ilioinguinal nerve, illustrating the presence of two muscle bellies and the proximity of the nerve (*) to peritoneum (^).

Rectus sheath block

Indications
- Umbilical and periumbilical surgery.

Contraindications
- General.

Anatomy
- The rectus muscles extend from the xiphisternum to the pubis.
- A fascial sheath encloses each rectus muscle. The sheath is formed by the combination of the aponeuroses of the lateral abdominal muscles (external oblique, internal oblique, and transversus abdominis).
- The posterior wall of the sheath is loosely connected to the rectus muscle.
- The rectus muscle is divided into three parts by intertendinous intersections. These are found at the level of the xiphisternum, at the umbilicus, and halfway between the two.
- The lateral border of the rectus muscle is called the semilunaris. In small infants it may be difficult to define.
- The rectus muscles meet in the midline—linea alba.
- The 9th–11th intercostals nerves penetrate the sheath to supply the periumbilical skin.

Technique
- Patient supine.
- When using a landmark technique the needle is inserted just medial to the semilunaris at the umbilical level. The needle is inserted at an angle of $60°$ aiming towards the umbilicus.
- If the semilunaris is not identifiable, then insert the needle 2–3 cm lateral to the umbilicus.
- The needle is felt to 'pop' as it passes through the anterior sheath into the rectus muscle. The needle tip needs to reach the space between the muscle and the posterior sheath as this allows optimal spread of LA. This is felt as a 'scratch' by gently moving the needle from side to side.
- The procedure is then repeated for the opposite side.
- The depth of insertion is not related to age or weight, in children under 10 years of age the needle should not be inserted beyond 1 cm.
- Volume of LA is 0.2–0.4 mL/kg/side.
- When using US (Fig. 7.2) the needle is guided precisely to the posterior sheath and a reliable block is produced using 0.1 mL/kg/side.

Complications
- Haematoma.
- Visceral puncture.

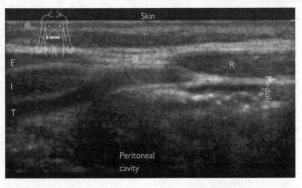

Fig. 7.2 Ultrasonographic appearance of the rectus sheath, external oblique muscle (E), internal oblique muscle (I), transversus abdominis muscle (T), rectus muscle (R) and semilunaris (SL).

Penile nerve block

Indications
- Circumcision.
- Distal hypospadias repair (discuss with surgeon).

Contraindications
- LA containing adrenaline.

Anatomy
- The ilioinguinal and genitofemoral nerves supply the penile base.
- The dorsal penile nerves (S2–4) supply the remainder of the penis.
- The dorsal nerves pass under the pubic ramus within the subpubic space.
- The subpubic space is divided into left and right compartments by the suspensory ligament.
- The anterior border of the subpubic space is formed by Scarpa's fascia.
- The dorsal penile arteries, superficial and deep veins are in the midline. The dorsal nerves run lateral to these vessels.
- The ventral branches of the dorsal penile nerves originate in the subpubic space.
- The dorsal penile nerves run in the 10 and 2 o'clock positions within the penile shaft.

Technique 1: subpubic block
- Advantage of this method is ↓ risk of neurovascular or corpus cavernosum damage.
- Patient supine.
- Locate the symphysis pubis in the midline
- The penis is pulled down ensuring the subpubic skin is taut.
- The needle is inserted just through the skin in the midline. Aim the needle posteriorly, 10° caudal and 20° lateral.
- A slight 'pop' is felt as the needle first breaches the superficial fascia, then a more definite 'pop' is felt on traversing the deep (Scarpa's) fascia at a depth of between 8–30 mm.
- Depth of insertion is independent of patient weight or age.
- Withdraw the needle to just under the skin and redirect it to the contralateral side.
- 0.25% levobupivacaine 0.1 mL/kg each side, maximum 5 mL each side. The volume injected is limited to ↓ the possibility of vascular compromise.
- Success rate may be improved by blocking the ventral penile nerves. LA is injected subcutaneously at the penile–scrotal junction.

Technique 2: ring block
- A simpler method.
- LA is injected subcutaneously around the base of the penis.

Complications
- Superficial haematoma.
- Deep haematoma potentially causing vascular compromise and ischaemia.

Ring block and digital nerve block

Indications
- Operations on fingers and toes e.g. nail bed repair.

Contraindications
- LA containing adrenaline.

Anatomy
- The digital nerves of the fingers are derived from the radial and ulnar nerves dorsally, and the median and ulnar nerves ventrally.
- Dorsal and ventral nerves on the medial and lateral aspect innervate each finger. They are positioned at 2, 5, 7, and 10 o'clock in relation to the phalanx.

Technique
- The needle is inserted lateral to the extensor tendon. The needle is directed subcutaneously along the side of the phalanx until the volar skin surface tents. The syringe is aspirated and, as the needle is withdrawn, LA is injected.
- The needle is removed and reinserted medial to the extensor tendon and the process repeated.
- 0.25% levobupivacaine 1–2 mL/side.
- When the operative site is at the base of the finger, a metacarpal block can be performed.
- The needle is inserted at 90° to the skin between the metacarpals approximately midway along the bone.
- It is advanced until resistance from the palmar aponeurosis is felt. After aspiration, LA is injected as the needle is withdrawn. The process is repeated on the other side of the finger.
- Toe and metatarsal blocks are performed in a similar manner.

Complications
- Ischaemia of the digit. This is prevented by avoiding adrenaline in the LA and limiting the volume injected.

Axillary brachial plexus block

Indications
- Hand, wrist or forearm surgery.

Contraindications
- General.

Anatomy
- Within the axilla the three cords form the four main nerves – median, musculocutaneous, radial and ulnar.
- The axillary and musculocutaneous nerves depart from the sheath around the level of the coracoid process.
- With the patient supine the classic nerve distribution in relation to the artery has the median and musculocutaneous nerves lying superior, the ulnar nerve inferior and the radial nerve posterior. However, US assessment in adults shows great variability in nerve distribution.

Technique
- The transarterial approach is not advised.
- Patient supine with elbow flexed and arm abducted to 90°. Hand rests on or is taped to pillow.
- The axillary artery is palpated as proximal as possible within the axilla.
- The needle of a nerve stimulator is inserted (with a slight cephalad angulation) just above the artery and then redirected below the artery.
- The initial insertion aims to produce a fascial click on entering the sheath, and stimulates the median nerve (wrist flexion and pronation, flexion of the first fingers should be observed). Half of the total volume of LA for the block is injected.
- Redirection of the needle again elicits a fascial click and stimulates the radial nerve (wrist and finger extension should be observed) with a current of 0.3–0.5 mA. The remainder of the LA is injected.
- A total volume of 0.5 mL/kg of LA (0.25% levobupivacaine with or without 1/200,000 adrenaline) is divided between the injection sites.
- When inserting a continuous nerve catheter a more cephalad needle direction will aid threading.

Complications
- Arterial puncture with possibility of vascular occlusion.
- Haematoma.
- Intravascular injection.
- Nerve damage.

Supraclavicular brachial plexus block

Indications
- Surgery on the elbow and upper arm.

Contraindications
- General.
- Contralateral phrenic or recurrent laryngeal nerve palsy.
- Relative—previous neck surgery, contralateral pneumothorax.

Anatomy
- The nerve roots of the plexus travel between the scalene muscles, forming the trunks in the lower half of the posterior triangle of the neck.
- The plexus lies slightly cephalad and posterior to the subclavian artery.
- The trunks become divisions prior to passing beneath the clavicle.

Technique
- The following description is of an US guided technique.
- Patient supine with the arm by their side, and head turned slightly away from side to be blocked.
- A head ring is useful to stabilize the head. In small children, a small roll between the shoulders improves access to the posterior triangle.
- When performing a right-sided block a right-handed anaesthetist should stand at the head of the bed with the US machine on the patient's right.
- A linear hockey stick transducer of 10 MHz plus is placed behind and parallel to the clavicle.
- Firstly, the subclavian artery lying on the first rib is identified; beneath the rib the cervical pleura and lung are visualized. The brachial plexus is located between the anterior and middle scalene muscles, superficial and posterolateral to the subclavian artery (Fig 7.3).
- The needle is inserted beneath the long axis of the transducer (an in-line technique) in a lateral to medial direction. This keeps the whole length of the needle visible allowing accurate real time guidance.
- The pleura should be visible on screen at all times.
- The needle is guided into the sheath (a 'click' will be felt).
- Initially 0.25–0.5 mL of LA is injected to ensure optimal needle tip position. If LA starts to spread within the sheath a total volume of 0.1–0.2 mL/kg (0.25% levobupivacaine with or without 1/200,000 adrenaline) is injected.
- Occasionally the inferior trunk does not come into contact with LA and the needle needs to be redirected to correct this.

Complications
- Pneumothorax.
- Intravascular injection.
- Nerve damage.
- Phrenic nerve palsy.
- Recurrent laryngeal nerve palsy and Horner's syndrome are common side effects.

The potential complications mean that this block should only to be performed by experienced paediatric regional anaesthetists, preferably under ultrasound guidance.

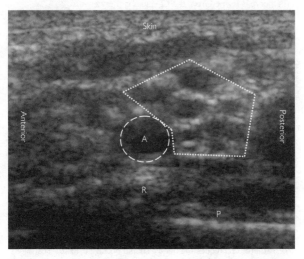

Fig. 7.3 Ultrasonographic appearance of the brachial plexus (dotted area) highlighting the proximity to the pleura (P), rib (R) and subclavian artery (A).

Femoral nerve block

Indications
- Fractured femur
- Surgery on anterior aspect of thigh, medial aspect of calf and ankle.

Contraindications
- General.

Anatomy
- The nerve is formed from the L2–4 lumbar nerve roots.
- It enters the thigh beneath the inguinal ligament, lateral to the femoral artery (Fig. 7.4).
- The nerve lies on the iliopsoas muscle and is deep to fascia lata and fascia iliaca.

Technique
- Patient supine.
- The needle is inserted perpendicular to the skin at a point 0.5 cm lateral to the femoral pulse and 0.5 cm inferior to the ilioinguinal ligament.
- The first 'click' felt is the fascia lata; this is followed by a second 'click' as the fascia iliaca is traversed.
- The accuracy of this technique may be improved by the use of a PNS. Contraction of the quadriceps is the desired end point.
- Volume of LA 0.3 mL/kg. Depending on the circumstances 0.25% or 0.5% levobupivacaine with or without adrenaline 1/200,000 can be used.
- If a 3-in-1 block is required then a greater volume (0.5 mL/kg) needs to be injected to allow medial and lateral spread (to block the lateral cutaneous and obturator nerves), cephalad spread towards the lumbar plexus is uncommon.
- For catheter techniques the needle should be angled 10–20° rostrally to allow threading of the catheter. No more than a few cm of catheter should be left beyond the bevel of the needle.

Complications
- Arterial puncture.
- Haematoma.
- Intravascular injection.
- Nerve damage.

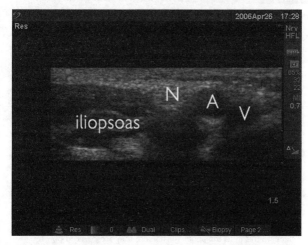

Fig. 7.4 Ultrasonographic appearance of the femoral nerve (N), femoral artery (A), femoral vein (V).

Fascia iliaca compartment block

This blocks the femoral, obturator, and lateral cutaneous nerve of thigh with a single injection. The success rate is higher than that for a 3-in-1 block. The injection site is distant from nerves or vessels and a PNS is not required.

Indications
- Fractured femur.
- Surgery on anterior and lateral aspect of thigh.

Contraindications
- General.

Anatomy
- The lumbar plexus forms the femoral, lateral cutaneous and obturator nerves.
- All three nerves pass through the iliac fossa in the potential space between the iliacus muscle and the fascia iliaca.
- The nerves become superficial at the inguinal ligament and pass beneath this in to the upper thigh. Here they are covered only by skin, subcutaneous fat, fascia lata, and the underlying fascia iliaca (which extends slightly beyond the iliac fossa beneath the inguinal ligament).
- Injection deep to the fascia iliaca at this point may result in spread of LA upwards in the potential space between fascia iliaca and iliacus and block the three nerves in the iliac fossa.

Technique
- Locate the ASIS and pubic tubercle. Divide the distance between these two points into thirds. Make a puncture in the skin 0.5 cm inferior to the junction of the medial two-thirds and lateral third of the line between the ASIS and pubic tubercle.
- The needle is inserted perpendicular to the skin. The initial 'click' is due to the fascia lata; a second 'click' is felt on passing through the fascia iliaca.
- Volume of LA 0.5–1.0 mL/kg. 0.25% levobupivacaine with or without adrenaline 1/200,000. Maximum 30 mL.
- If using a nerve catheter, angle the needle slightly rostral and thread the catheter 2–3 cm beyond the needle tip after the second click.

Complications
- Haematoma.

Ankle block

Indications
- Foot or toe surgery.

Contraindications
- General.

Anatomy
- The tibial nerve travels posterior to the medial malleolus, behind the posterior tibial artery. It supplies the medial heel, medial two-thirds of the sole and the plantar aspect of the medial three and a half toes.
- The sural nerve travels midway between the lateral malleolus and the calcaneum, supplying the lateral aspect of foot and little toe.
- The superficial peroneal nerve travels superficially over the lateral half of the ankle and the dorsal aspect of the foot. It supplies the dorsal aspect of foot and toes excluding the first web.
- The deep peroneal nerve is lateral to the anterior tibial artery and extensor hallucis longus tendon at the level of the malleoli. It supplies the first web space.
- The saphenous nerve passes anterior to the medial malleolus. It supplies the medial aspect of the ankle and foot.

Technique
- The posterior tibial nerve is blocked by inserting the needle posterior to the posterior tibial artery perpendicular to the skin.
- The sural nerve is blocked by inserting the needle at a point midway between the lateral malleolus and the calcaneum perpendicular to the skin.
- The deep peroneal nerve is blocked by inserting the needle lateral to the anterior tibial artery (at the intermalleolar level) perpendicular to the skin.
- The superficial peroneal is blocked by superficial infiltration between the two malleoli.
- The saphenous nerve is blocked by infiltration anterior to the medial malleolus in the region of the long saphenous vein.
- Blocks of the posterior tibial, sural, deep peroneal and saphenous nerves at the ankle require about 2 mL of LA for each. The wider infiltration to block the superficial peroneal may require 6–8 mL depending on the size of the child. 0.25% or 0.5% levobupivacaine is usually used.
- The total dose of LA not to exceed maximum recommended dose.

Complications
- Haematoma.
- Nerve damage.

Sciatic nerve block

Indications
- Surgery on the posterior aspect of the thigh, lateral aspect of lower leg, ankle and whole of foot.
- The saphenous nerve can supply sensation distal to the medial malleolus, up to the medial aspect of the great toe. Therefore, foot surgery may require a saphenous or femoral nerve block in addition to a sciatic nerve block.

Contraindications
- General.
- Relative—risk of compartment syndrome.

Anatomy
- The sciatic nerve is actually two nerves within a common fascial sheath. They are the tibial and common peroneal nerves, originating from the lumbar and sacral plexuses (L4, L5, and S1, S2, and S3 roots).
- On leaving the pelvis via the greater sciatic foramen, the sciatic nerve passes midway between the greater trochanter and ischial tuberosity.
- The nerve travels deep to the gluteus maximus muscle.
- The posterior cutaneous nerve of the thigh lies superficial to the sciatic nerve.
- The sciatic nerve divides into its two components approximately two-thirds of the way down the thigh. The level of division is variable.

Technique
- Patient supine with leg flexed at the hip.
- Locate the ischial tuberosity and greater trochanter. At a point midway between the two insert the needle perpendicular to the skin.
- A PNS needle is used and is inserted until plantar or dorsiflexion of the foot is elicited.
- 0.25 or 0.5% levobupivacaine with or without adrenaline 1/200,000 can be used depending on the circumstances. Volume is usually about 0.3 mL/kg.

Complications
- Nerve damage.

Popliteal nerve block

Indications
- Any operation below the knee when *combined* with a saphenous or femoral nerve block e.g. club foot surgery.
- Otherwise suitable for surgery on the lateral aspect of the leg, ankle and whole of foot.

Contraindications
- General.
- Relative—risk of compartment syndrome.

Anatomy
- The popliteal fossa is bound superiorly by the semitendinosus and semimembranosus tendons medially and the tendon of biceps femoris laterally. The inferior border is demarcated by the medial and lateral heads of gastrocnemius.
- The fossa is divided in two by the popliteal crease or intercondylar line.
- The popliteal artery is palpated at the apex of the fossa.
- The sciatic nerve is found superficial and lateral to the artery.
- The division into tibial and common peroneal nerves is variable, and can occur as proximal as the piriformis muscle.
- US is the only reliable means of locating the division of the sciatic nerve (Fig 7.5).
- An US study in children located the nerve division 32–76 mm proximal to the knee joint. The nerves were 7–18 mm deep to the skin.

Technique
- The patient is positioned prone or lateral (operative side uppermost).
- When using a PNS needle a line between the mid point of the popliteal crease and the apex of the popliteal fossa is identified.
- The popliteal artery is palpable at this point. The needle is inserted perpendicular to the skin just lateral to the arterial pulsation.
- Plantar flexion and inversion indicates tibial nerve stimulation, dorsiflexion and eversion indicates common peroneal nerve.
- The most reliable method of identifying the sciatic division is US and this improves the success rate of the block to virtually 100% with limited volumes of LA.
- 0.3–0.5 mL/kg of 0.25% or 0.5% levobupivacaine.

Complications
- Nerve damage.
- Vascular damage.

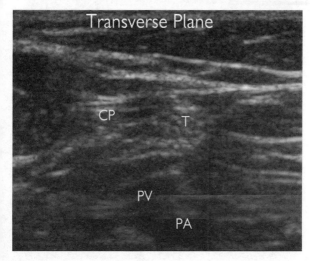

Fig. 7.5 Ultrasonographic appearance of the sciatic division: tibial nerve (T), common peroneal nerve (CP), lying superficial to the popliteal vein (PV) and artery (PA).

Regional anaesthetic techniques: central blocks

Graham Bell

Overview and safety

- Central blocks in children continue to ↑ in popularity in the UK. The reasons for this include:
  - Better appreciation of neonatal and paediatric pain and its long-term consequences.
  - A wish to avoid the side effects of opioids in vulnerable groups.
  - Improved postoperative infusion devices.
  - Accumulating evidence of safety in children.
- Normal practice is to perform regional blocks with the patient anaesthetized. This differs from adult practice but there is no evidence of a higher complication rate. Under general anaesthesia, the initial symptoms and signs of neurotoxicity are not evident. However, children less than 8 years old will not reliably report symptoms of toxicity even if awake. This makes the operator more reliant on monitoring, which must be applied prior to the procedure.
- An aseptic technique is required and is assumed for all the blocks described in this chapter.
- There is some evidence that young infants have a higher threshold for neurotoxicity of local anaesthetics but they may have a lower threshold for cardiotoxicity.
- Equipment and drugs for resuscitation must be immediately available wherever regional anaesthetic blocks are performed, with or without general anaesthesia.
- Clinical assessment of the extent of the block must wait until the patient is awake.
- Awake regional techniques remain popular for ex-premature neonates, children with muscular diseases who may tolerate general anaesthesia poorly and miscellaneous others such as patients known to be susceptible to malignant hyperthermia.
- Contraindications to central regional anaesthetic blocks depend on the block to be performed but fall into broad categories:
  - Patient or parent refusal.
  - Systemic sepsis.
  - Local sepsis at the needle insertion site.
  - Coagulopathy.
  - Some neurological diseases (relative).
  - Allergy to local anaesthetics.
- Consent should be obtained for all nerve blocks. This should include an explanation of common and serious risks. Consent may be verbal but it should be recorded in detail in the case records.

Pharmacology

- Age related differences in pharmacology and physiology must be considered for safe and effective practice.
- Central blocks may require the use of relatively high doses of local anaesthetic.
- In children, fibrous sheaths around nerves are not well developed and myelination is not complete until about 2 years of age. This makes immature nerves more sensitive to local anaesthetics and less concentrated solutions than are used in adults usually result in a dense block.
- The elimination half-life of amide local anaesthetics in neonates is at least twice the adult value; this reflects an ↑ volume of distribution and possibly a reduced clearance.
- Local anaesthetics are bound to plasma proteins, although α-1 acid glycoprotein has a high affinity for local anaesthetics, a larger mass of drug will be bound (albeit weakly) to albumin.
- Acidosis reduces the protein binding and therefore ↑ the proportion of free drug (responsible for toxicity).
- The choice of local anaesthetic for nerve block requiring a low mass of drug is purely a matter for personal preference. If there are patient factors such as hepatic impairment, anaesthetic factors such as potential for intravascular injection or rapid absorption, or surgical factors such as prolonged analgesic infusion requirements, it is prudent to use conservative doses or choose one of the less toxic single racemates.
- Less than 6 months of age, immature hepatic metabolism of amide drugs and reduced α-1 acid glycoprotein lead to higher free plasma levels of drug. The recommended dose in neonates is half the adult maximum, both for bolus doses and infusions. Halving the dose seems arbitrary but it does retain the same safety margin (on available pharmacokinetic evidence) for this higher risk group. Children over 6 months of age receive the same dose on a mg/kg as adults.

Bupivacaine

- Potent amide local anaesthetic.
- Hepatic metabolism produces slightly active metabolites which are significantly less toxic than the parent drug.
- Longer half-life than in adults and may accumulate with infusions.
- An infusion of 0.1% or 0.125% generally provides good postoperative analgesia.

Levobupivacaine

- Single stereoisomer S(-)-bupivacaine.
- Equipotent to but less toxic than racemic bupivacaine.
- Pharmacology is not yet fully studied but for practical purposes it is assumed to behave as bupivacaine.

Ropivacaine

- Amide local anaesthetic, single isomer.
- Similar potency but less toxic than bupivacaine.

- Maximum concentrations seen 30–115 min after injection perhaps due to local vasoconstriction by ropivacaine.
- This potential for vasoconstriction makes ropivacaine unsuitable for blocks of involving end-arterial blood supply.
- Maximum dose 2.5 mg/kg.

Prilocaine
- Should be avoided under three months of age due to ↑ risk of methaemaglobinaemia
- Maximum dose 5 mg/kg.

Table 8.1 Pharmacology of local anaesthetics commonly given in regional anaesthetic blocksc

	Maximum dose mg/kg	$t_{1/2}$ hours (under 6 months)	$t_{1/2}$ hours (over 6 months)	t_{max} minutes
Lidocaine	7 (10 with adrenaline)	?	2	25–45
Bupivacaine	2.5	2–7	2–5	15–30
Ropivacaine	2.5	5	2–5	30–115

Toxicity
- Often presents as cardiovascular collapse in children.
- Is treated initially using the APLS guidelines.
- ECG may show T wave morphology or ST segment changes.
- Bretylium is no longer available for the treatment of ventricular dysrhythmias.
- Magnesium (50 mg/kg over 15 min followed by infusion of 25 mg/kg/hour), phenytoin (5–10 mg/kg IV) amiodarone (5 mg/kg IV over 3 min followed by infusion of 5–15 mcg/kg/min), and intralipid 20% (1 mL/kg over 1 min, repeated every 3–5 min followed by infusion of 0.25 mL/kg/min) can all be used in the management of local anaesthetic toxicity. Individual departments will have a protocol for this with drug dosages.

Caudal epidural blockade

- This involves injection of local anaesthetic solution in to the epidural space below the termination of the spinal cord.
- The widespread popularity of the caudal approach to the epidural space is testament to its simplicity, efficacy, and safety.
- The technique is easier in children than in adults as:
  - The sacrum feels flatter and the angle of injection is easier, probably because the gluteal muscles are less bulky and the natal cleft lower.
  - The sacral hiatus is relatively large since there is less ossification around the sacrococcygeal membrane.

Indications

- Caudal epidural blocks may be used or intra- and postoperative analgesia for surgery up to the umbilicus in neonates and infants.
- The lower thoracic nerve routes are not blocked consistently in older children where it is restricted to sacral and lumbar nerve roots.
- Common indications include:
  - Circumcision
  - Hypospadias repair
  - Inguinal herniotomy
  - Orchidopexy
  - Ano-rectal surgery
  - Lower limb elective orthopaedic surgery
  - Lower limb plastic surgery.

Contraindications

- General contraindications to central blocks.
- Abnormal sacral anatomy. Local skin changes such as pigmentation, dimples, or hairy patches may be associated with spinal dysraphism or a tethered spinal cord and a caudal should not be attempted without confirmation of normal neuroanatomy.
- Mongolian blue spots are not a contraindication to caudal injection.

Anatomy

- The neonatal sacrum is composed of five cartilaginous sacral vertebrae that gradually ossify and fuse to form the adult sacrum.
- The sacral hiatus results from the failure of fusion of the posterior arches of the fifth, sometimes the fourth and occasionally the third, sacral vertebrae. This deficiency in the neural arch of the fifth sacral vertebra is covered by a ligamentous membrane called the sacrococcygeal membrane.
- Sacral anatomy changes with age.
  - It is wider from side to side in the toddler than the neonate.
  - Antero-posterior diameter also ↑ with age
  - In neonates and infants the pelvis is proportionally smaller than in adults and the sacrum is higher in relation to the iliac crests. As the pelvis grows the position of the sacrum relative to the pelvis descends to adult position by 4 years of age.

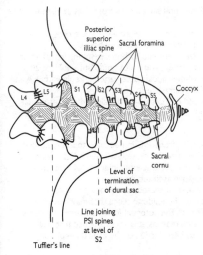

Fig. 8.1 Sacral anatomy in the neonate

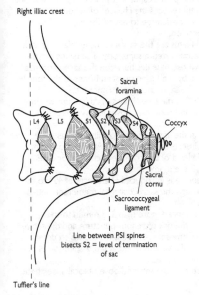

Fig. 8.2 Sacral anatomy at 8 years old

- • The termination of the dural sac ascends from S3/4 at birth to S2 by 3 years of age.
- • The posterior laminae begin to fuse around 7 years of age. The posterior wall is largely ligamentous until puberty.
- • Cartilage is progressively replaced by bone, resulting in reduction in the size of the hiatus. Bony fusion is not complete until late 20s.
- Hence, the dimensions of the caudal space vary markedly with age and between individuals of the same age.
- Sacral anomalies are found in 3–5% of individuals and can result in a reduced distance from the sacral hiatus to the dural sac.

Technique

- Hypodermic needles varying from 25G in neonates to 20G in older children can be used. Finer needles cause less trauma but have been implicated in accidental IV or subarachnoid injection of local anaesthetic following false negative aspiration tests.
- Styletted needles or cannulae are used increasingly to avoid transporting skin plugs into the epidural space that may contain bacteria or dermal cells with the potential for epidermoid tumour development. For the same reasons, it is good practice to make a small skin incision prior to introduction of the caudal needle or cannula.
- IV cannulae are frequently used. Once the membrane is pierced, the needle is withdrawn and the plastic cannula advanced into the epidural space. The blunt cannula tip reduces the chances of venous perforation, dural puncture or damage to neural tissue.
- Patient is in the lateral position.
- Landmarks for the sacral hiatus are the sacral cornuae inferiorly and the body of the fourth sacral vertebra superiorly. The hiatus can be considered as a triangle whose base lies between the sacral cornuae and whose apex is formed by the fusion of sacral bones of the fourth vertebra and covered by the sacrococcygeal membrane.
- With the hips flexed to 90° in the lateral position, a line drawn along the long axis of the femur and continued posteriorly will cross the midline at the level of the sacral cornuae.
- The caudal space tapers in the antero-posterior direction as the sacrococcygeal ligament inserts into the coccyx. An insertion point 5 mm or so rostral to the level of the cornuae is chosen for ease of locating the space through the ligament.
- The chosen needle or cannula is introduced at an angle of 45° to the sacrum and advanced through the sacrococcygeal membrane until a pop or loss of resistance is felt.
- A needle should not be advanced more than 2–3 mm in to the epidural space since this ↑ the risk of venous puncture and dural tap.
- The needle is left open to atmosphere for a few seconds to detect blood or CSF in the event of a venous or dural tap. Aspiration of fine epidural veins will often be negative.
- After a negative aspiration test, the selected dose of local anaesthetic solution is injected slowly.

Confirmation of correct needle placement
- Experienced operators rely on the distinctive physical end points.
- Much has been written about the relative merits of various test injections to diagnose intravascular injection. None are 100% sensitive or specific and so local anaesthetic should always be injected slowly with ECG monitoring in place.
- The whoosh test is the injection of saline or air into the caudal space with auscultation over the lower spine by an observer to confirm epidural injection. This will shortly give way to a more eloquent use of sound.
- Ultrasonography of the caudal space is simple, carries no risk of air embolism and effectively confirms injection in to the epidural space.

Dosage
- Bupivacaine is being replaced as the commonest drug for this block by levobupivacaine and ropivacaine.
- Concentration of bupivacaine or levobupivacaine is usually 0.25%. 0.5% is used to provide a dense sacral nerve root block lasting well in to the postoperative period (e.g. for hypospadias repair). 0.125% is often used under 6 months of age. Ropivacaine 0.2% is popular.

- Armitage produced the best known formula for volume of local anaesthetic required using a caudal injection to obtain a given height of block:
  - 0.5 mL/kg sacral nerve roots.
  - 1.0 mL/kg lower thoracic and upper lumbar nerve roots.
  - 1.25 mL/kg mid-thoracic (T6) nerve roots.

- There are problems with this formula. Although 0.5 mL/kg will consistently produce a sacral block, 1.25 mL/kg of local anaesthetic may result in erratic and occasionally alarming cephalad spread! For this reason it is more common to block thoracic dermatomes using a caudal catheter technique (📖 p.208) or an intervertebral epidural (📖 p.205).

- The Armitage guide is then simplified to:
  - Over 6 months 1 mL/kg of 0.25% bupivacaine will block upper lumbar nerve roots i.e. the groin in children less than 20 kg (above this weight the technique becomes inconsistent at blocking these nerve roots).
  - At all ages sacral nerve roots are blocked reliably by 0.3–0.5 mL/kg of solution.

Use of adjuncts to local anaesthetic solution
- Caudal analgesia in children has suffered a smorgasbord of additives.
- Opioids are effective but the potential for synergistic effects with systemic opioids on the respiratory centre have limited their use.

- When epidural opioids are used, the risk of respiratory depression is small but present for up to 12 hours after administration. This occurs particularly in infants and is exacerbated by systemic opioid administration. Nausea, itch, and urinary retention are more commonly encountered side effects and can be treated by small doses of systemic naloxone. The maximum doses of epidural opioids for infusion are morphine 5 mcg/kg/hour and fentanyl 0.4 mcg/kg/hour.
- Clonidine has some effect in prolonging caudal analgesia but this may result simply from its systemic sedative and analgesic effects.
- Ketamine is emerging as the most promising adjunct as it significantly prolongs the duration of caudal bupivacaine up to fourfold. The usual dose of ketamine for epidural use is 0.5 mg/kg. This must be a preservative-free preparation of the drug, as with all agents administered centrally.
- Adrenaline appears to add little to plain bupivacaine given caudally, and may be implicated in some cases of spinal cord ischemia when given into the subarachnoid space.
- Spinal opiates may produce respiratory depression up to 18 hours post administration and their use in children is rare.

Complications
- Failure—more common in children weighing less than 10 kg where difficulty in identifying the caudal hiatus occurs in about 10% of subjects.
- Urinary retention (almost always resolves without intervention).
- Motor block (i.e. inability to walk after day surgery).
- Dural puncture.
- Intravascular injection.

Epidural blockade

Has become popular because:

- Of ↑ attention to the requirements for effective analgesia in children.
- It often permits light anaesthesia, minimal opioid use, early extubation, and the avoidance of postoperative ventilation.
- The realization that postoperative outcome in some high risk cases is favourably influenced by epidural analgesia—open (rather than laparoscopic) fundoplication, severe respiratory disease undergoing abdominal surgery, neonates undergoing repair of oesophageal atresia.
- The availability of well made equipment of appropriate size.

Catheters manufactured for paediatric epidurals often have one end hole only and no side holes. They may not have identical depth markings to adult catheters and, in particular, they may lack a 20 cm mark.

Indications

- Epidural administration of local anaesthetics with or without opioids is used for intraoperative anaesthesia, usually as an adjunct to general anaesthesia, and for postoperative analgesia for thoracic, abdominal, or lower body procedures.
- Epidural anaesthesia is of most benefit after major surgery associated with protracted and severe postoperative pain.
- Despite enthusiasm, there is limited objective evidence that postoperative epidural analgesia after major surgery in children is more effective than IV opioid analgesia.

Contraindications

- General contraindications to central blocks.
- A ventriculo-peritoneal shunt is not a contraindication to epidural analgesia but meticulous attention to asepsis and consideration of prophylactic antibiotics would seem sensible.

Anatomy

- The depth of location of the epidural space is extremely variable. The formula depth = 1 mm/kg for identification of the lumbar epidural space in children over 1 year old, can be used as a rough guide.
- In young children the spinal cord terminates at a lower vertebral level than in older children and for the lumbar approach the preferred levels are L4/L5 or L5/S1.

Technique

- Almost identical to the technique used in adults apart from the fact that the child is anaesthetized.
- Loss of resistance to saline is preferred to loss of resistance to air which has resulted in air embolism and central neurological complications.
- The usual technique is loss of resistance to saline from a fluid filled syringe.

- The microdrip method also uses loss of resistance to an open saline drip, and allows both of the operator's hands to guide the Tuohy needle.
- Approach may be caudal, sacral intervertebral, lumbar, or thoracic.
- Cervical epidural analgesia has no place in children.
- The best angle for Tuohy needle insertion is 74° (pointing cephalad) in the lumbar region. The very steep angles used for adult thoracic epidurals are unnecessary in younger children.
- The paramedian approach is also possible. Here the needle is inserted slightly lateral to the midline, advanced to a lamina and the 'walked off' the superior edge of the lamina until the ligamentum flavum is reached.
- Checking of the catheter tip position may be by radiography, ultrasound in young children or by Tsui's methods of ECG morphology or electrical stimulation (🕮 p.208).
- Sacral intervertebral epidural block is possible because bony fusion of the sacrum is not complete in children. The easiest approach is at the S2/3 level just below the line joining the posterior superior iliac spines. Angulation of the needle is not necessary and a standard epidural technique is used. The distance to the epidural space is less than in the lumbar region because there is no lordosis at the sacral level.

Dosage

- There is no perfect formula for local anaesthetic dose.
- A reasonable initial bolus dose for a lumbar epidural is 0.7 mL/kg of 0.25% bupivacaine.
- For postoperative infusions, most centres use 0.1% or 0.125% as a standard concentration. More dilute solutions are effective if adjuncts are used.
- Maximum infusion rates of bupivacaine are 0.25 mg/kg/hour below 6 months of age and 0.4 mg/kg/hour in older children.
- Ropivacaine is usually infused as 0.2 mL/kg/hour of 0.2% solution (0.4 mg/kg/hour).
- Low dose opioids are commonly added to the local anaesthetic for epidural infusion and have a good safety record. A low dose would be morphine 1–5 mcg/kg/hour, fentanyl 0.1–0.5 mcg/kg/hour or
- diamorphine 5–25 mcg/kg/hour (if still available in the UK).
- Continuous saturation monitoring is required. Opioids will produce a degree of sedation—this should be monitored but is not necessarily a side effect as active children with epidural catheters can be difficult to manage.
- Patients with an epidural infusion are often nursed in an HDU, but many centres nurse them on surgical wards with observations and management carried out in accordance with an agreed protocol.

Complications

- Epidural block has fewer cardiovascular effects due to immaturity of the sympathetic system and lower vascular tone in small children.
- If hypotension does occur in the absence of bleeding then suspect a subarachnoid or subdural catheter site.
- Hypotension is more common over 8 years of age.

- Bloody tap, especially if there is IVC obstruction or excessive spinal flexion at the time of insertion.
- Leak around catheters. Neonatal epidural catheter sites leak. This is not so much a complication as a fact of life. The most effective way to manage this is to ignore it, especially if the block is effective. Dressings may need to be changed more frequently in neonates because of this leak.

Caudal catheter technique

- This is sometimes used to produce thoracic epidural blockade in an anaesthetized infant without having to perform an intervertebral approach.
- Fat in the epidural space of neonates and infants is loculated with distinct spaces between individual lobules.
- At this age, an epidural catheter introduced into the epidural space via the sacral hiatus can be threaded to the thoracic region of the epidural canal.
- The original Tuohy needle can be used to puncture the sacrococcygeal membrane, although this can be awkward. Alternatives include an IV cannula or a specifically designed blunt tipped introducer.
- The catheter is threaded up the epidural space to a distance estimated to correspond to the appropriate nerve roots for blockade. The catheter advances more easily in infants than older children or adults.
- The position of the catheter tip can be checked using radiological screening. An alternative approach uses electrocardiography. A specially devised epidural catheter with a metal hub to allow connection to an ECG display is flushed with saline and acts as a unipolar ECG electrode. The display of the (ECG) signal from the tip is compared with the ECG from a surface electrode positioned at the target segmental level. When the ECG traces are identical, the tip of the catheter is at the target level. Motor nerve root stimulation has also been used. A styletted epidural catheter with an ECG adapter cathode at the hub allows electrical motor root stimulation from the catheter tip using a peripheral nerve stimulator. Observation of the truncal motor response (in an unparalysed patient) during catheter advancement indicates the level of the catheter tip.
- Handheld ultrasound machines allow the catheter to be visualized as it is threaded up the epidural space. This technique may become more popular with these advances in ensuring accurate placement.
- A catheter introduced through the caudal hiatus reaches the desired thoracic position in 85% of premature neonates and 95% of term infants.
- It is less reliable with increasing age and the catheter often coils in the lumbar region. This is due to the development of the lumbar lordosis and the increasing density of epidural fat when lobules become more densely packed and are connected by fibrous strands.
- There is a greater risk of colonization of caudal epidural catheters (compared to thoraco-lumbar) with Gram-negative organisms but actual infections appear to be extremely rare with short term use (<72 hours).

Subarachnoid (spinal) blockade

This is less common than epidural blockade but is technically easy and carries a low risk of systemic toxicity from the small doses of local anaesthetic used.

Indications

Two groups are commonly considered for subarachnoid block:

- Ex-premature neonates who may prove difficult to extubate even after limited surgery. The classic operation involved is repair of inguinal hernia which is common in premature infants. There is evidence that these patients experience a lower rate of postoperative apnoea after spinal, compared with general anaesthesia. Apnoea may still occur after a spinal so postoperative monitoring is the same as for general anaesthesia.
- Older children with muscular or neuromuscular disease who are ↑ risk of the complications of general anaesthesia; performing a spinal block in these children is essentially the same as in adults, with a small amount of sedation, sensible 12-year-olds will cooperate sufficiently to allow successful spinal anaesthesia.

Spinals do not provide postoperative analgesia and something must be in place to prevent sudden severe pain as the block regresses.

Contraindications

- Procedures expected to last more than 1 hour (unless an epidural block is performed simultaneously).

Anatomy

- The spinal cord of the term neonate generally ends at the level of the L3 vertebra although it may extend as low as the L4 vertebra.
- The volume of cerebrospinal fluid in infants is 4 mL/kg (2 mL/kg in adults) with 50% being in the spinal canal compared with 25% in adults. These factors produce proportionately more dilution of local anaesthetic solution in the cerebrospinal fluid in children than in adults and contribute to the short duration of subarachnoid anaesthesia in children.
- The depth of the subarachnoid space in the lumbar region is approximately 10 mm at birth and 16 mm at 3 years.

Technique of neonatal subarachnoid blockade

- The technique is similar to adult subarachnoid block.
- Performed with the infant held in the sitting or the lateral position. This is largely a matter of personal preference. Care is taken to avoid flexing the neck and obstructing the airway.
- IV access is mandatory.
- A midline approach at L4/L5 or L5/S1 below the termination of the cord is easiest.
- Short pencil point needles are available. Excessively narrow needles are unhelpful as speed of recognition of CSF flow is important in these patients who will invariably attempt to move.

- The speed of onset in neonates is impressively fast. Similarly, the block wears off quickly, often regressing rapidly after 30–60 min. This is presumably partly due to the relatively greater CSF volume in neonates (📖 Chapter 1).
- It is common to perform a caudal block as well as a spinal to prolong the duration of analgesia. This then becomes, of course, a combined spinal epidural technique.
- Assessing the block is difficult. The response to cold spray can be useful, as may observation of paradoxical respiratory muscle movement and loss of response to a low amperage tetanic stimulus.
- Spread of the block is less predictable than in adults and high blocks are relatively common.
- The feet must not be raised above the head, e.g. when placing a diathermy pad, or a high block may be produced.
- Sedation is not given in this group because, like general anaesthesia, it carries the risk of postoperative apnoeas.

Dosage

- Heavy bupivacaine is recommended in a dose of 0.3–1 mg/kg = 0.07–0.2 mL/kg of 0.5% solution.
- Lidocaine is relatively contraindicated since it produces a very short duration of anaesthesia and is associated with transient neurological symptoms.

Complications

- Relatively high failure rate of 10–20%.
- Although hypotension is rare, bradycardia occasionally occurs.
- Post dural puncture headache (PDPH) is rare in neonates but persistent CSF leak has been described. Headache will not be reported but irritability or other behavioural changes should raise suspicion.
- In older children, the incidence of PDPH is relatively high and probably under-recognized.
  - Symptoms are more variable in children who may experience dizziness, nausea or hearing loss more than headache.
  - Bed rest probably only serves to delay onset of any symptoms.
  - The patient should be kept adequately hydrated and given simple analgesics. Caffeine may be of benefit.
  - Most PDPH resolve within 6 days with conservative management.
  - Prophylactic epidural blood patch is not recommended unless conservative management fails (0.3 mL/kg of blood is taken with full asepsis). Blood patch is associated with side effects—back stiffness, parasthesiae, and subdural haematoma.

Psoas (lumbar) plexus blockade

- This comprises a posterior approach to the lumbar plexus.
- The aim is to anaesthetize the lumbar plexus and some of the sacral plexus by injecting inbetween the quadratus lumborum and psoas major muscles.
- It produces analgesia in the distributions of the obturator and femoral nerves and the lateral cutaneous nerve of thigh with some upper branches of the sciatic plexus also affected.
- The distribution of this block is similar to that of a 3 in 1 block or an illiacus sheath (fascia iliaca compartment) block.
- May be a good choice following previous hip surgery as adhesions can limit the spread of local anaesthetic through tissue plains required for efficacy of a 3 in 1 block or an illiacus sheath block.

Indications
- Unilateral procedures on the hip, femur, thigh, or knee.

Contraindications
- General to central blocks.

Anatomy
- The anterior rami of the lumbar nerve roots (and T12) enter psoas and merge within it to form the psoas (lumbar) plexus and produce the ilioinguinal, hypogastric, obturator, femoral, and lateral cutaneous nerve of thigh.
- The plexus can be approached percutaneously through the quadratus lumborum and posterior part of the psoas muscle.

Technique
- The commonest technique uses a nerve stimulator so the patient is not paralysed. Alternatively, a loss of resistance technique is used which detects when the needle enters the psoas compartment.
- Patient positioned laterally with hips and knees flexed to 90°. Operative side is uppermost.
- Insertion point is identified 5 cm lateral from the spinous process of L4 then 3 cm caudal from this point (cm in adults, fingerbreadths in children). Alternatively, 2/3 of the distance down a line connecting the spinous process of L4 with the posterior superior iliac spine. Both techniques lead to the point close to where the intercristal line (superior borders of both iliac crests) intersects a paraspinous line passing through the ipsilateral posterior superior iliac spine.
- An insulated needle is inserted perpendicular to the skin and then advanced with a slight medial direction.
- The needle is advanced until it makes contact with the transverse process of L5, then 'walked off' the cranial border until either contractions of the quadriceps are visible (or a loss of resistance is felt as the needle exits the anterior edge of quadratus lumborum). Either of these end points should be reached not more than 20 mm deeper than contact with the transverse process.

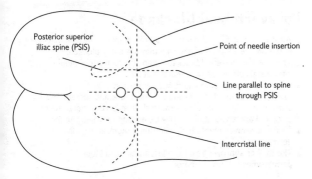

Fig. 8.3 Landmarks for psoas plexus block.

- A nerve stimulator is attached to the needle and correct positioning is determined by contractions in the quadriceps femoris muscles at about 0.5 mA.
- This is quite a deep block, with the end point one and a half times the depth of the epidural space.
- Local anaesthetic is injected, with immediate loss of contractions.
- A catheter may be introduced into this fascial space for continuous plexus block.

Dosage
- Relatively large volume of local anaesthetic is required to achieve the necessary spread.
- Bupivacaine 0.5% 2.5 mg/kg. Maximum volume of 30 mL. Levobupivacaine or ropivacaine also used.

Complications
- Epidural block from injection into a dural cuff or medial spread of the local anaesthetic.
- Retroperitoneal haematoma (rare)
- Dural cuff puncture and spinal anaesthesia (rare).

Paravertebral blockade

- After emerging from the intervertebral foramina, the spinal nerves run in the paravertebral space where they are easily blocked.
- Thoracic paravertebral blockade is an alternative to multiple intercostals blocks or to an epidural block.
- It has a low failure rate and few complications.
- The block will produce unilateral sympathetic and somatic block of spinal nerves immediately lateral to their exit from the vertebral column. Paravertebral block may be either thoracic or lumbar.
- Thoracic paravertebral block will usually block at least five dermatomes.
- The lumbar approach results in less spread and block of two dermatomes is more common.

Indications
- Unilateral procedures.
- Common indications for thoracic paravertebral block include thoracotomy and renal surgery.
- The lumbar approach is useful for hip and thigh surgery.

Contraindications
- General for central blocks.

Anatomy
- The paravertebral space is a wedge-shaped area that lies on either side of the vertebral column. It:
  - Is continuous with the intercostal space laterally.
  - Has parietal pleura as its anterior boundary.
  - Is limited medially by the lateral aspect of the vertebral body and intervertebral discs.
  - Is limited posteriorly by the transverse processes, the ribs, and the costotransverse ligament.
- Within this space, the spinal nerve root emerges from the intervertebral foramen and divides into dorsal and ventral rami. In addition, sympathetic fibres of the ventral rami enter the sympathetic trunk via the preganglionic white rami communicantes and the postganglionic grey rami communicantes in this space. Because of the multiple neural structures within this space, local anesthetics introduced here can produce unilateral motor, sensory, and sympathetic blockade.
- The thoracic paravertebral spaces communicate down to T12 where psoas is adherent. Below T12, the space is segmental.
- Local anaesthetic has the potential to spread in most directions after injection to the paravertebral space.

Technique
Thoracic paravertebral block
- The patient is positioned in the lateral position with the operative side uppermost.

- A Tuohy needle and loss of resistance syringe are usually used.
- The desired spinous process (usually T7–T9) is identified and the needle is inserted lateral to the spinous process. This lateral distance approximates to the distance between the tips of the spinous processes (1–2 cm). The depth is estimated by the formula $0.48 \times$ body weight/kg $+ 18.7$ in mm.
- The space is usually located with a loss of resistance technique through the costotransverse ligament. The end point is not as definite as with the epidural space.
- When the needle is advanced, it will often contact the transverse process. In this case, the needle is 'walked' off the superior aspect of the process into the costotransverse ligament and the loss of resistance is felt when this is penetrated.
- A single injection of local anaesthetic can be given through the needle or a catheter is introduced. This should not be threaded more than 3 cm in case the tip is pushed out of the paravertebral space.
- It is also possible to place a catheter in the paravertebral space under direct vision during surgery.

Lumbar paravertebral block

- The usefulness of this technique is limited by the segmental nature of the lumbar paravertebral space which prevents much spread of local anaesthetic to nerves above and below the injection site.
- Two spinal roots can be blocked at a time by injecting above and below any given transverse process, for example, L1 and L2 can be blocked in this way at the transverse process of L2 giving good analgesia for hip surgery.

Dosage

Usually 0.25% bupivacaine (or levobupivacaine or ropivacaine) 0.5 mL/kg. Postoperative infusions can be run but are not commonly used.

Complications

- Vascular puncture
- Pneumothorax (<1%)
- Horner's syndrome
- Epidural or spinal injection (rare).

Section 4

Elective surgery

Elective surgery

Day case, general, ENT, orthopaedic, neurosurgery, and maxillofacial surgery

Manchula Navaratnam

Day case surgery

- Children are excellent candidates for day case surgery.
- Current recommendations are that 50–70% of elective paediatric surgery be performed as day cases.
- Successful day case surgery requires a careful selection process, an experienced multidisciplinary team, appropriate facilities, and effective protocols for analgesia, discharge, and postoperative follow-up.

Selection and exclusion criteria

Should be clear and relevant to the unit with a focus on four key areas:
- The patient
- The procedure
- Anaesthetic considerations
- Social circumstances.

The patient

- Majority are healthy and free from chronic disease.
- Children with stable or well-controlled systemic disease e.g. asthma, epilepsy, malignancy, cerebral palsy are suitable.
- Children with asymptomatic, uncomplicated cardiac lesions e.g. small VSD or well children with surgically corrected cardiac lesions may be suitable with appropriate antibiotic prophylaxis against bacterial endocarditis.
- Children with insulin dependent diabetes mellitus (IDDM) or inborn errors of metabolism are unsuitable because of potentially complicated perioperative glycaemic control.
- Children with moderate or severe respiratory infection (📖 p.66) should be postponed.
- In the presence of a mild respiratory infection it is reasonable to proceed with surgery.
- Term infants >1 month of age can be treated on a day case basis for some procedures especially examination under anaesthesia i.e. no surgical procedure is carried out although many units have a lower age limit of 3 months.
- Preterm babies <50 weeks' postconceptual age are unsuitable candidates due to the risk of postoperative apnoea and the need for postoperative monitoring .The age at which these babies are no longer at risk is unclear but may be up to 60 weeks' postconceptual age or higher if there is chronic lung disease.

The procedure

- Preferably superficial and of short duration with postoperative pain managed by oral analgesics.
- Ideally should not involve a body cavity and last no longer than 1 hour.
- Not be associated with significant risk of postoperative haemorrhage.
- Suitability of adenotonsillectomy is debatable. As surgical techniques which reduce the incidence of postoperative haemorrhage are introduced this may become a common day case procedure.

Anaesthetic considerations

- Previous anaesthetic problems or a difficult airway may preclude day surgery but the decision depends on the individual patient and expertise of the anaesthetist and day care unit.
- Prolonged anaesthesia is associated with delayed recovery and complications such as nausea and vomiting.

Social circumstances

- Some units recommend that families should live no further than a 1-hour drive by car.
- Families should have access to a telephone and transport to return to the hospital if necessary.

Facilities and procedures

There are widely accepted quality standards for paediatric day case surgery. Key points include:

- An integrated admission plan incorporating an efficient pre-admission system.
- Specific written advice for the parent(s).
- Child should be admitted to a designated day case area with designated day case staff. Should not be mixed with acutely ill inpatients.
- Children should not be admitted or treated alongside adults.
- The environment should comply with child safety standards and be child friendly.
- Essential documentation should be completed before discharge to ensure efficient aftercare and follow up.

Anaesthetic considerations

- A streamlined assessment in advance of day surgery provides a more effective service.
- Popular methods include structured questionnaires and a nurse led pre-admission clinic with input from the surgeon and anaesthetist.
- Preoperative assessment by telephone allows staff to check that the child will attend, potential problems to be identified before admission, and advice on fasting to be emphasized.
- Clear verbal and written fasting instructions are essential. Liberal regimens for oral fluids reduce preoperative distress in patients and parents and improve perioperative behaviour.
- Sedative premedication in appropriate cases is not contraindicated. Oral midazolam 0.5 mg/kg to a maximum of 20 mg is not associated with delayed discharge.

Analgesia and discharge

Analgesia

- Good analgesia is essential for successful day case surgery.
- LA techniques should be used where possible and include topical, local infiltration, peripheral nerve blocks (📖 Chapter 7) and caudal epidural blocks (📖 Chapter 8).
- Peripheral nerve blocks include penile blocks for circumcision, ilioinguinal blocks for inguinal herniotomy, and greater auricular nerve blocks for otoplasty.
- Caudal epidural blocks can be used for many procedures below the umbilicus. Using dilute LA concentrations reduces the incidence of leg weakness. Adjuncts such as ketamine (0.5 mg/kg) or clonidine (1 mcg/kg) extend the duration of block although there is a risk of sedation and transient hypotension with clonidine.
- Paracetamol and NSAIDs enhance the quality of analgesia.
- Paracetamol is widely used either by preoperative oral loading 20 mg/kg or rectally after induction 30–40 mg/kg. IV paracetamol (15 mg/kg) may be a better alternative to the rectal route, which has erratic and unreliable absorption.
- NSAIDs such as ibuprofen 5–10 mg/kg or diclofenac 1 mg/kg are commonly given by mouth preoperatively or rectally after induction.
- Single perioperative doses of opioids such as fentanyl (1–2 mcg/kg) or codeine phosphate (1 mg/kg) are useful in certain cases. An antiemetic should be given if an opioid is used. Procedures requiring repeated opioid analgesia are not appropriate day cases.
- The mainstay of analgesia after discharge is paracetamol and NSAIDs. For some procedures, 3 or 4 doses of a weak opioid such as codeine phosphate to be administered by the parents at home with written advice can also be dispensed before the child is discharged.

Discharge criteria

- Protective airway reflexes intact and no respiratory distress or stridor.
- Stable vital signs and conscious level appropriate for individual child.
- No bleeding or surgical complications.
- No or minimal pain and PONV.
- Ambulation appropriate for child.
- Desirable (but not essential) that child is able to drink.
- Written and verbal instructions given with clear lines of contact to the hospital if required.
- Escort home by responsible adult in private car or taxi.

Audit and quality control

- The commonest problems requiring inpatient admission are PONV and severe pain.
- A widely quoted benchmark for admission is 1–2%.
- Regular audit should address cancellation, unplanned admissions, postoperative morbidity, and parent and child satisfaction.

General paediatric surgery

Considerations in paediatric general surgery

- Many (70–80%) procedures are undertaken on a day case basis.
- Most procedures involve the penile or groin areas.
- Multimodal analgesia is important with the use of LA techniques where possible.
- The use of laparoscopic techniques is increasing rapidly.

Circumcision

- Very common procedure.
- Involves removal of some of or the entire foreskin.
- Usually performed as a day case procedure.
- Indications are social or religious beliefs of the parent(s), balanitis xerotica obliterans, infection, phimosis, and paraphimosis.
- Patient supine with minimal blood loss.

Preoperative assessment

Patients are usually healthy. Respiratory infection is the commonest issue to be considered and a decision made on whether to proceed or defer ([Book] Chapter 3).

Anaesthetic technique

- Older boys are often anxious about circumcision and benefit from sedative premedication (midazolam 0.5 mg/kg; maximum 20 mg).
- Induction depends largely on age. In older boys, an IV induction is common. Chubby infants for religious/cultural circumcisions usually have an inhalational induction.
- Spontaneous ventilation with a LMA is the norm in older boys. Endotracheal intubation and IPPV may be preferable in infants.
- Maintenance is with volatile in oxygen and air or nitrous oxide.

Analgesia

Options for regional analgesia are a caudal epidural block ([Book] Chapter 8) or a penile nerve block ([Book] Chapter 7).

- A caudal block (0.3 mL/kg 0.5% levobupivacaine or similar) is often preferred in infants. Motor block is not an issue in these patients and effective penile blocks may be difficult to perform consistently in infants.
- In older boys, a penile nerve block is more common (0.1 mL/kg 0.25% levobupivacaine or similar each side). Motor block after caudal epidural is now a potential problem and the technique of penile nerve block is more consistently successful than in infants.
- In all cases, a NSAID is also given unless there is a contraindication.
- There is an incidence of failure to achieve an effective block with both caudal and penile nerve blocks. This is usually obvious during surgery and an opioid (morphine sulphate 100–150 mcg/kg IV, codeine phosphate 0.5–1 mg/kg IM, fentanyl 2–4 mcg/kg IV) should be given to ensure that the child does not emerge from anaesthesia with no effective analgesia.
- Lidocaine ointment can be smeared on the glans at the end of surgery to supplement the analgesia used.

Postoperative care

Oral intake is usually resumed soon after surgery. A combination of paracetamol 15 mg/kg oral 4-hourly, a NSAID e.g. ibuprofen 10 mg/kg oral 6-hourly and a weak opioid (such as codeine phosphate 1 mg/kg oral 4-hourly) is prescribed. Discharge is usually 2–4 hours postoperatively. Boys should have passed urine, be walking if appropriate and not be actively bleeding. Significant pain after discharge is the norm for 24–48 hours and the parents must be given advice on regular administration of analgesics at home. Many hospitals dispense some form of analgesia for the parents to use at home such as lidocaine ointment, ibuprofen or a weak opioid in addition to paracetamol.

Preputioplasty

- Preputioplasty, or dorsal slit with transverse closure, overcomes phimosis in children while conserving the foreskin.
- The narrowed preputial outlet is incised longitudinally and repaired transversely.
- Under these circumstances, preputioplasty is an alternative to circumcision that preserves the foreskin and causes less morbidity than circumcision.
- Performed in older boys since it is not an alternative to religious/cultural circumcsion in infants.

Preoperative assessment

As for circumcision.

Anaesthetic technique

- Sedative premedication if indicated.
- IV induction is the norm.
- Spontaneous ventilation with a LMA.
- Volatile in oxygen and air or nitrous oxide.

Analgesia

Effective analgesia is easier to provide than for circumcision.

- A penile nerve block with 0.1 mL/kg 0.25% levobupivacaine or similar (📖 Chapter 7) is almost always adequate. This need not be circumferential since the operation is restricted to the dorsum of the penis and only the dorsal penile nerves need to be blocked.
- A NSAID is also used unless contraindicated.

Postoperative care

Oral intake resumes soon after surgery. Paracetamol, NSAID and a weak opioid are prescribed although further analgesia is not usually required in hospital. Discharge is usually 2–4 hours postoperatively and pain at home is much less than after circumcision.

Hypospadias repair

- Hypospadias is a relatively common congenital defect (approximately 1:350 male births). Other congenital anomalies are rare and renal function is usually normal.
- It is characterized by an abnormal position of the meatus. The degree of hypospadias depends on the location of the opening on the penis. The defect may occur anywhere along the underside of the penis down to the scrotum. The penile skin does not form a normal foreskin around the shortened urethral tube resulting in a hood like effect.
- Chordee (a downward curve of the penis, especially when erect) is usually, but not always, associated with hypospadias.
- The aims of surgery are:
  - To create a neourethra with the meatus at the tip of the glans.
  - Release chordee if present.
  - Achieve adequate skin coverage.
  - Produce acceptable cosmesis.
- Surgical correction is usually performed during the first or second year of life.
  - Distal hypospadias is treated with a MAGPI procedure (meatal advancement and glanduloplasty) or urethroplasty.
  - Complex proximal lesions often undergo a staged repair.
  - Fistula formation may occur and require re-operation.
  - Occasionally graft tissue may be taken to repair larger defects—usually from buccal mucosa (sometimes from bladder mucosa).
  - The procedure requires a urethral or suprapubic catheter for 24–48 hours postoperatively to stop surgical oedema preventing urination.

Preoperative assessment

Boys are usually fit and healthy.

Anaesthetic technique

- Sedative premedication may be helpful if the boy is to have multiple procedures.
- Induction is usually inhalational in this age group.
- Surgery may last several hours and endotracheal intubation with IPPV is the norm although spontaneous ventilation with an LMA is often appropriate.
- Endotracheal intubation is required if buccal mucosa is used either with nasal tube or oral RAE positioned to one side of the mouth. A throat pack is placed in case of bleeding into the oral cavity.
- Maintenance is with volatile in oxygen and air or nitrous oxide.
- Erection can make surgery difficult and can be avoided with regional block and adequate depth of anaesthesia.

Analgesia
- Is best provided in most cases by a caudal epidural block (0.3–0.5 mL/kg 0.5% levobupivacaine or similar). Clonidine (1–2 mcg/kg) or preservative free ketamine (0.5 mg/kg) are useful adjuncts to extend the duration of the block (📖 Chapter 8).
- A penile nerve block (📖 Chapter 7) may be suitable if the hypospadias is minor and distal.
- A NSAID is also given unless contraindicated.
- In many cases a minor degree of postoperative sedation is desirable to stop the boy investigating the dressings or urinary catheter. For this reason a bolus of opioid (morphine sulphate 100–150 mcg/kg IV or codeine phosphate 0.5–1 mg/kg IM) is often given despite an effective caudal epidural block.

Postoperative care

Maintenance fluids are prescribed until oral intake is well established to ensure urine flow through the catheter. In most cases, a combination of paracetamol, a NSAID and an oral opioid provide adequate analgesia. After complex or major repairs an IV infusion of morphine sulphate or nurse controlled analgesia (📖 Chapter 6) can be used.

After complex repairs sutures are often removed under anaesthesia about 5 days postoperatively.

Inguinal hernia repair and hydrocele

- Inguinal hernias are common in children. The surgical approach and anaesthetic considerations for treatment of a hydrocele are almost identical to those for an inguinal hernia.
- Incidence of inguinal hernia is 1–3% (five times as common in boys as in girls), around 10% in premature infants, and 30% in children born at <28 weeks' gestation.
- During gestation, each testis migrates from the abdomen to the scrotum through the internal inguinal ring and inguinal canal. A diverticulum of peritoneum the processus vaginalis follows the testis in to the scrotum
- In 90% of people the processus vaginalis involutes and is obliterated. Persistent patency of all or part of the processus results in various inguinal conditions.
  - Inguinal hernia: obliteration of distal processus and patency of proximal processus
  - Hydrocele: obliterated proximal segment and patent distal segment
  - Encysted hydrocele of the cord: obliteration of both ends of the processus with a saccular dilatation in the middle.
- The majority of inguinal hernias are repaired as elective cases. Occasionally, especially in neonates and infants an urgent procedure is required to deal with an incarcerated or strangulated hernia.
- Laparoscopic repair is performed by some surgeons and will probably become a common technique.

Preoperative assessment

Most children for elective surgery are fit and healthy. Infants with incarcerated hernias may have been vomiting and be dehydrated or present an aspiration risk. Opioid analgesia has often been given to facilitate an attempt at manual reduction of the hernia. Premature infants present a number of challenges (📖 Chapter 15). Of particular interest is the degree of prematurity, respiratory function, oxygen requirements, and other congenital anomalies or intercurrent disease such as patent ductus arteriosus. Parents of premature infants are advised about the incidence of postoperative apnoeas and the likelihood of postoperative IPPV being required.

Anaesthetic technique

- For elective cases in healthy children induction as requested.
- Spontaneous ventilation with a LMA is the norm. Infants may be intubated. Laparoscopic repair requires endotracheal intubation and IPPV.
- Maintenance with volatile in oxygen and air or nitrous oxide.
- For repair of incarcerated hernias in infants, endotracheal intubation with IPPV is the norm. These are good candidates for a caudal epidural block and a NSAID if not contraindicated.

- The options for inguinal hernia repair in premature infants:
  - General anaesthesia with endotracheal intubation and IPPV.
  - Subarachnoid block with 0.3–1 mg/kg 0.5% heavy bupivacaine (📖 Chapter 8). This reduces the risk of postoperative apnoeas. The main limitation of this technique is technical difficulty resulting in a failure rate and its short duration of action in the region of 60 min. Some neonatal hernias are surgically difficult and repair takes over 60 min. If a subarachnoid block is used then some form of postoperative analgesia such as wound infiltration must be provided.
  - Caudal epidural block.

Analgesia

- For most children an ilioinguinal block with 0.3–0.5 mL/kg 0.25% levobupivacaine or similar (📖 Chapter 7) is the regional technique of choice.
- Many anaesthetists also ask the surgeon to infiltrate the wound with LA.
- In infants, where the aponeurosis of external oblique is not well developed, it may be more effective for the surgeon to block the ilioinguinal nerve under direct vision.
- A caudal epidural block can be used children up to 20 kg bearing in mind that it must extend to T12 and needs 1 mL/kg of 0.25% levobupivacaine or similar (📖 Chapter 8).
- In some older children, especially if they are overweight, an ilioinguinal block is insufficient and a bolus of opioid (morphine sulphate 100–150 mcg/kg IV, codeine phosphate 0.5–1 mg/kg IM, fentanyl 2–4 mcg/kg IV) plus an antiemetic is required to provide adequate analgesia.
- A NSAID is usually given if there are no contraindications.

Postoperative care

After elective repair oral intake usually resumes very quickly. A combination of paracetamol, NSAID and an oral opioid are prescribed. If an ilioinguinal nerve block had been performed then the child should be assessed for the presence of a femoral nerve block (5%) before walking unaided. The child is discharged 2–4 hours postoperatively.

Patients are usually kept in hospital overnight after repair of an incarcerated hernia. There is more swelling, bruising and pain with higher analgesic requirements than after elective repair.

Ex-premature infants up to 48–60 weeks' postconceptual age (depending on hospital protocol) stay overnight and require monitoring with a pulse oximeter and apnoea monitor for 12 hours postoperatively.

Orchidopexy

- Incomplete descent of the testis from its fetal abdominal position to the scrotum is found at the age of 12 months in 1% of term boys and 5% of premature boys.
- Orchidopexy is performed for both undescended and ectopic (these deviate from the normal path of descent after emerging from the external inguinal ring) testes.
  - Undescended testes may be high in the scrotum, in the inguinal canal or intra-abdominal.
  - Ectopic testes may be in the superficial inguinal pouch, the perineum, root of the penis, or femoral canal. Unlike an incompletely descended testis, the ectopic one is usually well developed and histologically normal.
  - There is an incidence of anorchia (absent testis) where the vas deferens ends blindly at the internal inguinal ring.
- The indications for surgery are to preserve fertility, reduce the incidence of testicular trauma and torsion and aid detection of a testicular tumour.
  - Orchidopexy is ideally performed during the second year (although many are done later than this) and is a common day case procedure.
  - It usually involves an inguinal incision and small scrotal incision.
  - The testis is located, any associated inguinal hernial sac is tied off, the testicular vessels are dissected out to ↑ their length and the testis is secured in a subcutaneous pouch in the scrotum.
  - If there is no testis palpable on examination (20%), the boy may undergo laparoscopy to determine if it is intra-abdominal or absent.
  - If the testis is very high or intra-abdominal then a laparoscopically assisted orchidopexy or a two stage procedure may be used—an initial laparoscopy to identify the position of the testis and bring it down into the inguinal canal. Six months later a further procedure is performed to position the testis in the scrotum.
- The main risk of surgery is testicular atrophy due to impaired blood supply.

Preoperative assessment

Most boys are fit and healthy. Since an undescended testis is more common in ex-premature boys some patients will have residual features of this, notably bronchopulmonary dysplasia with irritable airways and poor venous access. Older boys may be very anxious about the proposed surgery.

Anaesthetic technique

- Sedative premedication if indicated or requested.
- IV or inhalational induction depending on the child, their veins, and parental views.
- Spontaneous respiration with a LMA is common.
- Maintenance is with volatile in oxygen and air or nitrous oxide.

Analgesia
- For unilateral surgery, an ilioinguinal block with infiltration of the scrotal wound by the surgeon is commonly used.
- For bilateral surgery, a caudal block may be more appropriate.
- The testes have a sympathetic innervation that reaches the CNS at about T10. For this reason even with a good block for the incision, traction on the testis can produce laryngospasm or a bradycardia mediated by the vagus nerve. Because of this some anaesthetists give a bolus of opioid (morphine sulphate 100–150 mcg/kg IV, codeine phosphate 0.5–1 mg/kg IM, fentanyl 2–4 mcg/kg IV) plus an antiemetic to boys undergoing orchidopexy. Others prefer to intubate younger boys.

Postoperative care

Most boys resume oral intake rapidly. Paracetamol, a NSAID and an oral opioid are prescribed. Discharge is usually 2–4 hours postoperatively. Boys over about 5 years of age find the operation more painful than toddlers and also have a significant incidence of PONV. Some of these will not be fit for discharge on the same day because of pain, PONV, or both and need to stay overnight.

Pyeloplasty and nephrectomy

- Pyeloplasty is performed to relieve pelviureteric junction (PUJ) obstruction. This is usually due to an aperistaltic segment of ureter, from which the normal musculature is absent. The condition is congenital and is often diagnosed antenatally by ultrasound.
- PUJ obstruction is usually unilateral and not associated with renal impairment.
- Classical pyeloplasty is an open procedure using either a lateral (flank) renal or subcostal incision. Transabdominal or posterior approaches are also possible.
- Nephrectomy or hemi-nephrectomy is performed to remove all or part of a non-functioning kidney. Underlying pathology includes a multicystic dysplastic kidney, congenital renal dysplasia, severe reflux nephropathy, severe obstructive uropathy and Wilm's tumour (nephroblastoma).
- Pyeloplasty and nephrectomy are increasingly being performed laparoscopically.

Preoperative assessment

Most children are healthy with no features of chronic renal disease or fluid and electrolyte disturbances. Some children have underlying conditions that affect the anaesthetic technique. These include spina bifida, renal artery stenosis, polycystic disease, Wilms' tumour, or chronic renal failure. Considerations include anaemia, hyperkalaemia, fluid overload, hypertension, intercurrent drug treatment, and venous access. Patients have often had symptoms and illness for months and may have undergone multiple investigations and imaging with or without anaesthesia.

Bleeding in not usually a problem with pyeloplasty or nephrectomy but is more of a risk with hemi-nephrectomy or in kidneys with a duplex system. It is a major consideration in removal of a Wilms' tumour (📖 Chapter 10) which may have invaded locally or extended into the IVC. These patients should be cross matched.

Anaesthetic technique

- Sedative premedication if requested or indicated.
- Endotracheal intubation and controlled ventilation are usually required.
- Two IV cannulae are sited.
- For lateral renal incisions, older children are placed in a lateral position with the table broken while a flank roll is used in babies to allow access to the kidney. The lateral renal incision does not split muscle and analgesic requirements are less than for more extensive procedures using a lower abdominal incision.
- Maintenance is with volatile in oxygen and air or nitrous oxide. This can be supplemented with an infusion of remifentanil (0.25–0.5 mcg/kg/minute) or a bolus of opioid such as morphine sulphate 100–150 mcg/kg or fentanyl citrate 2–4 mcg/kg.

- An antiemetic such as ondansetron 100 mcg/kg IV is given.
- Maintenance fluids are required and there may be a need for volume replacement with crystalloid, colloid or blood.
- Open procedures are very suitable for a combined general and regional anaesthetic technique. A lumbar epidural will provide intraoperative blockade because of spread of LA bolus but will be too low to provide effective postoperative infusion analgesia. If a postoperative epidural infusion is planned, then a low thoracic catheter is required.

Postoperative care

Maintenance fluids are required for 12–24 hours. Many children start drinking during the postoperative evening after a retroperitoneal approach to the kidney. This is also the case after a laparoscopic procedure. Options for analgesia after an open procedure include an IV infusion of morphine sulphate, PCA or an epidural infusion of local anaesthetic and opioid (⌨ Chapter 6). Paracetamol, a NSAID (if renal function is normal) and an antiemetic are also prescribed. Patients usually progress to oral analgesics on the first postoperative day unless there has been extensive surgery as in resection of a Wilms' tumour.

For laparoscopic procedures, the wounds are infiltrated with local anaesthetic. The choice for postoperative analgesia is between an IV morphine infusion and PCA for 12–24 hours or a combination of oral paracetamol, NSAID and opioid.

Laparoscopy

- Advantages over open procedures include improved cosmetic results, reduced postoperative pain, fewer wound complications, and quicker recovery.
- An open technique is used to insert the first trocar and subsequent trocars are placed under direct vision to avoid visceral or vascular injury.
- CO_2 is used to insufflate the peritoneum and provide a good visual field for surgery.
- CO_2 is used because of its inability to support combustion and its minimal effects in the event of intravascular embolization.
- The paediatric abdominal wall is more pliable than that of adults and adequate visualization of the intra-abdominal contents is possible at lower intra-abdominal pressures (IAP) than in adult laparoscopic surgery.
- Procedures may be prolonged.

Table 9.1 Indications for laparoscopy in children

Diagnostic laparoscopy	Therapeutic laparoscopy
Acute abdomen	Appendicectomy
Impalpable testes	Fundoplication
Recurrent abdominal pain	Orchidopexy
Blunt abdominal trauma	Splenectomy
Tumour staging, biopsy, etc	Pyloromyotomy
Intersex anomalies	Inguinal hernia repair
Malfunctioning V–P catheters	Nephrectomy and hemi-nephrectomy
	Pyeloplasty
	Cholecystectomy
	Oesophageal atresia (thoracoscopic)
	Pull through for Hirschsprung's
	Adhesionolysis
	Oophorectomy and ovarian cystectomy
	Adrenalectomy
	Varicocele
	Porto-enterostomy
	Congenital diaphragmatic hernia repair

- The physiological effects of a pneumoperitoneum are usually clinically benign.
  - Pneumoperitoneum results in ↑ IAP, a cephalad shift of the diaphragm, and a ↓ in FRC.
  - ↓ in the FRC relative to closing volume predisposes to atelectasis, ventilation–perfusion inequalities, and hypoxia. Pulmonary compliance also ↓ and airway resistance ↑.
  - Infants and neonates, who have a high closing volume and high oxygen consumption, are more prone to developing hypoxia.
  - The reduction in FRC may be exacerbated by the Trendelenberg position.
  - The reverse Trendelenberg position, used for upper abdominal procedures, may improve respiratory compliance.
  - Cardiovascular changes are related to the ↑ IAP, absorption of the insufflating CO_2, patient positioning, and underlying cardiovascular status.
  - When intra-abdominal pressures are less than right atrial pressure (<10 mmHg) compression of the splanchnic vasculature ↑ venous return to the heart with an ↑ in cardiac output.
  - When IAP >15 mmHg, inferior vena caval compression reduces venous return and thus cardiac output. This effect is potentiated by hypovolaemia and the head up position.
  - Systemic vascular resistance (SVR) is ↑ by aortic compression and hypercarbia.
  - Provided the insufflating pressure is <12 mmHg any cardiorespiratory changes that do occur are usually within acceptable values.
  - Effects on ICP are complex. ↑ in ICP during laparoscopy have been reported in patients with ventriculo–peritoneal shunts despite a low IAP and a normal arterial pCO_2. Hypercapnia ↑ cerebral blood flow and may ↑ ICP, which is further ↑ in the head down position. An ↑ in IAP also tends to ↑ ICP. When these changes are combined with a fall in cardiac output and a rise in intrathoracic pressure, the possibility of a reduction in cerebral perfusion pressure exists.

Preoperative assessment

The scenario may vary from an elective procedure in a healthy child to an emergency laparoscopy to evaluate an acute abdomen in a premature neonate. History and examination to evaluate the patient's preoperative clinical status with investigations as appropriate. Assessment of co-morbidities e.g. sickle cell disease in child presenting with gallstones for cholecystectomy, cerebral palsy in a child for laparoscopic fundoplication. Blood is usually grouped and saved for major laparoscopic procedures.

Anaesthetic technique

- Premedication with an anticholinergic agent (glycopyrronium bromide 100 mcg/kg orally or atropine 40 mcg/kg orally) 60–90 min preoperatively may be used to prevent bradycardia associated with abdominal insufflation or manipulation of the viscera. Alternatively, these can be given intra-venously as and if required.
- Standard IV or inhalation techniques are used, including a rapid sequence induction when appropriate.
- Endotracheal intubation with controlled ventilation is usual for paediatric laparoscopy.
- Where possible, a cuffed tube is preferable. For uncuffed tubes, a size which allows only a minimal leak at 20 cmH$_2$O inspiratory pressure should be used in order to maintain adequate ventilation when peak inspiratory pressure (PIP) ↑ with abdominal insufflation.
- Due to the potential for respiratory changes exhaled tidal volume and PIP are monitored during insufflation.
- Hypoxia is usually overcome with supplemental oxygen and moderate PEEP.
- The risk of endobronchial intubation is ↑ by elevation of the diaphragm caused by ↑ IAP and the head down position, moving the carina cephalad. This should be suspected if there is an ↑ in airway pressure and a fall in SpO$_2$ at the time of insufflation or patient positioning.
- A nasogastric tube is often used to decompress the stomach in order to improve visualization of the abdominal contents and limit the potential for inadvertent damage during trocar placement.
- Nitrous oxide is avoided because of the potential for bowel distension, which may result in PONV or may make a surgical approach more difficult. Nitrous oxide can also ↑ the size of gas bubbles in the event of an air embolus.
- An infusion of remifentanil (0.25–0.5 mcg/kg/minute) is often used as an alternative to nitrous oxide to blunt the haemodynamic response to a pneumoperitoneum.
- For analgesia a multimodal approach is crucial and begins with pre-emptive infiltration of the trocar insertion sites with LA. Provided there are no contraindications, IV or rectal paracetamol and rectal diclofenac are also given before or after the procedure. With the use of remifentanil infusions, longer acting opioids, typically morphine sulphate 100–150 mcg/kg IV can be given towards the end of the procedure to ensure adequate analgesia in the early postoperative period. Neurologically or respiratory compromised patients should have opioids titrated once adequate spontaneous respiration is established. Prophylactic antiemetic agents are usually given.
- Environmental lighting may be suboptimal and space and access is at a premium.

Postoperative care

Following completion of the procedure CO_2 is evacuated from the peritoneal cavity to limit problems with postoperative pain, PONV, and diaphragmatic splinting. Early postoperative pain may be severe but analgesic consumption usually ↓ dramatically over 24 hours. For many procedures, a combination of oral paracetamol, NSAID, and opioid for 24–48 hours provides adequate analgesia. For major procedures or for abdominal surgery associated with peritonism and a postoperative ileus an IV infusion of morphine sulphate or PCA (📖 Chapter 6) rather than oral opioids are usually required for 12–24 hours. Maintenance fluids will also be required for these cases.

Fundoplication

- Failure of the lower oesophageal sphincter mechanism results in gastro-oesophageal reflux (GOR). This is normal during the first year of life before the sphincter mechanism is fully developed. When it occurs later and causes symptoms, treatment is required. Symptoms include vomiting, dysphagia, failure to thrive, apnoea, chronic cough, recurrent chest infections, and stridor.
- GOR is a common problem in children with muscular incoordination as in cerebral palsy or severe developmental delay.
- Diagnosis is based on the history and investigations including barium swallow, upper gastrointestinal endoscopy with biopsies, and oesophageal pH probe testing.
- Initial treatment for physiological reflux in infants and mild reflux in older children includes upright positioning, feed thickeners, prokinetic agents, and antacid drugs. Surgical treatment is indicated for failed medical treatment or to avoid the need for indefinite drug therapy.
- Fundoplication is the usual surgical procedure and has a success rate of 80–90%. The Nissen fundoplication with a 360° wrap is the commonest.
- Fundoplication usually improves respiratory symptoms related to GOR.
- Surgical options include an open procedure through an upper abdominal incision or a laparoscopic approach.

Preoperative assessment

Most children for fundoplication have severe cerebral palsy and many of the issues that go with this (📖 Chapter 15) including reflux with or without aspiration, ineffective upper airway reflexes, recurrent respiratory infections, epilepsy, contractures, poor nutrition, chronic anaemia, and poor venous access. When possible, preoperative drugs are continued during the perioperative period including anticonvulsants, prokinetic and antacid drugs. Many children salivate excessively and find it difficult to swallow saliva. They may have a hyoscine (anticholinergic) patch behind an ear.

Respiratory function is assessed and optimized with chest physiotherapy and bronchodilators if appropriate.

A preoperative FBC and U&E are often indicated since poor nutrition is common and gastric bleeding may have occurred. A sample is often sent for group and save. These samples may be omitted in stable patients undergoing a laparoscopic procedure by an experienced surgeon, not least because of the difficulty and distress involved in obtaining the samples from many children.

If the patient is to undergo an open procedure then the postoperative analgesic technique and the likelihood of postoperative IPPV are discussed with the parent/s. In most cases, a thoracic epidural infusion is the analgesic technique of choice. This reduces the requirement for admission to ITU and postoperative IPPV (from 15–20% to 5–10%) but in very impaired children, this is still a likely part of the postoperative course. It is very infrequent for a child to need ITU admission and IPPV after a laparoscopic fundoplication.

Anaesthetic technique

- Premedication can be prescribed for various reasons in this population—sedative, antisialogogue, antacid, or prokinetic.
- A rapid sequence induction is often considered because of the presence of gastric reflux but in many cases the practical difficulties of obtaining IV access, preoxygenation, and the frailty of many patients makes this impractical.
- If veins are easily accessible then an IV induction may be appropriate. In many cases, an inhalational induction is unavoidable and venous cannulation is performed in the anaesthetized patient.
- The patient is paralysed and endotracheal intubation is performed with or without cricoid pressure.
- Venous access if often a significant problem. Patients undergoing an open procedure will require this for 3–5 days and a central line is often inserted. The requirement for venous access is shorter after laparoscopic procedures and most patients resume oral intake the day after surgery.

- Maintenance is with volatile in oxygen and air or nitrous oxide. Nitrous oxide is not used during laparoscopic procedures. An infusion of remifentanil (0.25–0.5 mcg/kg/min) helps to reduce volatile requirements and provide cardiovascular stability. Alternatives are morphine sulphate 100–150 mcg/kg or fentanyl citrate 2–4 mcg/kg repeated if necessary. An antiemetic such as ondansetron 100 mcg/kg (max 4mg) IV reduces the likelihood of the child retching against the fundoplication in the early postoperative period.
- Precautions are taken to avoid strain on joint contractures, protect pressure areas and to avoid damage to fragile skin. Pressure areas need adequate padding.
- Children with cerebral palsy are particularly prone to hypothermia during surgery and a warming mattress and Bair Hugger® are used.
- If the child is to receive an epidural, this is best placed in the mid-thoracic region to provide optimal blockade of mid-thoracic dermatomes. There is a significant incidence of scoliosis in the cerebral palsy population and, in some cases, the epidural space cannot be reliably identified.
- Surgical stimulation during a laparoscopic fundoplication is low for most of the time except for the initial incisions, dissection of the crura, and passage of oesophageal bougies (if used by the surgeon). This combined with the head up position may cause hypotension needing a reduction in volatile agent or remifentanil or a bolus of IV fluid.

Postoperative care

Maintenance fluids are required. Blood samples for FBC and U&E are usually sent after open procedures. Anticonvulsant drugs are restarted as soon as possible.

Open fundoplication is associated with significant postoperative analgesic requirements for 2–4 days and a requirement for care in a high dependency or intensive care unit. Thoracic epidural analgesia (Ⓛ Chapter 6) provides effective analgesia for open procedures, preserves respiratory function, avoids over sedation, and allows effective chest physiotherapy. IV infusions of morphine sulphate are effective but large doses are required for several days and many patients become over sedated or suffer respiratory depression especially those with pre-existing neurological or respiratory disease. Paracetamol, NSAID (if no contra-indications) and an antiemetic are also prescribed.

The laparoscopic approach is associated with greatly reduced analgesic requirements and a shorter hospital stay. With infiltration of the incisions with LA, most children require an IV infusion of morphine sulphate (Ⓛ Chapter 6) for 12–24 hours plus paracetamol, NSAID, and an antiemetic. Alternatively, regular oral opioid may be prescribed rather than an intravenous infusion. They usually restart oral intake on the first postoperative day. Patients are usually cared for on a general surgical ward.

Ear, nose, and throat surgery

Considerations in paediatric ENT surgery

- The shared airway requires excellent communication between surgeon and anaesthetist.
- The anaesthetist is often remote from the airway.
- Many procedures are suitable as day cases.
- Large numbers of paediatric ENT procedures are performed, mostly in general hospitals rather than paediatric centres.
- Requires sound knowledge of anatomy, physiology, and pathology of the paediatric airway.
- Requires awareness of unusual conditions or syndromes associated with airway and intubation difficulties.

Myringotomy and grommets

- One of the commonest paediatric operations in the UK.
- Myringotomy refers to an incision in the tympanic membrane and suction of the middle ear secretions. This may be combined with placement of grommets (tympanostomy tubes).
- Used for treatment of recurrent otitis media and persistent middle ear effusions.
- Most commonly performed in infants and toddlers.
- Usually a short procedure in the supine position with the head turned to the side.
- Usually bilateral.
- An operating microscope is used and the magnified field of view requires an immobile patient.
- Most procedures are performed as day cases.

Preoperative assessment

There is a high incidence of respiratory symptoms in this patient group. In most cases the procedure goes ahead but there is an incidence of laryngospasm and hypoxia associated with it. A significant minority of patient have an underlying congenital condition notably Down's syndrome (☐ Chapter 15) that may present additional considerations.

Anaesthetic technique

- Method of induction as indicated or requested. There is a high incidence of inhalational induction because of the age of patients and difficult venous access.
- Airway management is with a face mask or LMA.
- Anaesthesia is maintained with volatile agent in oxygen and air or nitrous oxide.
- Spontaneous ventilation is the norm.

Postoperative care

Postoperative pain is unpredictable and variable ranging from no apparent distress to a howling, inconsolable child. Pain mainly results from trauma to the external auditory meatus and possibly acute pressure changes in the middle ear. Simple analgesics such as paracetamol and NSAIDS are sufficient. Some anaesthetists premedicate with analgesics—paracetamol or ibuprofen.

Tonsillectomy

- A common paediatric operation with two main indications:
  - Recurrent throat infections.
  - Adenotonsillar hypertrophy with upper airway obstruction with or without obstructive sleep apnoea (OSA).
- Patients with upper airway obstruction are generally younger than those undergoing surgery for recurrent infection.
- Preexisting condition may predispose to upper airway obstruction:
  - Congenital or acquired craniofacial abnormalities e.g. Pierre Robin, Treacher Collins, Down's syndrome
  - Neuromuscular disease e.g. cerebral palsy.
- Often combined with adenoidectomy. Adenoidectomy may be carried out as a sole procedure or, commonly, combined with insertion of grommets. Anaesthetic considerations are similar to those for tonsillectomy.
- Surgical technique:
  - Supine with the neck in extension—a small or moderate leak around the ETT can become a large leak with the neck extended
  - The mouth gag can cause obstruction, kinking or displacement of the ETT.

Preoperative assessment

Upper respiratory symptoms are common in this group and are not necessarily a contraindication to anaesthesia and surgery if the child is apyrexial and there are no chest signs on auscultation (📖 Chapter 3). Often due to adenoidal hypertrophy.

Children referred with OSA have a history of an abnormal sleep pattern with restlessness, snoring, and apnoeic pauses. These children may fail to thrive and develop facial abnormalities. Sleep studies show the frequency and duration of apnoeas and associated ↓ in arterial oxygen saturation. In severe chronic OSA, chronic hypoxia can result in pulmonary hypertension, cor pulmonale, and right heart strain (identified on an ECG). Obstructive symptoms do not resolve immediately after surgery. Children with OSA are at risk of postoperative apnoeas and hypoxia. Severe cases may require supplemental oxygen, a nasopharyngeal airway, and nasal CPAP, or intubation and admission to an ITU.

Anaesthetic technique

- In patients with OSA, sedative premedication should be avoided and opioids used cautiously. Other patients are premedicated as required.
- During induction (inhalational or IV) airway obstruction is possible. Usually alleviated with CPAP or insertion of an oral airway when depth of anaesthesia is sufficient.
- The airway must be secure and protected from soiling by blood and debris.

- Preformed 'south facing' RAE ETTs are the commonest for this operation, placed in the midline with the aid of a short acting muscle relaxant.
- Reinforced or armoured LMAs can be used in preference to an ETT. Use of the LMA makes positioning the mouth gag more difficult and requires particular care from the surgeon. Common problems include laryngospasm or obstruction during placement of the gag. The LMA is not usually suitable for children <3 years of age.
- In the UK, all surgical or anaesthetic airway equipment used in adenoidectomy or tonsillectomy is now disposable, single use only because of concern about transmission of prion diseases.
- Spontaneous ventilation or IPPV are both suitable with volatile agent in oxygen and air or oxygen and nitrous oxide.
- Multimodal analgesia includes a combination of paracetamol and opioids (codeine phosphate 0.5–1 mg/kg IM, morphine sulphate 100–150 mcg/kg IV, fentanyl citrate 1–2 mcg/kg IV). The use of NSAIDs is common in most UK hospitals despite concern about their effects on haemostasis.
- Antiemetics (ondansetron 100 mcg/kg (max 4mg) IV and/or dexamethasone 150 mcg/kg IV) are given. A bolus of IV fluid is commonly given to help reduce the incidence of PONV.
- Extubation is either 'deep' or 'awake' depending on preference although an awake extubation is safest for children with OSA.
- Patients are recovered in the head down lateral position.

Postoperative care

Oral intake usually resumes in the early postoperative period. A combination of paracetamol 15 mg/kg oral 4-hourly, ibuprofen 10 mg/kg oral 6-hourly, and codeine phosphate 1 mg/kg oral 4-hourly is commonly prescribed for postoperative analgesia. Most patients in the UK currently stay in hospital overnight. Day case tonsillectomy is, however, becoming more common and requires careful patient selection, meticulous surgical technique, and strict patient observation for haemorrhage in the immediate postoperative period. Overnight observation is recommended for patients:

- <2–3 years of age
- With OSA
- With craniofacial abnormalities
- With failure to thrive or significant obesity
- With hypotonia
- With chronic medical problems.

Examples of protocols for dealing with these issues in tonsillectomy are shown overleaf.

Summary of anaesthetic guidelines for 'day stay tonsillectomy' at The Children's Hospital at Westmead, Sydney

Patients
- 5 years of age or older.
- No significant history of respiratory obstruction.
- Indication for surgery: recurrent tonsillitis.
- Systemically well (ASA class I or II).
- No intercurrent illness.

Family
- 30 minutes road access to a hospital.
- Able to communicate with a good understanding in English.

Management
- Preoperative assessment and explanation of the procedure, approximately 1 week prior to surgery, if possible.
- Appropriate fasting.
- Preoperative paracetamol.
- General anaesthetic according to anaesthetist.
- IV narcotic.
- Prophylactic antiemetic regime—dexamethasone/ondansetron.
- Intraoperative IV fluids (Hartmann's solution approximately 20 mL per kg).
- 6 hour postoperative stay with ½ hourly pulse and respiratory rate for 4 hours then hourly for 2 hours.
- Blood pressure recorded hourly for 2 hours.
- Pulse oximetry until patient awake with hemodynamic and oximetry readings within normal ranges.
- Postoperative pain relief—paracetamol 15 mg/kg given every 4 hours while awake, codeine 0.5 mg/kg 4–6-hourly as required.

Summary of anaesthetic guidelines for 'adenotonsillectomy in children with OSA' at The Children's Hospital at Westmead, Sydney

Definitions:

Moderate or severe OSA includes at least two of:
- Hourly apnoeas 10–20 or more.
- Minimum saturations below 90%.
- Transcutaneous carbon dioxide ($TcCO_2$) measurements elevated 10–15 mmHg or more.

Recommendations for the postoperative care of these patients:

- Patients requiring postoperative endotracheal intubation will be admitted to an intensive care bed.
- The following will be admitted to a high dependency bed:
  - Patients with syndromes potentially affecting the airway (e.g. Downs, Treacher Collins, Pierre Robin) and moderate or severe OSA.
  - Patients requiring an artificial airway such as a nasopharyngeal airway.
  - Patients aged ≤12 months.
  - Patients with marked obesity or malnourishment (body mass index (BMI) more than or less than two standard deviations from the mean) and moderate or severe OSA.
- Patients without a recognized syndrome affecting the airway but with a diagnosis of moderate or severe OSA, will be admitted to a high acuity monitored bed in the ward.
- Patients with mild OSA will be admitted to a general ward bed, with the ability to monitor the patient as required.

Middle ear surgery

- Mostly mastoidectomy and tympanoplasty
- Mastoidectomy is performed to remove infected air cells within the mastoid bone usually caused by cholesteatoma. Cholesteatoma arises from migration of squamous epithelium in to the middle ear and comprises keratinizing squamous epithelium and accumulated desquamated epithelium that accumulates in the middle ear as a result of chronic middle ear infection. It erodes middle ear structures and remains a source of ongoing infection.
- This procedure is now relatively unusual because of the widespread use of antibiotics.
- Several surgical procedures may be performed:
  - Simple (or partial). The operation is performed through the ear or through an incision behind the ear. The surgeon opens the mastoid bone and removes the infected air cells. The eardrum is incised to drain the middle ear.
  - Radical mastoidectomy. The eardrum and most middle ear structures are removed, but the innermost small bone (the stapes) is left behind so that a hearing aid can be used later to offset the hearing loss.
  - Modified radical mastoidectomy. The eardrum and the middle ear structures are saved, which allows for better hearing than is possible after a radical operation. The wound is stitched around a drain, which is removed a day or two later.
- Tympanoplasty is performed to repair a persistent perforation in the tympanic membrane. A graft of temporalis fascia is usually taken and used to repair the defect.

Preoperative assessment

Patients are usually older children and generally healthy. They will often have had many anaesthetics and may be anxious. PONV is a potentially significant problem and requires a multimodal approach.

Anaesthetic technique

- Sedative premedication if indicated or requested.
- Induction as indicated or requested by patient or parents.
- Endotracheal intubation with spontaneous ventilation or IPPV.
- Maintenance with volatile in oxygen and air.
- Nitrous oxide is usually avoided. There is a high incidence of PONV after these procedures and it is contraindicated during tympanoplasty because of potential pressure changes in the middle ear during and after surgery.
- A 15–20° head up position and mild hypotension are usually used.

- A remifentanil infusion helps provide good operating conditions by providing moderate hypotension. It also reduces volatile requirements and avoids the need for relaxant. If function of the facial nerve during surgery is to be monitored (nerve stimulator or electromyography), then neuromuscular blockers are avoided (endotracheal intubation is aided by a short acting relaxant or remifentanil).
- TIVA is appropriate in older patients.
- Maintenance fluids and prophylactic antiemetic e.g. ondansetron 100 mcg/kg (max 4mg) IV.
- The surgeon usually infiltrates LA and adrenaline superficially to produce vasoconstriction.
- Morphine sulphate 100–150 mcg/kg IV to provide analgesia and sedation in the early postoperative period.

Postoperative care

A combination of paracetamol 15 mg/kg oral 4-hourly, ibuprofen 10 mg/kg oral 6-hourly, and an oral opioid—codeine phosphate 1 mg/kg oral 4-hourly or morphine sulphate 200–300 mcg/kg oral 4-hourly—is prescribed along with an antiemetic. IV maintenance fluids are required until oral intake is resumed.

Bronchoscopy

- Indications for bronchoscopy fall into two groups:

Diagnostic	Therapeutic
Recurrent pneumonia	Foreign body removal
Tracheo-oesophageal fistula	Mucus plugs e.g. cystic fibrosis
Airway obstruction	Lobar collapse
Laryngomalacia	Refractory atelectasis
Haemoptysis	Balloon dilatation
To obtain biopsy or brushings	Stent insertion
Failure to wean from ventilator	Laser treatment

- Most patients have some degree of respiratory compromise.
- Signs and symptoms include stridor, wheeze, hoarseness, recurrent infection, cyanosis, persistent cough, dyspnoea, and tachypnoea.
- Rigid or flexible bronchoscope:
  - The Storz ventilating bronchoscope is the most common rigid bronchoscope used in paediatrics.
  - Consists of a metal tube with a removable optical telescope.
  - Holes in the wall allow ventilation of the contralateral lung when the distal end of the bronchoscope is positioned in a bronchus (Fig 9.1).
  - The side arm has a 15 mm attachment for an anaesthetic T-piece circuit (Fig 9.2).
  - Ventilation occurs between the lumen of the bronchoscope and the outer surface of the telescope.
  - The telescope occupies most of the internal diameter of smaller bronchoscopes and impedes ventilation in infants.
  - With the telescope in place, a closed system exists and allows controlled ventilation but the cross sectional area of lumen through which the infant can breathe is reduced.
  - Using too large a bronchoscope leads to compression of tracheal mucosa and postoperative oedema with the risk of stridor.
  - Venturi bronchoscopes are commonly used in adults but in paediatrics should be limited to patients weighing >40 kg because of the risk of barotrauma. Ventilation occurs via jet insufflation with oxygen and entrained air using a Sanders injector. Anaesthesia is maintained with IV agents. CO_2 retention is a greater problem with this method.
  - Fibreoptic bronchoscopes have a greater field of vision than rigid scopes and their smaller diameter allows access to the distal airways.
- The smallest diameter of fibreoptic bronchoscope in general use has an ED 1.8 mm distally and 2.2 mm proximally.

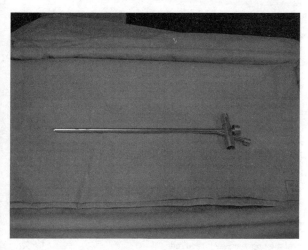

Fig. 9.1 Storz rigid ventilating bronchoscope. Note distal side holes for ventilation of the contralateral lung.

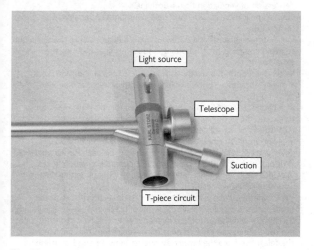

Fig. 9.2 Storz bronchoscope. Close up of proximal end.

Previous anaesthetic charts provide useful information regarding laryngo-scopy, airway obstruction, size of ETT and any difficulties encountered.

Careful history and examination focusing on airway and respiratory system e.g. how do symptoms change with position, crying, and feeding.

Specific investigations may be indicated e.g. CXR for suspected foreign body aspiration, CT for lower airway obstruction.

Anaesthetic technique

Rigid bronchoscopy

- Avoid sedative premedication if there is evidence of airway obstruction or respiratory compromise.
- An anticholinergic (atropine 10–20 mcg/kg or glycopyrronium bromide 5–10 mcg/kg) is usually given intravenously at induction for an antisia-logogue effect and to prevent bradycardia from airway manipulation.
- Spontaneous ventilation is maintained in children with possible airway obstruction and in diagnostic procedures where functional assessment of the upper airway is required.
- Inhalational induction with sevoflurane or halothane in 100% oxygen. Sevoflurane provides a more rapid induction but causes more depression of ventilation than halothane.
- Gentle application of CPAP will help overcome upper airway obstruction.
- Dense topical anaesthesia of the larynx is fundamental to the technique to avoid coughing, breath holding, and laryngospasm during the examination.
- When the depth of anaesthesia is adequate topical lidocaine (up to 4 mg/kg) should be sprayed on the epiglottis, larynx, and between the vocal cords.
- The patient is positioned supine with a support beneath the scapulae to extend the neck and push the trachea anteriorly.
- Anaesthesia is maintained with volatile in 100% oxygen given from a T-piece circuit attached to the side port of the bronchoscope. Alternatively, total IV anaesthesia (TIVA) can be used for maintenance. Propofol with or without remifentanil suppresses airway reflexes, provides rapid emergence, and ↓ pollution of the operating theatre atmosphere with anaesthetic agents.
- When the telescope is introduced, the cross sectional area of the bronchoscope is reduced and the work of breathing may be significantly ↑. This is a significant problem in infants where narrow bronchoscopes are used. Adequate gas exchange may require intermittent removal of the telescope from the bronchoscope to allow a period of uninter-rupted ventilation.
- If assisted ventilation is used a long time constant may be needed to avoid air trapping.
- Dexamethasone (250 mcg/kg IV) may be given to reduce postoperative airway oedema.

Fibreoptic bronchoscopy

- Generally as for rigid bronchoscopy.
- The method of airway management depends on the indications for the examination. If laryngomalacia is possible then a facemask (fitted with an angle piece modified for passage of a bronchoscope) with spontaneous ventilation is required to allow examination of the larynx during normal breathing. Under these circumstances, an LMA will distort the larynx and may impede movement of the vocal cords. Examination of the trachea can be done through an LMA. Examination of the bronchial tree and/or broncho-alveolar lavage allows the use of an ETT if indicated.
- When a facemask or LMA is used, spontaneous ventilation is maintained and CPAP used to aid management of airway obstruction. The endoscopist may want to examine the airway with and without CPAP to assess it effects as in tracheomalacia.
- An appropriately sized LMA allows the passage of a larger fibrescope than with a tracheal tube.
- If a spontaneous ventilation technique is used then LA is applied to the larynx via the injection port of the fiberscope to provide topical anaesthesia before the fibrescope passes through the larynx.

Postoperative care

Oral paracetamol and possibly a NSAID will provide adequate analgesia. IV fluids and antibiotics may be indicated depending on the situation. Patients should remain nil by mouth for 2 hours after topical anaesthesia to the larynx. Further doses of steroid and nebulized adrenaline may be necessary if the patient has postoperative stridor. Patients require arterial oxygen saturation monitoring for at least 2 hours to detect hypoxia secondary to hypoventilation. Temperature is measured in case of pyrexia secondary to bacteraemia from the investigation.

Microlaryngeal surgery

- Indicated for laryngeal papillomatosis and congenital or acquired anatomical laryngeal lesions such as laryngomalacia and laryngeal web.
- Performed using a suspension laryngoscope and operating microscope.
- Patients often present for repeated procedures and may have significant airway obstruction.
- Many have a tracheostomy.
- Similar anaesthetic principles apply as for bronchoscopy.
- Spontaneous ventilation with volatile agent in oxygen and topical anaesthesia is a common technique.
- Often involves laser surgery to the airway and the relevant precautions that go with this.
- Camera and video display allow the anaesthetist to observe the airway and surgical field.

Preoperative assessment

Many patients present with significant obstructive symptoms especially from recurrent papillomatosis and may develop total airway obstruction after induction of anaesthesia.

Anaesthetic technique

- If the child has a tracheostomy then a standard anaesthetic technique is used with induction as requested by the child. The tracheostomy is connected to the anaesthetic circuit and spontaneous ventilation or IPPV used.
- If there is no tracheostomy then sedative premedication is avoided.
- An inhalational induction with sevoflurane or halothane in 100% oxygen is performed.
- The larynx is sprayed with lidocaine (up to 4 mg/kg) to ensure dense topical analgesia.
- Options for maintenance include:
  - Endotracheal intubation and IPPV. A narrow ETT is used to allow visualization of the larynx. However, the view of the larynx is impaired and other techniques are often preferred.
  - Spontaneous ventilation of volatile in oxygen through an ETT (placed through the nose or via dedicated channel in the suspension laryngoscope) with the distal end in the oropharynx above the laryngeal inlet so as not to obscure the surgical field.
  - Apneoic insufflation where the child is paralysed and volatile and oxygen insufflated through an ETT placed as above. Arterial CO_2 rises during apnoea and during prolonged procedures surgery is interrupted to allow a period of IPPV. There is also pollution of the operating theatre atmosphere with volatile agent.
  - A propofol infusion can be used to supplement anaesthesia, ensure lack of awareness, and reduce pollution.
  - Jet ventilation combined with TIVA in a paralysed patient. This has a risk of barotrauma.

Postoperative care

Oral paracetamol and possibly a NSAID will provide adequate analgesia. IV fluids and antibiotics may be indicated depending on the situation. Patients should remain nil by mouth for 2 hours after topical anaesthesia to the larynx. Further does of steroid and nebulized adrenaline may be necessary if the patient has postoperative stridor. Patients require arterial oxygen saturation monitoring for at least 2 hours to detect hypoxia secondary to hypoventilation.

Orthopaedic surgery

Considerations in paediatric orthopaedic surgery

- The majority of children are well with an isolated orthopaedic condition but some orthopaedic conditions are associated with syndromes and neuromuscular disorders.
- For many conditions, repeated general anaesthetics will be necessary for a mixture of surgical procedures, plaster application, plaster changes and removal of metalwork.
- Tourniquets are commonly used and awareness of the issues they raise is important.
- Scoliosis surgery is extensive with an emphasis on proper patient positioning, controlled haemodynamics, and intraoperative neurophysiological monitoring.
- Many procedures are suitable for regional anaesthetic techniques.

Developmental (congenital) dislocation of the hip (DDH)

- This term refers to a dislocated or dislocatable (unstable) hip at birth. About 1.5% of children have unstable hips at birth but only about 1 in 400 children (UK) require treatment. A small number of children have an irreducible fixed dislocation at birth called a teratologic dislocation.
- 4–5 times more common in girls than boys, after breech delivery and in those with a family history. The left hip is affected most commonly. Variable incidence in different parts of the world.
- Ideally, this condition is detected in the neonatal period by screening (Ortolani and Barlow tests). In the UK, ultrasound is used only in children with risk factors although it is routine in some countries.
- Sadly, late presentation is relatively common and classically occurs around 1 year of age soon after the child starts walking with a painless limp and leg shortening or occasionally later still.
- Infants usually spend some time in Pavlik harness or gallows traction before undergoing an arthrogram and closed reduction under general anaesthesia. The hip is manipulated in to a reduced position with the femoral head congruous with the acetabulum. This is often combined with a percutaneous adductor tenotomy. A lower body plaster cast (hip spica) is applied. Depending on local practice the spica is changed (under general anaesthesia) at roughly monthly intervals for a period of 2–3 months.
- Older children will often require an open reduction of the hip (usually through a groin incision) followed by a series of hip spicas. A proportion of these children will require further surgery including pelvic and/or femoral osteotomy.
- Children who present at 3–4 years may undergo open reduction combined with femoral shortening (osteotomy) and internal fixation through a lateral thigh incision or a pelvic osteotomy.
- The most feared surgical complication is avascular necrosis of the hip.

Preoperative assessment

There may be other congenital anomalies that are relevant to anaesthesia. In many cases, the child is starting a series of procedures that will all require general anaesthesia and it is important to establish a rapport with the parents. Preoperative blood tests are rarely required unless there is an associated disease and blood transfusion is not likely unless associated pelvic or femoral surgery is anticipated.

Anaesthetic technique

Arthrogram and closed reduction of dislocated hip

- This is normally performed in infants detected by the screening programme and takes about an hour.
- An inhalational induction is the norm. Venous access is usually difficult and, since this must be restricted to the upper limbs, the chances of success are higher in an anaesthetized patient.

- Analgesia is not usually necessary unless an adductor tenotomy is performed when LA can be infiltrated at the operative site.
- If the hip cannot be reduced manually and an open reduction becomes necessary then either a bolus of morphine sulphate (100 mcg/kg IV is given or a caudal epidural injection (1 mL/kg 0.25% levobupivacaine) performed before the operation starts.

Open reduction of dislocated hip
- Usually performed in older children.
- Premedication is helpful since the child will attend for repeated anaesthetics and anything to reduce the distress associated with this is useful.
- Induction as indicated bearing in mind that venous access must be in the upper body. A number of patients require an internal jugular line because a cannula cannot be sited in the hands or arms. There is morbidity from this and, for this reason, unless the venous access is easy it may be preferable to use an inhalational induction and attempt venous cannulation under optimal conditions in the anaesthetized child.
- Endotracheal intubation and IPPV are the norm. In older children, an LMA and spontaneous ventilation combined with an epidural can be used. Maintenance is with volatile in oxygen and nitrous oxide or air. The addition of a remifentanil infusion reduces volatile requirements.
- An epidural technique is commonly used for analgesia. In children up to 10–15 kg, a caudal epidural injection (1 mL/kg of 0.25 levobupivacaine or equivalent) will block the inguinal dermatomes. In older children, a lumbar epidural is preferable (0.3–0.5 mL/kg 0.5% levobupivacaine or equivalent will provide a dense block) (📖 Chapter 8). This is combined with a NSAID and an opioid (morphine sulphate 100 mcg/kg).
- If an epidural catheter is left *in situ* some centres fashion a window in the back of the hip spica to allow access.

Change of hip spica
- Usually performed as a day case. This involves removing the current hip spica, washing the lower body, application of another spica, and a check pelvic radiograph to ensure that the hip remains reduced. The whole procedure takes 40–60 min.
- Sedative premedication should be considered if repeated anaesthetics are distressing the child.
- Induction as indicated.
- Endotracheal intubation and IPPV is the norm in infants. In older children an LMA and spontaneous ventilation is appropriate.
- There are several changes in patient position during this procedure so close attention to the security of the ETT or LMA and IV cannula is required.
- The child is exposed during this procedure and small infants can become hypothermic. The operating theatre temperature should be raised and patient temperature should be monitored.
- Analgesia is not usually required.

Postoperative care

Closed reduction

Oral intake usually resumes immediately. Paracetamol and an NSAID are prescribed for initial discomfort in the spica. If the child vomits, the hip spica may be compressing the abdomen and a window may need to be cut over the abdomen.

Open reduction

IV fluids are required until oral intake resumes. Options for postoperative analgesia are an epidural infusion (📖 Chapter 6), an IV morphine infusion (📖 Chapter 6) or oral opioid (morphine sulphate 200–300 mcg/kg 4-hourly or codeine phosphate 1 mg/kg 4-hourly) on a regular or as required basis. Paracetamol and an NSAID are also prescribed.

Congenital talipes equinovarus (clubfoot)

- This is one of the most common congenital orthopaedic abnormalities requiring surgery in infancy.
- Incidence is 1–3:1000 live births in the UK; 50% are bilateral and the male: female ratio is 2.5:1.
- The majority of children are healthy although neuromuscular disorders or other conditions such as arthrogryposis or cerebral palsy may be present. Minor abnormalities of the lower spine are relatively common in association with this condition.
- The condition comprises a mixture of bony abnormalities, joint deformity, subluxation within the foot, and muscle imbalance between the plantar flexion/inversion group and the dorsiflexion/eversion group. The result is adduction of the forefoot, varus, and equinus of the hind foot. The aim of treatment is to obtain a plantigrade foot with reasonable shape and function.
- Conservative treatment using strapping or serial plasters is adequate in 30–50% of cases depending on the criteria used to define successful outcome.
- For the remainder, corrective surgery and repeated changes of plaster with manipulation is undertaken before the child begins to walk. The primary operation is usually performed between 3–9 months of age and varies from a limited medial soft tissue release through extensive posterior and medial tendon lengthening to bony surgery with or without K-wire fixation.
- Further procedures (tendon transfers and osteotomies) are required later in childhood in about 25% of cases.
- Primary surgery usually takes about an hour for each foot and is performed in the supine or prone position depending on the surgical approach and technique.

Preoperative assessment

Particular attention should be paid to the possibility of a lower spine abnormality if caudal epidural blockade is planned. There may be a congenital neuromuscular disease that is relevant to anaesthesia.

Anaesthetic technique

- An inhalational induction is usual in infants. In older children undergoing secondary surgery sedative premedication should be considered and induction performed as indicated or requested.
- IV access is placed in the upper body if possible. This is essential in the case of bilateral procedures. Venous access may be difficult and a small number of children require an internal jugular line.
- Endotracheal intubation with IPPV is the norm in infants and if the child is to be positioned prone an armoured ETT should be used.
- Maintenance is with volatile in oxygen and air or nitrous oxide.

- Tourniquets are used and may contribute to hyperthermia (reduced heat loss distal to the tourniquet) especially if they are bilateral and inflated at the same time. Bilateral tourniquets should not be deflated simultaneously so that exposure to metabolites from the ischaemic limbs is staged.
- Options for regional analgesia are a caudal epidural to block sacral dermatomes (0.3–0.5 mL/kg 0.5% levobupivacaine or equivalent) (📖 Chapter 8), a lumbar epidural with catheter or a sciatic nerve block. The popliteal approach to the sciatic nerve is useful for this distal procedure (📖 Chapter 7). A NSAID is also given perioperatively.
- If regional techniques are contraindicated or unsuccessful then a bolus of morphine sulphate (100–150 mcg/kg) is given with a NSAID.

Postoperative care

Maintenance fluids are required until the infant resumes feeding. Pain may be severe after bilateral or extensive procedures and in these cases an epidural infusion or an intravenous infusion of morphine sulphate is required (📖 Chapter 6) combined with a NSAID and paracetamol. For less extensive surgery, a combination of paracetamol, NSAID and oral opioid is effective.

Femoral osteotomy

- Performed for three main indications:
  - Perthe's disease where it is performed to improve congruity between the femoral head and acetabulum.
  - A part of the treatment of late DDH where it is carried out to reduce femoral anteversion and, if necessary, to shorten the overgrown femur and reduce pressure on the reduced femoral head.
  - As part of the treatment of cerebral palsy where it is usually combined with reduction of a dislocated hip and often a pelvic osteotomy to reshape the acetabulum.
- There are a variety of less common indications.
- Undertaken through a lateral approach. The femur is usually fixed with a blade plate.
- Hemorrhage is not usually a major problem unless combined with other procedures as in cerebral palsy.

Preoperative assessment

Children with Perthe's disease are usually healthy. Children with late DDH have often undergone several previous procedures and may be anxious or uncooperative. Premedication should be considered. Parents may be despondent at the need for further surgery after a real or perceived failure of the neonatal screening programme.

In cerebral palsy there are many issues to consider (☐ Chapter 15) including respiratory function, regurgitation, possible impairment of protective airway reflexes, epilepsy, and medication. Drugs are given as normal on the morning of surgery. A blood sample should be sent for group and save.

Anaesthetic technique

- Premedication if required.
- An inhalational induction may be easier in young children or in cerebral palsy. Older children usually prefer an IV induction.
- Endotracheal intubation with IPPV is common and maintenance is with volatile in oxygen and air or nitrous oxide. An infusion of remifentanil is very useful to reduce volatile requirements and provide moderate hypotension with a reduction in blood loss. In healthy older children, notably the group with Perthe's disease undergoing an isolated femoral osteotomy, a LMA, and spontaneous ventilation may be appropriate.
- Blood loss is variable. This can usually be replaced with crystalloid or colloid. Blood transfusion is needed occasionally especially if a pelvic osteotomy is performed concurrently.
- Options for 'single shot' regional analgesia include:
  - Caudal epidural block in younger children.
  - Lumbar epidural block.
  - Psoas plexus block (☐ Chapter 8).

- A three in one block (this has a significant failure rate for this operation).
- The fascia iliaca compartment block (📖 Chapter 7) has a high success rate and a long duration of action.
- A lumbar epidural followed by a postoperative infusion can also be used and is particularly indicated in children with severe cerebral palsy where the femoral osteotomy is combined with pelvic surgery. In these patients, postoperative muscle spasm may be extremely painful. These children are often sensitive to opioids and a morphine infusion may produce significant respiratory depression.
- If regional techniques are contraindicated or unsuccessful then intraoperative opioid (morphine sulphate 100–200 mcg/kg or fentanyl 2–4 mcg/kg) is given. Remifentanil can also be used intraoperatively with a bolus of morphine given before emergence from anaesthesia.

Postoperative care

Maintenance fluids are usually required overnight. If a 'single shot' regional technique is used then an IV infusion of morphine sulphate or PCA should be instituted for when this wears off (📖 Chapter 6) and combined with paracetamol and a NSAID. If an epidural catheter has been sited then an epidural infusion of local anaesthetic with opioid can be given in the appropriate setting. Intravenous or epidural analgesia is usually required for 24–72 hours depending on the extent of surgery.

Pelvic osteotomy

- This is usually indicated as part of the treatment of a dislocated hip:
  - As part of the treatment of late DDH to improve acetabular cover of the femoral head (Salter innominate osteotomy, Pemberton acetabuloplasty, Dega pelvic osteotomy).
  - The Chiari medial displacement osteotomy is performed in older children as a salvage procedure in a hip where anatomical reduction cannot be achieved.
  - Also used in treatment of hip dislocation associated with severe cerebral palsy (Dega or Pemberton procedures).
- Often performed in association with another procedure such as reduction of the dislocated hip or femoral osteotomy.

Preoperative assessment

Children with late DDH have often undergone several previous procedures and may be anxious or uncooperative. Premedication should be considered. Parents may be despondent at the need for further surgery after a real or perceived failure of the neonatal screening programme.

In cerebral palsy there are many issues to consider (📖 Chapter 15) including respiratory function, regurgitation, possible impairment of protective airway reflexes, epilepsy, and medication. Drugs are given as normal on the morning of surgery. A blood sample is sent for group and save.

Anaesthetic technique

- Induction as requested or indicated.
- Endotracheal intubation and IPPV are the norm.
- A urinary catheter is helpful in most patients especially teenagers who may suffer urinary retention postoperatively and if epidural infusion analgesia is planned. Measuring urine output also helps in the assessment of circulating volume.
- In view of the significant blood loss at least two IV cannulae of adequate gauge to support significant volume replacement are required. In some patients with poor venous access, especially in cerebral palsy, an internal jugular line is required to provide adequate access. This also provides an opportunity to monitor CVP during and after surgery.
- Maintenance with volatile in oxygen and air or nitrous oxide. A remifentanil infusion will reduce volatile requirements and provide moderate hypotension.
- TIVA is appropriate in older children.
- For a combined general and regional technique a lumbar epidural is necessary and can be used for an infusion postoperatively.
- If an epidural is not used then a generous dose of morphine is required.

- Blood transfusion is sometimes required in the cerebral palsy patients who tend to have combined procedures, suffer considerable blood loss and may have a degree of anaemia preoperatively.
- These patients are also prone to hypothermia during extensive procedures even when a warming mattress, warm air blanket and IV fluid warmer are used.

Postoperative care

If the child is hypothermic active warming with a warm air blanket (Bair Hugger® type) is continued in the recovery area. Maintenance fluids are required for 24–48 hours. FBC and U&E are checked if there has been significant blood loss or a blood transfusion.

For most patients postoperative epidural analgesia is the analgesic technique of choice for 48–72 hours. This is supplemented with paracetamol and regular NSAID if no contraindications. Once the epidural is discontinued oral opioid analgesia is required—codeine phosphate 1 mg/kg oral 4-hourly or morphine sulphate 200–300 mcg/kg oral 4-hourly.

Scoliosis

Idiopathic scoliosis

- Accounts for 70% of cases.
- Early onset or infantile (<5 years of age) or late onset adolescent types.
- Occurs mainly in adolescents with severe curves more predominant in girls.
- With severe curvature, the chest cavity can become narrowed resulting in a restrictive lung defect. This is rarely significant for curves <65°. Severe respiratory compromise probably only occurs in curves >100°.

Neuromuscular scoliosis

- Associated with myopathies e.g. Duchenne and upper and lower motor neuron diseases e.g. cerebral palsy, spinal muscular atrophy.
- Respiratory function may be further compromised by inability to cough, bulbar palsy leading to recurrent aspiration, and reduced ventilatory capacity.
- Scoliosis tends to involve most of the thoracolumbar spine.
- There is a higher incidence of complications including perioperative haemorrhage and respiratory failure than in idiopathic scoliosis.

Other

- Congenital scoliosis is associated with congenital vertebral abnormalities e.g. spina bifida and other defects especially renal and cardiac. High incidence of underlying cord abnormalities including tethering.
- Neurofibromatosis.
- Mesenchymal diseases e.g. dwarfism, Marfan's, rheumatoid arthritis, osteogenesis imperfecta.
- Trauma such as vertebral fracture or irradiation.

Posterior approach

- Most common approach.
- The patient is prone and the spinous processes and interspinous ligaments are removed and the facet joints destroyed.
- Pedicle screws or laminar hooks are used for multilevel fixation and two contoured rods are used to correct the deformity in all planes.
- For smaller children or those with bones unable to support laminar hooks (most patients with neuromuscular curves) Luque rods and sublaminar wires are used.
- Bone graft is applied to the entire fusion area after instrumentation and correction of the deformity.
- The instrumentation provides stability enabling early postoperative mobilization before bony fusion is complete.

Combined approach

- A combined anterior and posterior approach is used in more severe and rigid curves or where there is a need to prevent anterior growth.
- The two procedures may be staged over 1–2 weeks or done as one operation.

- Staged approaches are associated with less morbidity and mortality in high-risk patients.
- For the anterior approach a large thoraco-abdominal or flank incision is made followed by retroperitoneal dissection. Surgical access may be aided by single lung ventilation especially in larger children.
- For some congenital curves, an anterior approach alone is used.

Complications

- Complications of scoliosis surgery include major neurological injury, blood loss, coagulopathy, venous air embolism and postoperative visual loss.

Preoperative assessment

A multidisciplinary approach is ideal preferably in a preoperative clinic that allows sufficient time for discussion.

Medical assessment should focus on cardiorespiratory function. Exercise tolerance, ability to cough, and frequency and severity of chest infections are important.

Routine spirometry may show a moderate restrictive defect. Postoperative ventilation is rarely indicated unless the defect is severe (FVC <30% predicted) or two-stage surgery is undertaken on the same day. Arterial blood gases are indicated in severe cases. Hypercapnia is an indicator that the child may require chronic ventilatory support postoperatively and is usually seen in patients with severe early onset idiopathic scoliosis or a myopathy.

Cardiac involvement may complicate conditions associated with scoliosis e.g. cardiomyopathy and dysrhythmias in Duchenne muscular dystrophy or aortic and mitral valve abnormalities in Marfan's syndrome. Preoperative ECG, echocardiogram, and review by a cardiologist are required in these children.

Assessment of cardiorespiratory function may be difficult in some patients e.g. a patient with severe cerebral palsy may be wheelchair bound and unable to perform spirometry.

Full blood count is checked and blood cross matched.

Anaesthetic technique

- In the absence of contraindications, sedative premedication with oral midazolam 0.5 mg/kg to a maximum of 20 mg may be used to facilitate a smooth induction.
- Following gaseous or IV induction routine monitoring is initiated.
- Armoured ETTs are usually used for posterior fusions. Double lumen tubes or an endobronchial blocker may be needed for anterior fusions in older children. IPPV is used.
- Maintenance of anaesthesia is with volatile in air and oxygen combined with an infusion of remifentanil or with TIVA using propofol and remifentanil infusions. The choice depends on personal preference and the requirements for monitoring evoked potentials.

- Large bore venous access is required and central venous access is indicated in patients with difficult peripheral access, those having combined procedures, or where inotropic support may be needed.
- An arterial line for monitoring and blood sampling is sited.
- A urinary catheter is inserted.
- Particular attention to patient positioning and temperature maintenance is required.
- Temperature preserving mechanisms include the use of a warming mattress, a forced warm air blanket, and warmed IV fluids with monitoring of core temperature.
- Patients undergoing thoracotomy for anterior release are placed in the lateral position.
- The prone position is used for posterior fusions. This necessitates teamwork and meticulous care. The arms should be positioned in no more than 90° of abduction or forward flexion. Avoid compression of the axilla, ulnar nerves at the elbow, and lateral cutaneous nerves in the upper thigh. Free movement of the abdomen is needed to allow for adequate ventilation and to avoid elevated venous pressure, which could contribute to bleeding. Eyes must be protected and free from external pressure.
- Blood loss and coagulopathy:
  - This is related to the duration of surgery and the number of segments fused, the underlying pathology, and the surgical technique.
  - Patients with neuromuscular disease are at ↑ risk because they often have longer, more complex procedures with osteopenic bone that is more prone to bleeding.
  - Strategies to reduce blood loss include ensuring free abdominal movement, the use of antifibrinolytics and the use of cell salvage.
  - Induced hypotension and haemodilution (to reduce blood loss) may be used but are not pursued vigorously because of concerns about spinal cord perfusion.
  - Cell salvage is used in high-risk patients although in small patients allogenic transfusion is often needed before there is enough processed blood from cell salvage.
  - Aprotinin (a proteolytic enzyme inhibitor acting on plasmin and kallikrein to inhibit fibrinolysis) can be used in high-risk patients by giving a loading dose of 15,000 KIU/kg over 20 min and 7500 KIU/kg/hour for the duration of the operation.

Spinal cord monitoring

The risk of spinal cord injury is 0.3–0.6%. Ischaemic injury is the most common cause and the motor pathways supplied by the anterior spinal artery are most vulnerable. Intraoperative spinal cord monitoring has been developed to ↓ the risk of neurological injury.

Wake up test

This allows sufficient emergence from anaesthesia to test lower limb motor function. Loss of function may be irreversible and if the test is positive the surgeon is obliged to remove all the implants. Patient movement during emergence may result in accidental extubation or loss of IV access.

Somatosenory evoked potentials (SSEPs)

This involves stimulation of a peripheral nerve (usually the posterior tibial) and the detection a spinal response with epidural electrodes or a cortical response with scalp electrodes. It only monitors the dorsal sensory pathways and not the vulnerable anterior motor pathways. An amplitude fall of more than 50% is usually regarded as significant. There is an incidence of false negative recordings i.e. spinal cord damage occurs despite the detection of SSEPs.

Motor evoked potentials (MEPs)

This involves stimulating the motor cortex with transcranial electrical impulses and signal detection from muscles as a compound muscle action potential (CMAP) or at spinal level with epidural electrodes. The technique monitors the anterior cord. Compound muscle action potentials can also be generated by surgical manoeuvres that result in irritation of nerve roots or cord concussion.

Anaesthetic considerations for reliable spinal cord monitoring

- Volatiles and propofol depress SSEPs and MEPs in a dose dependent manner.
- Ketamine and etomidate may enhance recordings.
- Nitrous oxide profoundly depresses SSEPs and MEPs unless epidural recordings are used.
- Muscles relaxants reduce background noise and enhance SSEP recordings. Profound muscle relaxation abolishes CMAPs but not epidural MEPs.
- Bite blocks are recommended when using CMAP monitoring to prevent biting on the endotracheal tube and tongue lacerations.

A typical anaesthetic for MEP monitoring is sevoflurane (0.4–0.7 MAC) and a high dose infusion of remifentanil without nitrous oxide or muscle relaxants. A propofol infusion can be used instead of volatile.

Postoperative care

Respiratory complications including atelectasis are common. A chest drain is required after anterior surgery to drain the resulting pneumothorax and haemothorax. Admission to intensive care for IPPV may be required in some patients especially if there is limited preoperative respiratory function or if two-stage surgery is performed on the same day. Careful fluid management is required with hourly urine measures, assessment of volume status and appropriate replacement of ongoing losses. An effective analgesic regimen is essential to facilitate frequent physiotherapy and early mobilization. Multimodal pain management includes opioids, LA techniques, and NSAIDs.

There are various options for the provision of postoperative analgesia:
- A typical analgesic regimen would be an IV infusion of morphine sulphate 20–60 mcg/kg/hour with regular paracetamol, NSAID and antiemetic. Alternatively, PCA with a bolus dose of 20 mcg/kg morphine sulphate and background infusion of 10–20 mcg/kg/hour can be used.
- Spinal (subarachnoid) opioid can be used e.g. morphine sulphate 5 mcg/kg to a maximum of 300 mcg administered by the anaesthetist after induction or by the surgeon. If this route is not feasible caudal morphine 50 mcg/kg to a maximum of 3 mg can be given.
- For posterior fusions an epidural catheter placed by the surgeon under direct vision and tunnelled subcutaneously from the surgical wound can be used for a continuous infusion of LA. For anterior corrections a catheter can be placed in the paravertebral space underneath the reconstituted parietal pleura.
- Ketamine can be used for patients with continuous pain or excess sedation from morphine.

Neurosurgery

Considerations in paediatric neurosurgical anaesthesia

- Requires knowledge of cerebral physiology and an understanding of the pathology of individual patients.
- Assessment of preoperative neurological status (conscious level, presence of raised ICP, focal signs, cranial nerve function, and airway protective reflexes) and perioperative control of ICP are important.
- Patients often present for repeated procedures and may have significant co-morbidities.
- The cranium is regarded as a closed box:
- Brain tissue 80%.
- Cerebral blood volume (CBV) 10%.
- CSF 10%.
- Brain tissue is relatively incompressible and changes in CSF volume act as an initial buffer against ↑ ICP. When changes in CSF volume can no longer compensate, ICP ↑. In infants and young children, gradual changes in ICP can be compensated for by expansion of sutures and fontanelles.
- Clinical features of raised ICP include vomiting, irritability, seizures, lethargy, a bulging anterior fontanelle, and increasing head circumference.
- ICP in neonates and infants is usually 2–5 mmHg (adults 8–18 mmHg).
- In normal conditions, ICP is more dependent on cerebral blood flow (CBF) and CBV than CSF production.
- CBF is regulated by metabolic demands of the brain, arterial pCO_2 and arterial pO_2, and is subject to autoregulation.
- Children have a higher cerebral metabolic rate than adults and CBF is higher (100 mL/min/100 g compared with 50 mL/min/100 g in adults). Values for newborns and premature infants are less (40 mL/min/100 g).
- Autoregulation occurs over a wide range of systemic pressures (50–150 mmHg) and the lower limit is related to normal mean arterial blood pressure (as low as 45–50 mmHg in the newborn).
- In premature neonates, autoregulation is impaired and CBF is proportional to arterial pressure.
- Damaged areas of brain lose their autoregulation and are prone to the intracerebral steal syndrome.

Ventriculo-peritoneal (V-P) shunt insertion

- Performed for hydrocephalus caused by an abnormal accumulation of CSF within the cranium.
- Hydrocephalus can be congenital (e.g. aqueduct stenosis, myelomeningocele, Arnold–Chiari syndrome) or acquired (infection, intraventricular haemorrhage, tumour).
- In communicating hydrocephalus, there is flow of CSF between the ventricles and a pathway into the subarachnoid space. Flow is obstructed after leaving the ventricles (e.g. after meningitis).
- In non-communicating hydrocephalus, there is obstruction to the CSF flow within the ventricular system proximal to the subarachnoid space.
- Excess CSF causes dilatation of the ventricles, damaging the brain and causing enlargement of the cranium.
- Progressive hydrocephalus is diagnosed by increasing head circumference.
- Hydrocephalus occurs in over 80% patients with myelomeningocele
- The classical clinical picture of an enlarged head, bulging fontanelles, and engorged veins with 'sun setting' eyes is rarely seen and is a late sign.
- Hydrocephalus is usually treated by diverting CSF using a shunt with a low-pressure valve from the ventricles to the peritoneum (ventriculo-peritoneal shunt).
- An alternative treatment for non-communicating hydrocephalus is a surgical or endoscopic third ventriculostomy (surgical connection between the third ventricle and the subarachnoid space). This bypasses some intraventricular obstructions to CSF flow such as aqueductal stenosis. Ventriculostomy avoids the common complications of shunt infection and blockage.
- In premature babies with hydrocephalus from intraventricular haemorrhage, the CSF protein content is high which may lead to blockage of VP shunts. These babies are better managed with repeated ventricular taps either directly or after insertion of an access device (Rickham reservoir) until the CSF protein content falls.

Preoperative assessment

General considerations as mentioned previously. Assessment and recording of baseline neurological status is required (assessed regularly on the ward since rapid deterioration can occur).

Problems associated with raised ICP include vomiting, dehydration, reduced conscious level and potentially a risk of pulmonary aspiration. A high proportion of patients are ex-premature infants with the complications of prematurity—bronchopulmonary dysplasia, an oxygen requirement, and difficult venous access. An important sign of raised ICP in neonates is a tendency to apnoeic episodes.

Children often present for repeated revisions and may have other co-morbidities especially cerebral palsy and/or epilepsy. Children with chronic shunt infections become anaemic due to poor oral intake and bone marrow depression.

Anaesthetic technique

- If an IV cannula is present or can be placed without distressing the child then an IV induction is performed. An inhalational induction is often the more realistic option in infants.
- Intubation and controlled ventilation is required.
- Maintenance is with volatile in oxygen and air or nitrous oxide.
- Analgesia is usually provided with fentanyl 1–2 mcg/kg although this may need to be reduced or omitted (if LA infiltration is adequate) in ex-premature infants weighing <5 kg.
- Temperature maintenance may be difficult especially in ex-premature infants.
- Blood loss is usually small and invasive monitoring not usually required.
- Cardiovascular changes may occur at any time and are related to changes in ICP e.g. hypotension at the time of the CSF tap especially if blood pressure and ICP were previously raised.

Postoperative care

Postoperative analgesia is provided by wound infiltration with LA by the surgeon, paracetamol 15 mg/kg oral 4-hourly, and codeine phosphate 1 mg/kg oral 4-hourly (0.5 mg/kg <6 months of age).

Pre-term babies and those with neural tube defects need postoperative monitoring for apnoeas. Preoperative respiratory support may need to be ↑ postoperatively e.g. oxygen therapy to nasal CPAP, nasal CPAP to endotracheal intubation, and IPPV.

Baclofen pump insertion

- Motor spasticity arises from damage to the descending inhibitory control in the spinal cord and can be a major problem in children with conditions such as cerebral palsy.
- Baclofen is an agonist at gamma-aminobutyric acid B receptors and acts in the spinal cord to inhibit release of excitatory neurotransmitters. It is used to reduce pain associated with muscle spasms and may delay the development of contractures.
- Oral baclofen improves spasticity but its clinical use is limited by systemic side effects such as somnolence, confusion, ataxia, and urinary frequency.
- Intrathecal baclofen reduces spasticity at lower doses than oral baclofen and has fewer side effects.
- A trial to assess patient response is usually performed before insertion of a pump. For the trial a subarachnoid catheter is inserted under general anaesthesia and used to administer intrathecal baclofen for 48–72 hours while the response is assessed.
- The pump and drug reservoir system are placed in a subcutaneous pocket in the lateral abdominal wall. A catheter is inserted percutaneously via a Tuohy needle into the subarachnoid space and connected to the pump by subcutaneous tunnelling.
- Baclofen is instilled into the reservoir percutaneously and the system has external programming.
- The main complications are infection (5%) and catheter problems such as disconnections or fracture.
- There has been a marked ↑ in the number of children requiring general anaesthesia for insertion of intrathecal baclofen pumps over the last decade.

Preoperative assessment

In cerebral palsy there are many issues to consider (⌨ Chapter 15) including respiratory function, regurgitation, possible impairment of protective airway reflexes, epilepsy, and medication. Normal drugs are usually given preoperatively and premedication is prescribed as indicated—antisialogogue, sedative, antacid. Venous access may be difficult. The child has often had several anaesthetics previously.

Anaesthetic technique

- Induction depends on child or parent preference, ease of venous access, and any specific indications such as risk of gastric reflux and aspiration.
- Endotracheal intubation and IPPV are the norm.
- The patient is placed in the lateral position.
- Most patients have cerebral palsy of varying degrees of severity and so relevant issues should be addressed such as padding of pressure points, care with contractures, temperature maintenance, and precautions against aspiration.

- Analgesia is provided by a bolus of opioid (morphine sulphate 100–150 mcg/kg; fentanyl 2–4 mcg/kg) and LA infiltration of the incision.
- At the end of surgery, the implanted pump is purged over 40 min to prime the combined dead space of both the pump and the implanted catheter.

Postoperative care

Maintenance fluids are required until oral intake resumes. Drugs are administered as normal. A combination of paracetamol, NSAID and oral opioid are prescribed.

A ↓ in spasticity is usually noted within 24–48 hours after starting the infusion. Overdose of baclofen may present suddenly or insidiously and may be manifest as drowsiness, respiratory depression, rostral progression of hypotonia, or loss of consciousness.

Abrupt withdrawal from oral or intrathecal baclofen may result in seizures, hallucinations, disorientation, dyskinesias, and itching, with symptoms lasting up to 72 hours.

Craniotomy

- Most common indication is tumour resection.
- CNS tumours are the second most common form of malignancy in children.
  - Posterior fossa is the site of 60%.
  - Peak incidence is between 1–8 years.
  - Comprise astrocytomas 30%, medulloblastomas 30%, brainstem gliomas 30%, ependymomas 7%.
- Other indications include epilepsy, head injury, vascular lesions and craniosynostosis.

Preoperative assessment

Accurate assessment of neurological status includes evidence of raised ICP, altered conscious level, and focal findings e.g. cranial nerve palsies. Bulbar palsies may have led to aspiration and lung damage. Dehydration may be present secondary to vomiting. Multisystem pathology is rare in children with CNS tumours.

Blood for FBC, U&E and cross match should have been taken.

Sedative premedication is usually avoided. Consider an antisialogogue in infants and in children being positioned prone to dry secretions and provide cardiovascular stability.

Anaesthetic technique

- An IV induction is usually preferred if the child has a raised ICP. In some circumstances, a smooth inhalational induction is preferable to a traumatic IV one and the choice will depend on the age of the child, degree of cooperation and ease of venous access.
- The sympathetic response to laryngoscopy and intubation can be attenuated, if desired, with a bolus of short acting opioid e.g. fentanyl or remifentanil and an adequate depth of anaesthesia. A neuromuscular blocker is usually given to provide optimal conditions for intubation.
- A reinforced armoured ETT is used to prevent kinking and should be securely fixed with waterproof tapes that are not loosened by secretions and fluids.
- Reinforced ETTs have thicker walls than normal ETTs and the internal diameter may need to be 0.5 mm smaller than predicted by age. Check for bilateral lung expansion with head in neutral position and in the intended surgical position. This is particularly important when a degree of cervical flexion is intended which can result in endobronchial intubation.
- Maintenance of anaesthesia is directed towards providing good operating conditions and rapid awakening at the end of surgery to allow neurological assessment.

- Maintenance is with volatile in oxygen and air or nitrous oxide (concerns about nitrous oxide include ↑ in CBF, ICP, and the size or pressure within intracranial air spaces). An infusion of remifentanil (0.25–0.5 mcg/kg/minute) reduces the requirements for volatile agent and provides a moderate degree of hypotension with cardiovascular stability. TIVA with propofol and remifentanil is a good technique in older children. Hypertension from inadequate anaesthesia should be avoided.
- An infusion of a potent opioid attenuates or abolishes the pressor response to stimulating episodes including insertion of the pins of the head rest, skin incision (reduced by infiltration of LA), opening of the dura, and wound closure. Alternatively, a bolus is given prior to these events.
- IPPV to normocapnia helps to maintain an acceptable ICP.
- Hyperventilation is reserved for acute rises in ICP.
- Two secure cannulae suitable for rapid fluid administration are required.
- Mannitol, furosemide, steroids, and antibiotics are given according to local protocol or at the request of the surgeon.
- Profound induced hypotension is rarely used.
- Hypertension may result from direct stimulation of cardiovascular centres in the brainstem and the surgeon should be informed of significant changes or of dysrhythmias.

Monitoring

- Capnography not only gives an indication of adequate ventilation but also serves as a monitor for venous air embolism that can occur in any neurosurgical case especially if the patient becomes hypovolaemic.
- Direct arterial pressure monitoring is used for major cases.
- If CVP monitoring is required, the femoral route may be the most appropriate.
- A urinary catheter is usually inserted and is essential for long cases, where mannitol or diuretic has been given, where high urine output is anticipated (e.g. craniopharyngioma) or significant bleeding is possible.

Positioning

- Most intracranial surgery occurs with the patient supine and the head turned to one side.
- A low cerebral venous pressure is ensured with a moderate head up position and the jugular vessels free from compression.
- Positioning may be harder in small children because of their relatively short necks and large heads, which may lead to kinking of the neck veins.
- The prone position (e.g. for posterior fossa surgery) necessitates meticulous care to ensure the abdomen is free from compression (adverse effects on venous pressure as well as ventilation) and the orbits and pressure points are protected.
- Use of the sitting position is rare because of concern about venous air embolism. The incidence of this is lower in children than in adults due to a less negative intracranial venous pressure. Advantages of the sitting position include better anatomical orientation, less bleeding, lower ICP, and lower incidence of postoperative cranial nerve damage. Postural hypotension is rare in children but they should still be moved gradually to the full sitting position over a few minutes.

Fluid balance
- A degree of fluid restriction is usual to avoid cerebral oedema. Despite this concern, the priority is to maintain adequate circulating blood volume for cerebral perfusion.
- 0.9% saline is usually the maintenance fluid of choice.
- Glucose containing fluids can be avoided during the first 24 hours after surgery in older children since hyperglycaemia is associated with worse neurological outcome after brain injury. However, small children are more prone to hypoglycaemia and close monitoring of blood glucose should guide administration of dextrose containing solutions if required.
- Hyperosmolar or hypo-osmolar fluids should not be used as these can exacerbate cerebral oedema.
- Measurement of blood loss can be difficult and fluid and blood replacement is guided by clinical assessment, urine output and serial measurements of haematocrit.

Postoperative care

The majority of patients will be extubated at the end of the procedure. Early neurological assessment is performed followed by regular assessment in a HDU. Maintenance fluids are prescribed. Analgesia is provided by a combination of infiltration of surgical sites with LA, paracetamol 15 mg/kg oral 4-hourly, a weak opioid such as oral codeine phosphate 1 mg/kg oral 4-hourly. NSAIDs may be withheld in the early postoperative period because of effects on platelets. For major procedures, an IV infusion of morphine sulphate, NCA or PCA may be used (□ Chapter 6).

Arterio-venous malformation embolization

- AVMs can present at various stages depending on their size and blood flow.
  - If the malformation is large, the child may be in high output cardiac failure.
  - In infants there may be increasing head size from hydrocephalus.
  - Fitting.
  - Older children may present with neurological deficit from the effect of vascular steal.
- The clinical condition of the patient predicts the specific risks of the procedure.
- Some lesions are associated with high mortality and morbidity rates regardless of whether treatment is surgical or by interventional radiology e.g. aneurysm of the vein of Galen.
- Interventional radiology and embolization of these lesions is the treatment of choice if feasible. Emboli of various substances including coils and glue are positioned in a feeding artery. Success depends on the number of feeding vessels and several sessions may be needed.
- Risks of the procedure include intracerebral bleeding, movement of the embolus, pulmonary artery emboli and ischemia to vital areas.

Preoperative assessment

As well as a general assessment, the baseline neurological function is noted. The child is assessed for evidence of high output cardiac failure.

Anaesthetic technique

- Procedures are performed in the neuroangiography suite. This is often not an ideal place for induction of infants and the insertion of invasive monitoring. It may be preferable to anaesthetize small children in a normal anaesthetic room and then transport them to the angiography suite.
- Patients should be intubated and ventilated to normocapnia.
- Limited patient access requires long extensions for IV access and ventilator tubing.
- Invasive monitoring is usually indicated. There may be cardiovascular instability with hypertension, bradycardia and dysrhythmias due to direct stimulation or dramatic alterations in blood flow to the malformation. The procedure is usually performed via an angiography catheter inserted into a femoral vessel. These catheters are relatively large in small children.
- Repeated flushing of the angiography catheter may result in hypervolaemia especially in infants.
- These are technically demanding procedures that may be prolonged. The angiography suite often has limited space for anaesthetic equipment, subdued lighting, and a cool ambient temperature.

- Monitoring and maintaining core temperature is important especially during prolonged procedures.
- IV contrast media is iodine based and carries a small risk of anaphylactic reactions. The recommended maximum dose of contrast media is 4 mL/kg. Contrast media is hyperosmolar and produces an initial volume overload followed by dehydration after an osmotic diuresis. IV fluids are required. Contrast media may also interfere with the clotting mechanisms.
- Blood loss estimation may be difficult and blood should be available.

Postoperative care

Sometimes admission to an ITU for a brief period of IPPV is appropriate especially if the child is hypothermic or has been transported between hospitals. Most of the postoperative assessment is directed to the detection of new neurological deficit. Maintenance fluids are required. Fluid balance must be monitored, a FBC performed, and electrolytes measured in view of the administration of flush solution. Femoral puncture sites are observed for bleeding and, if an artery was used, then perfusion of the leg is assessed regularly.

Maxillofacial and craniofacial surgery

Considerations in paediatric maxillofacial and craniofacial surgery

- Involves a wide range of congenital and acquired conditions in children of all ages.
- There are often associated problems with the airway and/or endotracheal intubation.
- May involve complex and prolonged procedures in infants.
- Major problems are related to a difficult airway, temperature control, and blood loss.
- Many patients require multiple procedures and anaesthetics over a number of years. There may be psychological morbidity as a result of these and concerns about self-image.
- These operations are usually performed in centralized, multidisciplinary units and there is a considerable burden of travel and time away from home for some families.

Mandibular surgery

- Surgery may be required to correct congenital or developmental facial deformities e.g. mandibular hypoplasia.
- Patients often have syndromes associated with difficult airways e.g. Treacher Collins.
- Procedures are complicated and carried out by teams of surgeons and anaesthetists in specialist centres.
- Surgery ranges from advancement osteotomies to extensive reconstruction.
- In some cases bone or cartilage grafts are taken from the iliac crest or ribs.
- The jaws may be wired together at the end of surgery.

Preoperative assessment

As well as the normal assessment of general health and intercurrent illness particular attention is paid to the airway and indicators of potential difficulties with airway maintenance or endotracheal intubation. Any previous anaesthetic history is vital and as this may have often taken place elsewhere it should be part of the initial outpatient surgical appointment to enquire about anaesthetic issues in other hospitals and if indicated obtain copies of the relevant anaesthetic charts.

The presenting syndrome, if any, may give an indication of likely airway difficulties. Patients may be difficult to intubate due to limited mouth opening or mandibular hypoplasia and it may also be difficult to maintain a patent airway under anaesthesia.

Micrognathia is the most common cause of difficult intubation and is associated with several developmental anomalies. The commonest combination of difficulty, if any, is for the patient to have an adequate airway but be difficult to intubate. Respiratory function is usually normal. The anaesthetist should be competent in the use of various aids to laryngoscopy and fibreoptic endotracheal intubation.

Anaesthetic technique

- Mandibular surgery is usually performed in children over the age of 5 years and an IV induction is appropriate unless difficulty with the airway or endotracheal intubation is anticipated.
- Endotracheal intubation and IPPV are the norm. A fibreoptic procedure is performed if necessary (☐ Chapter 5).
- A nasal ETT is usually required.
- For some procedures, a tracheostomy is performed before the operation starts.
- Maintenance of anaesthesia is with volatile in oxygen and air or nitrous oxide. An infusion of remifentanil 0.25–0.5 mcg/kg/min reduces volatile requirements, produces moderate hypotension, contributes to cardiovascular stability, and contributes to a rapid and smooth emergence from anaesthesia. TIVA is appropriate in older children.
- Bleeding may be a significant problem and adequate IV access is sited.

- A throat pack is used and is removed prior to extubation or before the end of surgery if the jaws are being wired together.
- Eyes should be padded and protected.
- The length of surgery may contribute to hypothermia and a warming mattress or a warming blanket should be used.
- There is a possibility of pneumothorax when a rib graft is used.
- Bradycardia may be caused by traction on the maxilla via the trigeminal-vagal reflex arc.

Postoperative care

Patients are usually extubated at the end of the procedure unless surgery is prolonged or has involved extensive manipulation of the pharyngeal mucosa. Patients with high risk for airway oedema are kept intubated and admitted to ITU for 24–48 hours. A nasopharyngeal airway may be useful postoperatively for airway maintenance and as an access route for suctioning. If the jaws are wired, the position of the wires should be noted prior to extubation and wire cutters must be available. Maintenance fluids are prescribed.

Analgesia is provided by a combination of paracetamol 15 mg/kg oral 4-hourly, ibuprofen 10 mg/kg oral 6-hourly, and codeine phosphate 1 mg/kg oral 4-hourly. An IV infusion of morphine sulphate (📖 Chapter 6) for 24 hours may be easier if the jaws are wired. An antiemetic e.g. ondansetron 100 mcg/kg (max 4mg) IV 8-hourly is prescribed and should be given regularly if the jaws are wired.

Craniofacial surgery

- Craniosynostosis refers to premature closure of cranial sutures resulting in dysostoses with abnormal bone growth. The abnormalities produced are scaphocephaly (sagittal suture fusion), plagiocephaly (one coronal or lamboid suture fusion), brachycepahaly (coronal suture fusion), oxycephaly (coronal and sagittal suture fusion), and trigonocephaly (metopic suture fusion).
- Estimated incidence is 1:2000 live births.
- The faciocraniosynostoses (much rarer) are more complex conditions with abnormalities of the skull and facial development (particularly midfacial hypoplasia). There are usually multiple suture stenoses with ocular malposition, proptosis and respiratory difficulties. These patients often have a syndrome including other congenital anomalies especially syndactyly. Syndromes include Apert's, Crouzon, and Pfeiffer's.
- These conditions:
  - May cause raised ICP in untreated cases especially in those with multiple suture involvement.
  - Papilloedema secondary to raised ICP can cause visual impairment.
  - There may be preoperative respiratory problems in the faciocraniosynosotoses and respiratory function is optimized prior to definitive surgery by treatment of choanal atresia or use of CPAP.
- Surgery is performed to relieve ICP, correct deformity, and improve appearance. Frontocranial remodelling is required to restore the normal anatomy of the forehead and cranial vault and allow normal growth of the brain. Facial advancement techniques are used for midface hypoplasia.
- Simple cases usually undergo surgery in the first year of life.
- In complex cases an operation on the frontal and cranial part of the malformation is usually also performed between 4–12 months of age. The facial retrusion is corrected later—in severe cases, before school age, around 5 years. In moderate cases, after final dentition appears, around 12 years of age.
- In most cases, a late advancement of the upper teeth through an oral approach (Le Fort I) will be necessary in adolescence, as well as various further aesthetic procedures (eyelids, chin, forehead) to obtain the best possible final result.
- Blood loss may be large and the oculo-cardiac reflex may be triggered by orbital dissection.

Preoperative assessment

Most paediatric centres have a craniofacial team and a comprehensive multidisciplinary assessment process. Thorough airway assessment is essential and involves a detailed history including feeding difficulties, failure to thrive, sleep disturbance, daytime somnolence and developmental difficulties. A team approach to optimize ENT and respiratory care including overnight sleep studies to assess upper airway obstruction with or without OSA is required in patients with maxillary hypoplasia.

Preoperative improvement of the airway using choanal dilatation with or without bony dissection, nasal stenting, nasopharyngeal airways, and nocturnal nasal CPAP is often required in the faciocraniosynostoses.

Tracheostomy may be needed in those with severe airway problems to provide a patent airway and provide time for growth before planned surgical intervention. Most complex children will have had anaesthetics for preoperative procedures such as MRI, CT, or choanal dilatation and the records will give useful information about any difficulties with the airway, endotracheal intubation or venous access. Blood is cross matched.

Anaesthetic technique

- Sedative premedication can be given to children without respiratory compromise or raised ICP.
- In many cases, an inhalational induction is preferred partly because the child undergoes many anaesthetics and partly because if there are limb anomalies venous access may be difficult.
- The commonest combination of airway difficulty, if any, is for the patient to have a difficult airway but be easy to intubate. Endotracheal intubation may be difficult but in most cases is straightforward.
- Children with maxillary hypoplasia may develop airway obstruction after induction. Marked proptosis may make it difficult to form a seal with a facemask.
- Endotracheal intubation and IPPV are necessary. The type of ETT depends on the planned surgery but is usually either an armoured or preformed tube. Secure fixation of the tube is essential and for maxillary osteotomies mandibular intradental wiring is the most secure method. A throat pack may be needed.
- For the more major procedures an arterial line, femoral venous line, and urinary catheter are required.
- Positioning may be difficult and it is important to avoid cerebral venous congestion by excessive neck rotation. Pressure area care must be meticulous and may require a foam or gel mattress.
- A moderate head up position is usually employed.
- A balanced anaesthetic technique to provide cardiovascular stability includes a combination of opioid and volatile agent. A remifentanil infusion 0.25–0.5 mcg/kg/min is useful.

- Hypotensive anaesthesia may be used but is not usually pursued vigorously because of concerns about cerebral perfusion in the head up position in the presence of a raised ICP.
- The amount of blood loss varies with the type of surgery but may be very large especially in infants undergoing complex procedures. The majority occurs during the first part of the surgical procedure (skull incision, craniotomy) and in the postoperative period.
- Blood loss may be may be torrential from large abnormal veins and most of the perioperative morbidity is related to intraoperative haemorrhage. At least two free flowing cannulae should be sited and secured. Meticulous monitoring and maintenance of normovolaemia is essential. Cell salvage is a useful method of reducing perioperative transfusion requirements.

Postoperative care

Most patients are extubated and nursed in an HDU. In some patients a period of IPPV is required especially after facial surgery. Maintenance fluids are prescribed. After major procedures, blood loss may continue into the postoperative period and babies may lose 10% of the blood volume into a drain or head bandages. For these cases, regular assessment of the cardiovascular system is required and a series of full blood counts is performed. Blood is transfused if indicated.

Analgesia is provided by a combination of paracetamol 15 mg/kg oral 4-hourly, ibuprofen 10 mg/kg oral 6-hourly (if bleeding is not a concern), and codeine phosphate 1 mg/kg oral 4-hourly. Pain scores are surprisingly low despite presence of marked head and facial swelling and bilateral black eyes.

Ophthalmology, plastics, oncology, radiology, thoracic, and dental surgery

Andrew Morrison

Ophthalmic surgery

- Unlike adult ophthalmic surgery where many procedures can be preformed with local anaesthesia, children require a general anaesthetic.
- Most patients are healthy and present no unusual anaesthetic challenges.
- A small number do have underlying conditions which may affect the anaesthetic technique.
- Most patients and procedures are suitable for treatment on a day case basis.
- Intraocular pressure (IOP) (normal 10–20 mmHg) is affected by anaesthesia in a number of ways.
  - Most induction and maintenance agents ↓ IOP by 20–30% (3–6 mmHg).
  - Ketamine probably ↑ it slightly. Its effect may be dose dependent with doses over 5 mg/kg producing an ↑.
  - Opioids have no effect or produce a small ↓.
  - Non-depolarizing neuromuscular blockers have no effect or produce a small ↓.
  - Suxamethonium causes an ↑ of about 8 mmHg with a return to baseline after 5–7 min.
  - IOP is ↑ by pressure on the eye from a face mask, laryngoscopy, endotracheal intubation, and insertion of a LMA. Coughing and upper airway obstruction also ↑ IOP.
- The oculocardiac reflex is a trigeminal-vagal reflex triggered by traction on the extraocular muscles (especially the medial rectus which has up to six times the mass of the lateral rectus), manipulation of the globe and an ↑ in intraorbital pressure. Sudden or strong traction has more effect than gentle progressive traction. The response is usually a sinus bradycardia. Junctional rhythms, atrioventricular block, atrial and ventricular ectopics can also occur. It is particularly common during strabismus (squint) surgery. The reflex weakens with repetition of the stimulus or the application of topical LA. The reflex can be prevented by giving atropine (20 mcg/kg IV) or glycopyrronium bromide (10 mcg/kg IV) before the surgical stimulus.
- Because of restricted access to the airway during surgery, endotracheal intubation (usually with a south facing RAE ETT) is very common. The reinforced LMA is also used, especially for older children, to avoid paralysis and coughing on an ETT at the end of surgery.
- PONV is extremely common after paediatric ophthalmic surgery.
- Topical drugs are a prominent part of ophthalmic surgery and anaesthesia. The commonest indications are pupillary dilatation and analgesia. Phenylephrine 2.5% is an α adrenergic agonist and cyclopentolate 1% is structurally similar to atropine. Amethocaine drops are used to provide topical analgesia and a preparation of diclofenac sodium for topical ophthalmic use is available (although not licensed for use in children). Systemic effects from these drugs are rare but possible. Systemic absorption mostly occurs after passage through the nasolacrimal duct and absorption from the pharyngeal mucosa.
- A requirement for multiple anaesthetics is a feature of many paediatric ophthalmic conditions.

Ophthalmology

Examination under anaesthesia and intraocular pressure measurement

It is uncommon for children under 5 years of age to be able to tolerate any significant eye examination, especially the measurement of intraocular pressure.

Preoperative assessment

Problems with anaesthesia in this group of children are more likely to be due to related conditions affecting the airway or a body system. History and examination will indicate concerns and potential problems.

- Metabolic: diabetes, mucopolysaccharidoses, hypercalcaemia, galactosaemia
- Infections: herpes simplex, CMV, rubella
- Syndrome: Apert's, Marfan's, Sturge–Weber, Lowe, Crouzon's syndromes
- Others: congenital myotonic dystrophy, sickle cell disease.

Anaesthetic technique

- Aim is to provide optimal examination conditions without altering IOP.
- For a general examination where IOP is not a concern:
  - IV or inhalational induction are both appropriate.
  - A LMA can be used for airway maintenance to allow the surgeon unrestricted access.
  - Anaesthesia is maintained with volatile in oxygen and air or nitrous oxide.
- If IOP is a concern:
  - The measurement is often taken after induction with ketamine 1–2 mg/kg IV or 5–10 mg/kg IM (atropine 20 mcg/kg or glyco-pyrronium bromide 10 mcg/kg are often given simultaneously to minimize the excess secretions produced by ketamine) before airway stimulation or further drug administration.
  - Since most anaesthetic drugs lower IOP a falsely low reading may be recorded after induction with drugs other than ketamine.
  - The unpopularity of IM injections and concern about emergence phenomena with ketamine mean that many anaesthetists prefer not to use it. If volatile or IV agents are used then the minimum to produce a still child is used and the IOP is measured as soon as possible.

Anaesthetic factors affecting IOP

- All inhalational agents cause a dose-related ↓ in IOP (due to a combination of relaxation of extraocular muscles, reduced aqueous production, ↑ drainage, and indirect effects via CNS depression).
- Ketamine probably has a dose related effect with an ↑ when doses over 5 mg/kg are used.

- Propofol and other IV induction agents, ↓ IOP in the presence of normocapnia.
- Opioids either have no effect or reduce IOP slightly.
- Atropine given parenterally has no effect.
- Non-depolarizing muscle relaxants either have no effect or reduce IOP slightly.
- Ganglion blockers reduce IOP.
- Hypertonic solutions (mannitol, dextran) reduce IOP.
- Hypoxia and hypercapnia cause an ↑ in IOP.
- Hypothermia reduces IOP.
- Suxamethonium ↑ IOP (by up to 8 mmHg) which returns to normal after 5–7 min. It is relatively contraindicated for use where perforation of the globe is suspected. Mechanisms include:
  - Contraction of extraocular muscles
  - ↓ aqueous drainage due to a change in angle of the anterior chamber (this cycloplegic action is seen in eyes where extraocular muscles have been detached)
  - Choroidal vascular dilatation.

Postoperative care

If ketamine has been used emergence phenomena such as hallucinations or unpleasant dreams may be a problem. Children are traditionally recovered in a dimly lit space and are not stimulated or disturbed. Oral intake is resumed rapidly and analgesia is rarely required.

Strabismus

- Misalignment of the visual axis is common (3–5% of the population), and strabismus surgery is the most common paediatric eye operation performed.
- ♂:♀ ratio 1:1

Aetiology

- Usually idiopathic, occasionally secondary to trauma, infection, inflammation (muscle palsies).
- Associated with family history, prematurity, CNS disorders (cerebral palsy, meningomyelocele with hydrocephalus).

Presentation

- Patients may have occult myopathies. There is a three fold ↑ in the incidence of masseter spasm in children anaesthetized for strabismus surgery. There is possibly also an ↑ (but still very low) risk of malignant hyperthermia. Suxamethonium is usually avoided.

Treatment

- Correction can be achieved by recession (lengthening), resection (tightening or shortening) or transposition of any, or combinations of the extraocular muscles (four recti and two oblique).
- In older children an adjustable suture is occasionally used (the final position is achieved using LA eye drops at 24–48 hours after surgery) to reduce the incidence of malposition.

Preoperative assessment

Most patients are healthy children. Premedication is prescribed if required.

Anaesthetic technique

- Induction as preferred or requested.
- Unless there is a specific indication, airway management can be with either an ETT or a LMA.
- SV or IPPV as preferred or indicated.
- Maintenance with volatile in oxygen and air. TIVA may reduce the incidence of PONV in older children.
- The surgeon may apply topical adrenaline to produce conjunctival vasoconstriction and reduce bleeding. There is systemic absorption and the ECG should be observed closely for a period.
- Forced duction testing is used to distinguish a paretic muscle from one with restricted motion. The surgeon manipulates the eye into the normal axis by traction on the sclera. The test is not possible if there has been administration of suxamethonium (causes contraction of extraocular muscles) in the previous 20 min. Non-depolarizing muscle relaxants do not interfere with testing.

- Oculocardiac reflex (see above) Tension on extraocular muscles can produce vagal stimulation and bradycardia. Prevented by atropine 20 mcg/kg or glycopyrronium bromide 10 mcg/kg.
- Analgesia is provided with topical tetracaine, NSAID, paracetamol. Fentanyl citrate 1–2 mcg/kg IV or codeine phosphate 1 mg/kg IM improve analgesia and provide some postoperative sedation but ↑ the risk of PONV.
- PONV is common (50–75%) after strabismus surgery. It is common to use two agents with different mechanisms of action e.g. ondansetron 100 mcg/kg (max 4mg), dexamethasone 100–200 mcg/kg. Combinations of antiemetics can reduce the incidence of PONV to approximately 5%.

Postoperative care

Children may be very distressed by the eye patch and restricted vision. Oral intake is usually resumed early in the postoperative period. A combination of paracetamol, NSAID and an oral opioid is prescribed. PONV may require a further antiemetic of a different class from the one(s) given during anaesthesia e.g. cyclizine 1 mg/kg IV if ondansetron and dexamethasone have already been given. The IV cannula is usually left in place postoperatively in case IV antiemetic is required. Most patients are treated as day cases.

Cataract extraction

- Cataract is a major worldwide cause of morbidity—1 child becomes blind every minute predominantly in developing countries. Of the 1.5 million blind children in the world, 85% live in Africa or in Asia.
- Paediatric cataracts can be classified as congenital (present at birth), infantile (develops during the first 2 years), or juvenile (later onset), although many infantile and juvenile cataracts have been present since birth.

Aetiology

- Hereditary (75%): autosomal dominant, usually otherwise well. Occasionally as part of syndrome e.g. Lowe's oculo-cerebro-renal syndrome (X linked recessive), Down's (Trisomy 21), Edwards, Cri du chat.
- Metabolic: glucose-6-phosphate dehydrogenase deficiency, galactosaemia, hypoglycaemia, hypocalcaemia in infancy.
- Trauma: blunt or penetrating, usually unilateral.
- Inflammation: uveitis (juvenile chronic arthritis).
- Tumour: (retinoblastoma).
- Intrauterine infection: rubella, CMV, toxoplasmosis, toxocariasis.
- Radiation: total body for leukaemia.
- Steroids: chronic use.

Treatment

- Surgery usually involves intraocular lens implantation done early (as young as 4 weeks old in some centres) to allow retinal stimulation and visual development. Surgery takes 30–60 min.
- Higher incidence of complications than in adults. Glaucoma (lifetime follow-up required), uveitis, iris damage or prolapse, endophthalmitis (bacterial infection), thickening of posterior lens capsule requiring further surgery (up to 90%), retinal detachment.

Preoperative assessment

Implications of the underlying condition for anaesthesia e.g. mucopolysaccharidosis and airway management, prematurity, Down's syndrome. The surgeon will prescribe drugs to produce mydriasis usually topical phenylephrine 2.5% and cyclopentolate 1%.

Anaesthetic technique

- Should ensure a motionless eye and avoid raised IOP. A smooth induction and emergence without coughing is desirable.
- IV or inhalational induction is appropriate.
- Usually endotracheal intubation (south facing RAE ETT) and IPPV to avoid hypercapnia.
- Maintenance of anesthesia with volatile in oxygen and air. Nitrous oxide is often avoided to reduce the risk of PONV. An infusion of remifentanil (0.1–0.25 mcg/kg/minute) reduces volatile requirements and is associated with a smooth emergence from anaesthesia. TIVA is often used in older children.

- Avoid a high F_IO_2 in premature neonates.
- Antiemetics are given to minimize the effects of vomiting on IOP. It is common to use two agents with different mechanisms of action e.g. ondansetron 100 mcg/kg, dexamethasone 100–200 mcg/kg.
- Analgesia usually involves topical tetracaine drops, a NSAID, and paracetamol. A dose of opioid e.g. fentanyl citrate 1–2 mcg/kg IV, codeine phosphate 0.5–1 mg/kg IM may be given to provide a combination of analgesia and mild postoperative sedation.

Postoperative care

Oral intake is usually resumed early in the postoperative period. A combination of paracetamol, NSAID, and an oral opioid e.g. codeine phosphate 1 mg/kg 4-hourly is prescribed. PONV may require a further antiemetic of a different class from the one(s) given during anaesthesia e.g. cyclizine 1 mg/kg IV if ondansetron and dexamethasone already used. The IV cannula is usually left in place postoperatively in case IV antiemetic is required. Most patients are treated as day cases. Specific care for an underlying syndrome may be required e.g. respiratory support in Pompe's disease.

Glaucoma

- Glaucoma is characterized by elevated IOP resulting in reduced capillary blood flow to the optic nerve with eventual loss of optic nerve tissue and function.
- Bilateral in 75% of cases. Incidence 1:10000 births (congenital glaucoma) and ♀:♂ ratio 65%:35%.
- Primary congenital glaucoma is due to failure of development of trabecular drainage channels for aqueous humour.
- Secondary glaucoma is due to blockage of existing drainage channels. It develops as a result of:
  - Infection.
  - Inflammation.
  - Trauma to the eye e.g. uveitis, iritis, or following surgery for congenital cataracts.
  - Some rare syndromes may also lead to glaucoma. Axenfeld–Reiger has an inherited tendency for abnormal formation of the iris and margin of the cornea. Aniridia (bilateral iris hypoplasia) is associated with genitourinary abnormalities e.g. Wilms' tumour (20%) and mental retardation. In Sturge–Weber syndrome (neurocutaneous angiomata) intraocular angiomas cause raised intraocular pressure and mechanical obstruction to the angle of the eye.
- Primary glaucoma is more common below the age of 3 years while after this secondary glaucoma predominates.

Treatment

- Medical treatment:
  - Acetazolamide (15–30 mg/kg/day oral in 3 or 4 divided doses) is a carbonic anhydrase inhibitor and suppresses aqueous production. It occasionally causes a metabolic acidosis. Topical β adrenergic blockers are sometimes used in conjunction with acetazolamide.
- Surgical treatment:
  - Examination under anaesthesia and measurement of IOP is carried out. If indicated, a definitive procedure is then performed. Glaucoma surgery aims to prevent blindness by reducing the IOP.
  - Trabeculectomy: a new drainage channel is created to drain aqueous from the intraocular anterior chamber to extraocular sub-Tenon's space, covered only by conjunctiva. Fluid accumulates in the subconjunctival layer and is absorbed. This may be combined with intraoperative application of antifibrotic agents (mitomycin C or 5-fluorouracil) to reduce the fibrotic response to surgery.
  - Aqueous shunt surgery with drainage tubes may be performed to achieve the same effect.
  - Trabeculotomy: a fine probe inserted into Schlemm's canal creates a new drainage channel.
  - Goniotomy: a gonioscope is used to visualize the anterior chamber, an incision is then made in the trabecular meshwork to allow drainage. Occasionally the superficial layer of cornea is removed to improve the view into the angle of the eye.
  - Laser treatment aimed at the ciliary body can help to reduce the production of aqueous.

Preoperative assessment

Is directed at the implications of any underlying cause of glaucoma. Children are either starting a series of many anaesthetics and examinations or are in the course of this process. Many will be anxious and require sedative premedication.

Anaesthetic technique

- Should avoid raised intraocular pressure (IOP). A smooth induction and emergence without coughing is desirable.
- IV or inhalational induction is appropriate. Most anaesthetic agents lower IOP, as does a calm or premedicated patient. Ketamine probably ↑ it slightly. Suxamethonium is avoided because of a definite ↑.
- IOP is usually measured after induction and before airway manipulation such as laryngoscopy and endotracheal intubation.
- Usually endotracheal intubation (south facing RAE ETT) and IPPV to avoid hypercapnia.
- Maintenance of anaesthesia with volatile in oxygen and air. Nitrous oxide is often avoided to reduce the risk of PONV. An infusion of remifentanil (0.1–0.25 mcg/kg/min) reduces volatile requirements and is associated with a smooth emergence from anaesthesia. TIVA is often used in older children.
- Antiemetics are given to minimize the effects of vomiting on IOP. It is common to use two agents with different mechanisms of action e.g. ondansetron 100 mcg/kg (max 4mg), dexamethasone 100–200 mcg/kg.
- Analgesia usually involves topical tetracaine drops, a NSAID, and paracetamol. A dose of opioid e.g. fentanyl citrate 1–2 mcg/kg IV, codeine phosphate 0.5–1 mg/kg IM may be given to provide a combination of analgesia and mild postoperative sedation.
- Extubation without coughing or straining.

Postoperative care

Oral intake is usually resumed early in the postoperative period. A combination of paracetamol, NSAID and an oral opioid e.g. codeine phosphate 1 mg/kg 4-hourly is prescribed. Pain is more of a problem than after some other paediatric ophthalmic procedures.

Plastic surgery

Lumps and bumps

- Of superficial lumps excised in infants and children, approximately 1% are malignant.
- About four-fifths of the malignant lesions can be recognized by:
  - Presentation as a neonate.
  - A history of rapid or progressive growth.
  - Skin ulceration.
  - Fixation (immobility).
  - Presence of a firm mass >3 cm in diameter.
- Although 5–10% of benign lumps will regress spontaneously, 90% persist or slowly enlarge and are excised for cosmetic reasons, to prevent late infection or inflammation and to avoid missing a malignancy.
- Superficial lumps include lipomas, haemangiomas, lymph nodes, naevi, dermoid cysts, calcified hair follicles, and rarely skin cancers such as malignant melanoma.

Neck lumps

- Can be diagnostic challenge. Cervical lymphadenopathy is the commonest cause (25–30%).
- Divided into infective, inflammatory, or congenital (embryological) masses.

Branchial remnants

- Cysts, sinuses, or cartilaginous tags. Remnants of the folding over of branchial arches in utero (Greek branchia = gills).
- Commonly present as preauricular tags of cartilage or pits.
- Formal excision required.
- Unless infected do not present airway problems.

Thyroglossal derivatives

- The thyroid is derived from the posterior third of the tongue and migrates during fetal life to the adult position anterior to the trachea. Several anomalies may result from this migration. Rarely, no migration occurs, and the thyroid develops entirely at the back of the tongue—a lingual thyroid. More common are thyroglossal cysts, ectodermal remnants that develop along the line of descent of the thyroid gland. Defective migration can leave the thyroid anywhere along this path.
- Midline swelling. Moves on swallowing and tongue protrusion.
- Excision.
- Assessment of the airway is required.

Cervicofacial dermoids

- The soft tissues of the face are formed by the convergence of the frontal, maxillary, and mandibular processes. Cystic swellings known as dermoids may occur along the lines of fusion. The commonest site for this phenomenon is at the upper lateral part of the forehead (an external angular dermoid). In the neck they are submental.
- A midline submental swelling. May rarely affect the airway.

Cystic hygroma
- Hamartomatous lymphatic swellings that result in a multicystic mass which infiltrates tissue planes.
- 60%+ found in the neck. Transilluminate.
- Antenatal diagnosis means the newborn may require intubation.
- Pharynx and larynx can be infiltrated and cause upper airway obstruction.

Sternomastoid tumour
- A lump in the middle third of the sternocleidomastoid muscle.
- Caused by stretching and muscle damage during delivery.
- Often detected weeks after birth as a lump ± torticollis.
- Physiotherapy and manipulation to minimize the torticollis is the treatment.

Cervical lymphadenopathy
- Stable, non-tender and enlarged cervical lymph node.
- Usually a reaction to infection, rarely neoplasia e.g. lymphoma.

Cervical lymphadenitis
- Swollen, tender and inflamed lymph node.
- Bacterial usually streptococcal or staphylococcal.
- Occasionally mycobacterium with a lengthy history.
- Drainage indicated if no response to antibiotics.
- Infective swellings are occasionally large causing distortion of the airway or reduced mouth opening due to trismus.

Most operations are quick but occasionally there is a need for frozen section tests or more extensive surgery than planned.

Preoperative assessment

Usually unremarkable. Occasional parental anxiety about possible malignancy. Rarely potential airway complications during anaesthesia.

Anaesthetic technique
- Inhalational or IV induction depending on patient/parent preference, child's veins and likely ease of cannulation.
- In most cases a LMA is used with SV.
- Maintenance of anaesthesia with volatile in oxygen and air or nitrous oxide.
- In most cases, the surgeon infiltrates LA with adrenaline to provide analgesia and contribute to haemostasis.
- A NSAID can be added if desired.

Postoperative care

Usually straightforward. Paracetamol and a NSAID for analgesia. PONV rare. Most children eat and drink quickly and are discharged a couple of hours postoperatively.

Otoplasty

- Performed for prominent ears ('bat ears') and microtia, the two most common congenital ear malformations. Both conditions can be unilateral or bilateral.
- Prominent ears are not usually associated with other malformations. Surgery aims to correct the specific area of prominence by reshaping the antihelical fold through an elliptical incision behind the ear.
- Microtia can be part of hemifacial microsomia with associated malformations such as an asymmetric mandible and potential airway problems. Surgery is reconstructive and often involves harvesting costal cartilage as part of the procedure.
- Complications: haematoma, asymmetry, infection, prominent scar.
- Age: 6 years and over.
- ♂:♀ ratio 2:1.

Preoperative assessment

Most patients are healthy children. A small number of patients with microtia are difficult to intubate conventionally (they usually have an easy airway) and may require fibreoptic endotracheal intubation (📖 Chapter 5). Sedative premedication if indicated.

Anaesthetic technique

- In these older children, an IV induction is usual unless airway problems are anticipated.
- Airway management with an armoured LMA or south facing preformed (RAE) ETT. ETT indicated if costal cartilage is to be harvested for ear reconstruction.
- IPPV or SV as preferred.
- Maintenance with volatile in oxygen and air or nitrous oxide (avoid if costal cartilage is harvested—small risk of pneumothorax).
- There is a significant incidence of PONV after otoplasty. An antiemetic e.g. ondansetron 100 mcg/kg (max 4mg) IV should be given.
- Maintenance fluids. A 20 mL/kg bolus is often given to reduce the incidence of PONV.
- Analgesia is provided by some combination of:
  - Infiltration with local anaesthetic and adrenaline (also helps with haemostasis).
  - Greater auricular nerve block. 2 mL 0.5% bupivacaine ± adrenaline is injected superficially at the junction of the posterior body of sternocleidomastoid and a line drawn laterally from the superior border of the cricoid cartilage. The nerve (from superficial cervical plexus C3), becomes superficial at this point before running up to supply the external ear and mastoid. A useful block for otoplasty and mastoid surgery.
  - Opioid: morphine sulphate 100–150 mcg/kg, fentanyl citrate 2–4 mcg/kg IV or codeine phosphate 0.5–1 mg/kg IM. Opioid administration is weighed against the high incidence of PONV.
  - NSAID: e.g. diclofenac sodium 1 mg/kg rectally.
  - Paracetamol: 15 mg/kg IV or 40 mg/kg rectally.

Postoperative care

Usually straightforward. Maintenance fluids until drinking and PONV is not a problem. If PONV occurs a different antiemetic from that given in theatre is used. A combination of oral paracetamol, a NSAID and opioid e.g. codeine phosphate 1 mg/kg 4-hourly is prescribed for analgesia. CXR after costal cartilage harvest to exclude pneumothorax. There is a low incidence of postoperative haemorrhage requiring exploration. Straightforward otoplasty for prominent ears is often performed on a day case basis.

Cleft lip and palate

- Commonest congenital abnormalities of the orofacial structure. Embryologically, clefts arise because of failure of fusion or breakdown of fusion between the nasal and maxillary processes and the palatine shelves that form these structures at 6–8 weeks of gestation.
- They are a diverse and variable group of congenital abnormalities:
  - Cleft lip and palate occurs in 1:600 live births.
  - Isolated cleft palate occurs in 1:1000 live births.
  - More common in far Eastern populations.
  - Cleft lip alone (15%), cleft lip and palate (45%), and isolated cleft palate (40%).
  - ♂:♀ ratio is 2:1 for cleft lip and palate and 1:3 for isolated cleft palate.
  - Often occur as isolated deformities. Can be associated with other anomalies, especially isolated cleft palate.
- Cleft lip may be either unilateral (left > right, either side more common than bilateral) or bilateral and is frequently associated with cleft palate or clefts in the alveolus.
- Cleft palate ± cleft lip may be:
  - Submucous (occult) mildest form, no visible cleft, non-union of palatal muscles.
  - Incomplete—soft palate cleft.
  - Complete—soft and hard palate cleft. May include the alveolar portion of the maxilla. Increasing severity of cleft predicts ↑ risk of respiratory complications postoperatively.

Aetiology

Both genetic and environmental components.

- Cleft palate may be inherited as an autosomal dominant condition with variable penetrance. Family history in a first degree relative increases the risk by a factor of twenty.
- Environmental factors include maternal epilepsy, infection, drugs (steroids, benzodiazepines, anticonvulsants), and possibly folic acid deficiency.
- Cleft lip and palate occurs as part of over 100 syndromes including:
  - Pierre Robin sequence—cleft palate in 80%, retrognathia, posteriorly displaced tongue
  - Treacher Collins syndrome (cleft in 28%)
  - Klippel–Feil syndrome (cleft in 15%)
  - Stickler syndrome
  - Down's Syndrome
  - Hemifacial microsomia (Goldenhar)
  - Velocardiofacial syndrome
  - Stickler syndrome
  - Fetal alcohol syndrome.
- Associated with:
  - Congenital heart disease (5–10%)
  - Upper respiratory tract infection and chronic otitis media
  - Subglottic stenosis.

Treatment

- Cleft lip is usually repaired at 3 months which allows time for diagnosis of other congenital conditions.
- Type of repair depends on the extent of available tissue, and usually involves advancement of a mucosal flap. Complex repairs of bilateral cleft lip and nasal floor simultaneously are occasionally performed, sometimes requiring nasal stents that may cause airway obstruction.
- Cleft palate is repaired at 9–12 months (prior to speech development).
- Goals are cosmesis, normal speech, and normal dental development.
- Operation involves mobilization of lateral tissue to allow midline closure. This includes apposition of the levator palati muscles, which are required to elevate the soft palate, occluding the nasopharynx and preventing 'rhinolalia' (nasal speech).

Preoperative assessment

Associated conditions which may affect anaesthesia or airway management. If there is any evidence of recent or incipient respiratory infection the procedure is usually deferred since the airway may be marginal postoperatively. Chronic airway obstruction or obstructive sleep apnoea ↑ the risk of postoperative airway problems. Overnight arterial oxygen saturation is measured preoperatively. If episodes of hypoxia occur then referral for a formal sleep study may be made. There may be physiological anaemia at 3–6 months of age. Blood is grouped and saved although significant blood loss is rare.

Anaesthetic technique

- Sedative premedication is not usually given.
- Inhalational induction. Antisialogogue if desired.
- Endotracheal intubation is required. This is usually uneventful but occasionally techniques for management of the difficult airway and intubation are required (📖 Chapter 5). A south facing preformed ETT (RAE) is usually used.
- Throat pack for cleft lip repair.
- IPPV common but SV feasible depending on the anaesthetic technique and preference. Maintenance with volatile in oxygen and air or nitrous oxide. Remifentanil reduces volatile requirements and promotes rapid emergence from anaesthesia.
- Maintenance fluids. Volume replacement if required.
- Temperature maintenance is not usually a problem.
- For cleft palate repair:
  - A mouth gag is used. It is important to check for kinking or obstruction of the ETT while this is being positioned. Communication with surgeon to attain a mutually satisfactory position.
  - A roll or bolster may be placed under the shoulders to extend the neck and improve surgical access.
  - A tongue suture is sometimes placed to be used postoperatively to pull the tongue forward and relieve airway obstruction.

- 10% will develop some evidence of airway obstruction especially if the repair is tight or the palate has been lengthened. Surgeon may place a nasopharyngeal airway at the end of surgery.
- Gentle suction under direct vision is performed without damaging the repaired palate.
- Aim for smooth emergence and extubation. Crying and agitation may precipitate bleeding.
- Awake extubation.

Analgesia

Depends on anaesthetic and surgical preference and is provided by some combination of:

- Infiltration with LA and adrenaline (usually done to improve haemostasis).
- Opioid: morphine sulphate 100–150 mcg/kg, fentanyl citrate 2–4 mcg/kg IV or codeine phosphate 0.5–1 mg/kg IM.
- Infraorbital nerve block for cleft lip repair. The infraorbital nerve is a terminal branch of the trigeminal nerve. It supplies sensory innervation to the skin and mucous membrane of the upper lip and lower eyelid, the skin between them, and to the side of the nose. It lies halfway between the midpoint of the palpebral fissure and the angle of the mouth, approximately 7.5 mm from the side of the nose. The nerve is blocked by inserting a needle perpendicularly to the skin and advancing it until bony resistance is felt. The needle is then withdrawn slightly and 1–2 mL of 0.5% bupivacaine + 1:200000 adrenaline is injected after performing a negative aspiration test. The needle should not enter the infraorbital foramen.
- NSAID e.g. diclofenac sodium 1 mg/kg rectally.
- Paracetamol 15 mg/kg IV or 40 mg/kg rectally.

Postoperative care

Pulse oximetry without supplementary oxygen to detect airway obstruction. Maintenance fluids until feeding (often very early in the postoperative period). A combination of paracetamol, NSAID and codeine phosphate 1 mg/kg 4-hourly orally is usually prescribed. A low dose IV infusion of morphine sulphate (☐ Chapter 6) is used in an HDU setting in some centres. After palate repair, early postoperative complications include haemorrhage which may require exploration (rare) and upper airway obstruction. This may be due to upper airway narrowing, blood clot, tongue swelling from retraction by the mouth gag or inadequate mouth breathing. Airway obstruction may require a nasopharyngeal airway or endotracheal intubation and IPPV. Patients at high risk of postoperative airway obstruction e.g. severe Pierre Robin syndrome may be admitted to ITU intubated for ventilation for 24–48 hours until oedema and swelling have resolved.

Syndactyly

Congenital failure of fingers to separate. Can involve two or more fingers.
- It is 'complete' if fusion extends to the finger tips.
- It is 'complex if there is fusion of phalanges, 'simple' if not.
- Incidence 1:2500.
- ♂:♀ ratio 2:1.
- Can also affect toes.

Aetiology

- Failure of differentiation during first trimester.
- Family history in up to 50%.
- Apert's syndrome (craniosynostosis, midface hypoplasia, cleft palate, small nares, syndactyly, learning difficulties in 30%).
- Epidermolysis bullosa.
- Polydactyly.
- Poland syndrome (absence or underdevelopment of pectoralis muscle on one side plus syndactyly of the ipsilateral hand).

Treatment

Early repair around 12 months of age gives the best aesthetic and functional results.
- Several staged procedures are usually required for complex syndactyly.
- A full thickness graft is often necessary to cover defects and is usually taken from the thigh.
- Digits may be pinned to prevent contractures.
- Morbidity—scarring and contractures requiring revision, infection.

Preoperative assessment

Previous anaesthetic history. Presence of a syndrome especially Apert's that may present airway difficulties. Sedative premedication (unless airway problems) since children usually undergo a number of procedures for this and associated conditions.

Anaesthetic technique

- Inhalational induction is common. Patients are usually toddlers, venous access is difficult and in Apert's syndrome there may be a difficult airway.
- Airway management with a LMA or ETT. An ETT is preferable for longer complex cases.
- SV or IPPV are both appropriate.
- Maintenance of anaesthesia with volatile in oxygen and air or nitrous oxide.
- Tourniquet.

Analgesia

Options for analgesia are:
- Opioid: morphine sulphate 100–150 mcg/kg IV, fentanyl citrate 2–4 mcg/kg IV.
- Brachial plexus block (📖 Chapter 7) for complex procedures.
- In both cases a NSAID e.g. diclofenac sodium 1 mg/kg rectally improves the quality of analgesia.

Postoperative care

Maintenance fluids until drinking. A combination of paracetamol, a NSAID, and an oral opioid such as codeine phosphate 1 mg/kg 4-hourly is prescribed. A further general anaesthetic will probably be required about a week later for removal of sutures and change of dressing.

Free flap surgery

- Reconstructive free flap surgery is used for large wounds not amenable to linear (primary) closure.
  - It involves the transfer of free tissue flap (usually musculocutaneous possibly with bone) to a site of tissue loss where its circulation is restored with microvascular anastomoses.
  - A muscle flap produces a better appearance than a skin graft and provides a better defence against infection.
  - Flap surgery is uncommon in children. When necessary the defect is usually caused by trauma.
  - Flap success rate is better than in adults (better vessels, increased blood flow).
  - The principles of anaesthesia for flap reconstruction also apply to reimplantation surgery (digits or limbs).
- Surgery involves:
  - Elevation of the flap and clamping of vessels.
  - Primary ischaemia as blood flow ceases and intracellular metabolism becomes anaerobic.
  - Reperfusion as the arterial and venous anastomoses are completed and the clamps released. Ideally, re-establishment of blood flow reverses the transient physiological derangement produced by primary ischaemia.
  - Secondary ischaemia occurs after a free flap has been transplanted and reperfused. This period of ischaemia is more damaging to the flap than primary ischaemia. Flaps affected by secondary ischaemia have intravascular thrombosis and interstitial oedema. Local fibrinogen and platelet concentrations are ↑. Skin flaps can tolerate 10–12 hours of ischaemia but irreversible changes in muscle occur after 4 hours.
- Causes of flap failure:
  - The arterial anastomosis may be inadequate, in spasm, or thrombosed.
  - The venous anastomosis may also be defective, in spasm, thrombosed, or compressed.
  - Oedema reduces flow to the flap and may be a result of excessive crystalloids, extreme haemodilution, trauma from handling, or a prolonged ischaemia time. Flap tissue has no lymphatic drainage and is therefore susceptible to oedema.
- Surgery is prolonged (6–12 hours) with several incisions. There may be significant blood and fluid losses as well as heat loss. Hypovolaemia, vasoconstriction and hypothermia reduce blood flow to the flap and contribute to flap failure. Aim to provide the flap or reimplanted tissue with the best possible environment to re-establish blood supply. Optimum blood flow to the flap requires vasodilatation, a good perfusion pressure and low viscosity.
- Vasodilatation. Vessel radius is the most important determinant of flow to and within the flap. Adequate vasodilatation requires:
  - Normothermia. Hypothermia causes vasoconstriction and a rise in haematocrit and plasma viscosity.

- Normovolaemia or mild hypervolaemia. Vasoconstriction due to an under replacement of fluid losses may occur. Bleeding and insensible fluid losses occur at both the donor site and the recipient site. Modest hypervolaemia ↑ cardiac output, ↓ sympathetic vascular tone, and dilates the vessels to the flap.
- Spasm of the transplanted vessels may occur after surgical handling and local vasodilators such as papaverine may be applied by the surgeon.
- Sympathetic blockade. The ideal block for this is an epidural followed by a postoperative epidural infusion. Other advantages of epidural analgesia include a reduction in intraoperative bleeding and rapid postoperative recovery. Alternatives, depending on the recipient site, are brachial plexus block and interpleural block. Good analgesia reduces the level of circulating catecholamines and the vasoconstrictor response to pain.
- Perfusion pressure:
  - A good perfusion pressure is needed for flap survival.
  - Usually attained by adequate depth of anaesthesia and fluid administration.
- Viscosity:
  - Haemodilution to a haematocrit of 30% improves flow by reducing viscosity. Further reductions in haematocrit do not provide much more advantage.
  - If the haematocrit falls further, the marginally improved flow characteristics from a lower viscosity may be offset by a reduction in oxygen delivery.
- The end result is usually an anaesthetic incorporating regional and general anaesthesia. Regional block may be continued postoperatively as effective analgesia will help to prevent vasoconstriction of small vessels.

Preoperative assessment

Background to the surgical condition and previous experiences with anaesthesia and analgesia are important to know. The child is likely to have had several related procedures already. Presence of coexisting medical conditions. FBC, U&E, cross match. Sedative premedication is usually given.

Anaesthetic technique

- Induction as preferred.
- Endotracheal intubation and IPPV. Avoid hypocapnia which causes vasoconstriction.
- Maintenance with volatile in oxygen and air or nitrous oxide. Supplementation with remifentanil 0.25–0.5 mcg/kg/hour reduces volatile requirements and provides a mild degree of hypotension.
- Standard monitoring plus arterial line, central venous pressure, urine output and core and peripheral temperature.
- Arterial blood gases and haematocrit are measured throughout the case.

- If possible, an appropriate regional block to cover the recipient site and provide sympathetic block is performed.
- These are long procedures and great care in positioning limbs and joints and protection of pressure areas and corneas is required.
- As the flap is mobilized, moderate hypotension provides good operating conditions and reduces blood loss. Titrated volatile agent is ideal as it provides direct vasodilatation.
- Strict attention to fluid input is required. Maintenance fluids, replacement of insensible losses and replacement of bleeding should be considered. A haematocrit of around 30% is usually regarded as ideal, provided cardiac output is maintained. Excess fluid (especially crystalloid) will accumulate in the flap causing swelling and obstruction to venous drainage.
- Central and peripheral temperatures are monitored aiming for a difference of less than 2°C as an indication of a warm, well filled and vasodilated patient. Ambient theatre temperature is ↑ and a warming mattress, warming blanket, and fluid warmer are used.
- By the time the flap is reperfused, the patient should be normothermic, vasodilated and slightly hypervolaemic ('*warm and wet*') with a cardiac output higher than normal.
- Vasodilators or inotropes are rarely required.
- Smooth emergence prevents sympathetic stimulation and vasoconstriction.

Postoperative care

Maintenance fluids. Boluses of colloid, if required, to maintain CVP and urine output. Postoperatively frequent checks are performed on the flap. If nursing staff notice ischaemia or congestion in the flap early, it may be salvageable. Postoperative regional techniques are becoming more common. Epidural infusion analgesia (⌨ Chapter 6) is ideal for lower limb flap surgery. A combination of an epidural infusion of LA to provide analgesia and vasodilatation for the recipient site and an IV morphine infusion or PCA for the donor site may be required depending on the exact procedures performed.

Femoral nerve, fascia iliaca compartment or '3 in 1' nerve blocks (⌨ Chapter 7) can help with pain from donor sites on the thigh (skin is often harvested from here to cover muscle flaps). Paracetamol, a NSAID, and an antiemetic are also prescribed.

Oncology

- About 1500 new cases of childhood cancer are diagnosed each year in the UK. The risk for an individual child of being diagnosed before the age of 15 is about 1:500. (1:1600 for leukaemia, 1:2200 for CNS tumours and 1:1100 for all other cancers combined).
- Of all paediatric cancers, 30% are leukaemias (acute lymphoblastic leukaemia (ALL) and acute myeloid leukaemia (AML)), 20% involve the CNS, 7% are neuroblastomas, 6% non-Hodgkin's lymphoma, 6% Wilms' tumour (nephroblastoma) and 5% Hodgkin's lymphoma.
- Anaesthesia is frequently required for procedures such as tumour biopsy, tumour resection, vascular access devices, lumbar puncture, intrathecal chemotherapy, bone marrow aspiration and imaging during periods of extreme physiological and emotional stress for both parent and child.
- Significant input from anaesthetists is required for acute and chronic pain management and pain management during palliative care.
- Patients are immunosuppressed for much of the time and may not mount a typical response to infection. Presentation of infections may be subtle and atypical. Rectal drugs are avoided in case of bacteraemia.
- There is often a thrombocytopenia. IM injections are avoided and epidural and caudal injections require careful consideration.

Leukaemia

- ALL is the most common (80% of leukaemias and 25% of all childhood cancer). Highest incidence is around 2–3 years old. It is 30% more frequent in boys than in girls. AML comprises 15% and chronic myeloid leukaemia <4% of paediatric leukaemias.
- Clinically: lethargy, fever, malaise, signs of marrow failure (petechiae, pallor, and ecchymoses) and pain due to marrow infiltration. Anaemia, neutropenia, and thrombocytopenia may be present.
- Treatment: aims to treat symptoms and signs of the disease at presentation, treat the leukaemia and treat the complications of therapy. Three phases:
  - Induction (of remission): lasts approximately 4 weeks. There is a high rate of tumour cell death (tumour lysis syndrome).
  - Consolidation: involves additional prolonged treatment ± intrathecal chemotherapy ± cranial radiotherapy.
  - Maintenance: comprises pulses of chemotherapy (over two to three years) to continue remission, and eradicate the leukaemia.
- Survival: ALL 5 year survival is around 80%. Acute non-lymphocytic leukaemia is around 55% increasing to 67% with bone marrow transplantation.

CNS

- CNS tumours are the most common solid tumours in children (20%).
- Around 40% are astrocytomas (usually low grade) and medulloblastomas. Ependymomas and gliomas comprise most of the remainder.

- Clinical presentation: depends on the location of the tumour. Infratentorial tumours may present with signs of increased intracranial pressure (headache, nausea and vomiting, nystagmus, ataxia or cranial nerve lesions). Supratentorial lesions may present with seizures, hemiparesis, ↑ ICP.
- Treatment: includes surgery (biopsy, excision, debulking, shunt procedures for ↑ ICP), chemotherapy, radiotherapy and occasionally molecular or immunotherapy.

Lymphomas

- Lymphoma is the third most common malignancy in childhood.
- Non-Hodgkin's lymphoma comprises a diverse group of cancers arising from lymphocytes. It accounts for 60% of paediatric lymphomas, is twice as common in boys and the incidence remains constant between the ages of 3–14 years. Proliferation of immature lymphoid cells outside bone marrow is common.
  - 30% are T cell lymphoblastic lymphomas (very similar to ALL)
  - 50% are B cell lymphomas
  - 20% are large cell lymphomas whose origin can be from T cells, B cells or indeterminate.
  - T cell NHL tends to manifest in the anterior mediastinum and is associated with airway compression, pleural effusions and large vessel vascular compression (SVC syndrome).
  - B cell NHL manifests most commonly in the abdomen, leading to pain, distension, ascites and intestinal obstruction.
  - Treatment is similar to ALL. Remission in 90% of children. Five year survival is approximately 80%.
- Hodgkin's lymphoma is less common (5% of all childhood cancer).
  - The incidence rises from 2 years onwards to peak between 15–30 years old. Firm cervical or supraclavicular lymphadenopathy is typical (up to 60% will also have enlarged mediastinal nodes).
  - Staging 1 to 4 depends on the sites of lymphadenopathy (1 = single region, 2 = two regions on same side of diaphragm, 3 = spread across diaphragm, 4 = disseminated) plus 'A' for absence of symptoms or 'B' for presence (night sweats, fever, weight loss).
  - Treatment: comprises chemotherapy and radiotherapy.
  - Survival: depends on grading. 5-year survival in Grade 1A is 90–95%; grade 4 is 65%.

Chemotherapy

- All chemotherapy agents have adverse effects.
- Anthracyclines (doxorubicin) causes cardiac side effects including: acute atrial and ventricular dysrhythmias and cardiac failure (with long-term use in conjunction with other chemotherapy agents). Bleomycin can cause interstitial pneumonitis and fibrosis. Cisplatin is nephrotoxic.
- Mucositis. Chemotherapy induced oral mucositis (erythema, oedema, atrophy and ulceration of the oral mucosa) develops to some extent in 40% of children on treatment In those being prepared for haemopoietic stem cell transplant it may be as high as 75%. Mucositis is often reported as the most debilitating aspect of treatment. It may extend through the entire GI tract.

- Treatment: cautious oral debridement, decontamination (nystatin, clotrimazole, chlorhexidine), prevention of trauma and bleeding (maintain platelets > 20000/mm^3).
- Pain management: oral care and rinses will help. Many children will require parenteral opioid infusions, NCA or PCA. Adjuncts should be added with care but may include ketamine, gabapentin, and clonidine. NSAIDs are relatively contraindicated (GI erosion, effects on platelets).

- Tumour lysis syndrome occurs during the initial induction phase of chemotherapy (especially the first 5 days). Lysis of tumour cells releases the intracellular contents into the circulation – ↑ K$^+$, ↑ PO$_4$, ↑ uric acid. Precipitation of uric acid and calcium phosphate in renal tubules may cause renal impairment. ↓ Ca^{2+} (bound with phosphate) → tetany. Hyperkalaemia → cardiac dysrhythmias. Treatment involves maintaining hydration, allopurinol, and diuretics.

Lumbar puncture, intrathecal drugs, bone marrow aspiration, and trephines

- Oncology and haematology patients undergo many invasive procedures over a number of years.
- Lumbar puncture may be diagnostic or therapeutic. Performed during the induction and consolidation phases of chemotherapy.
- Many children will tolerate, and some prefer, conscious sedation (provided by non-anaesthetists in some centres, using midazolam, ketamine or propofol) rather than general anaesthesia.

Preoperative assessment

Examine the child for evidence of toxic side effects:
- Cardiac: cyclosphosphamide, adriamycin, doxorubicin (dysrhythmias, cardiac failure), radiation (cardiomyopathy).
- Respiratory: respiratory tract infection is common (fever may not be evident), bleomycin, cyclophosphamide, methotrexate (pulmonary toxicity).

Most children and parents have a preference for the method of induction and this should be used unless there is a clinical contraindication. FBC ± U&E are checked preoperatively. In leukaemia, a normal platelet count may not mean normal function. There is no consensus as to a safe level for lumbar puncture. If less than $<50000/mm^3$, a platelet infusion may be needed before lumbar puncture.

Anaesthetic technique

- Induction can be inhalational or IV as preferred by the child.
- Patients frequently have indwelling vascular access (Hickman, portacath, or a peripherally inserted central line). An aseptic non-touch technique should be used when handling these devices for induction of anaesthesia. For anything other than a brief procedure a peripheral cannula is inserted to reduce handling of the indwelling venous access. If an indwelling central line is accessed it must be flushed with the locally agreed heparin solution to maintain patency.
- The airway is usually maintained by face mask or LMA. Maintenance of anaesthesia is with volatile in oxygen and air or nitrous oxide.
- Lumbar puncture is performed by oncology staff. The anaesthetist should not be involved as both operator and anaesthetist. Anaesthetists do not perform intrathecal injections of chemotherapeutic drugs. There is a local register of staff permitted to prescribe, check, and administer intrathecal chemotherapy drugs and procedures to avoid incorrect administration. Fatalities have occurred after errors in this field e.g. intrathecal vincristine and only staff on the register should be involved in the process.
- Intrathecal drugs: cytarabine, methotrexate, thiotepa, gentamicin, vancomycin and hydrocortisone may be given intrathecally.

- Antiemetic e.g. ondansetron 100 mcg/kg (max 4mg) IV if intrathecal chemotherapy is given.
- Bone marrow aspirates and bone trephines are usually taken from posterior superior iliac region with the patient lateral or semi-prone. Postoperative pain is moderate. LA can be infiltrated at the aspiration sites.

Postoperative care

The anaesthetic and procedure usually have little effect on the child. If the child is newly presented and unwell the postoperative care is determined by the clinical condition. Patients receiving maintenance therapy are treated as day cases. There is an incidence of post lumbar puncture headache, especially in older children, which may require a period of bed rest and regular oral analgesics.

Insertion of Portacath or Hickman line

- Patients for insertion of long-term vascular access usually have a severe chronic illness that requires repeated IV administration of drugs, fluids, or other supportive therapy.
- The biggest groups are patients with cancer requiring chemotherapy and intestinal failure requiring parenteral nutrition. Haemophiliacs usually have a portacath inserted for daily administration of factors at home.
- Hickman lines have a cuff at the skin exit site that helps secure the catheter and acts as a barrier to infection.
- Portacaths are connected to an access device called a port. The port comprises a chamber with a metal base plate and a hub or dome with a silicone membrane. This is implanted subcutaneously and accessed percutaneously by puncturing the overlying skin with a Gripper® device or Huber point needle (non-coring so little damage is caused to the membrane) for administration of drugs and fluids or sampling.
- Fully implanted devices (portacaths) have a lower rate of infection.
- The commonest site is an internal jugular vein accessed directly or via the external jugular. Subclavian veins are occasionally used but other sites are rare.
- Insertion is performed in theatre using fluoroscopic guidance.
- Insertion in children is usually performed as an open procedure with two incisions—one over the vein being used and one in the axilla or on the anterior chest wall. The catheter is tunnelled subcutaneously between the two and either implanted subcutaneously (Portacath) or brought out externally (Hickman).
- A percutaneous technique can be used with ultrasound guidance. Pneumothorax (1–2%) and arterial puncture (6%) are risks of the percutaneous technique.
- Many children undergo multiple procedures because of changes in their clinical condition or loss of catheters to infection (25%), thrombosis, wound infections (15%), or systemic bacterial or yeast infections that colonize the catheters.

Preoperative assessment

Patients range from very fit with minimal anaesthetic problems e.g. haemophiliac boy having a portacath inserted for administration of factors at home to near moribund with a complex disease and multiple organ impairment. Clotting is checked in patients at risk of a coagulopathy. Platelets need to be adequate in patients receiving chemotherapy. Haemophiliacs need cover with recombinant factor VIII as advised by haematology (🔲 pp.544–545).

Anaesthetic technique

- IV or inhalational induction depending on clinical state and venous access. May have an IV cannula *in situ*.
- Endotracheal intubation with IPPV is the commonest technique. A LMA and SV are appropriate in well older children.
- Maintenance is with volatile in oxygen and air or nitrous oxide. Nitrous is contraindicated for percutaneous procedures because of the risk of pneumothorax.
- Patients are positioned in the Trendelenberg position with the head turned to the side away from the access site ($\downarrow$ FRC, $\downarrow$ compliance). May require IPPV especially in infants.
- The main intraoperative complication is bleeding from the venotomy that can be difficult to control.

Analgesia

- Infiltration of wounds with 0.25% or 0.5% bupivacaine depending on patient weight and maximum dose. An opioid is often required (morphine sulphate 100–150 mcg/kg or fentanyl citrate 2–4 mcg/kg) particularly for a portacath where there is dissection down to the rib cage to find a firm surface for the base plate of the port. NSAIDs are usually relatively contraindicated because of the underlying condition.

Postoperative care

Largely determined by the underlying condition—fluids, oxygen etc. For analgesia, a combination of paracetamol 15 mg/kg oral 4-hourly and codeine phosphate 1 mg/kg 4-hourly oral is commonly used.

Bone marrow harvest

- Performed to obtain stem cells which can be transfused (bone marrow transplant) as treatment for:
  - Haematological tumours (leukaemia, Hodgkin's lymphoma).
  - Solid tumours (Wilms', retinoblastoma, neuroblastoma).
  - Fanconi syndrome (marrow failure).
- Bone marrow (autologous from the patient or allogenic from a suitable donor) is harvested, frozen, stored and then reinfused (after high dose chemotherapy) to re-establish cell production.

Preoperative assessment

For an autologous harvest, the patient must be well enough to be anaesthetized safely and undergo the procedure. FBC, U&E results must be acceptable and cardiac and respiratory function good enough. For allogenic donation consent from adults is straightforward. When the donor is a child (often a sibling of the patient) there is the ethical quandary of exposing the donor child to risk with no personal benefit in order to treat another child.

Anaesthetic technique

- A harvest is usually performed in the prone position. May take 60–90 min.
- ETT and IPPV are the norm.
- Maintenance of anaesthesia is with volatile in oxygen and air or nitrous oxide.
- A bone marrow harvest is extensive (up to 10% of patients marrow) and may render the donor hypovolaemic and anaemic. Fluid replacement is required. If blood transfusion is required this must be delayed until the harvest is complete or harvested marrow will be contaminated with transfused red cells.
- Multiple punctures are made and analgesia is required—morphine sulphate 100–150 mcg/kg IV or fentanyl citrate 2–4 mcg/kg IV as well as an antiemetic such as ondansetron 100 mcg/kg IV.

Postoperative care

IV fluids until oral intake resumes. Oral analgesia—paracetamol 15 mg/kg 6-hourly and codeine phosphate 1 mg/kg 4-hourly with a NSAID if no contraindications.

Wilms' tumour (nephroblastoma)

The most common intra-abdominal malignant tumour in children:

- Incidence is 0.8:100000.
- Makes up 6–8% of paediatric solid tumours.
- Mean age at presentation is 3.5 years and 90% present before 8 years of age.

Aetiology

- Sporadic gene mutations account for 90%.
- 1.5% of cases are familial.
- 10% are associated with syndromes e.g. Beckwith–Weidemann, isolated hemihypertrophy, Trisomy 18, Denys–Drash, WAGR (Wilms', aniridia, GU malformation, mental retardation).

Presentation

Presents most often as a painless mass in the abdomen or flank. There may also be:

- Pain
- Haematuria (30%) → anaemia
- Fever
- Anorexia
- Nausea and vomiting
- Hypertension in 50% of cases (↑ renin produced by renal cortex trapped within tumour or compressed adjacent to it, acts on angiotensinogen → angiotensin I → (converted in lungs) angiotensin II → vasoconstriction and polydypsia → hypertension).

Investigations

- Abdominal ultrasound.
- CT or MRI of abdomen and chest to look for pulmonary metastases, IVC, or atrial thrombosis or vascular extension of tumour).

Treatment

- Treatment is surgical resection and staging followed by chemotherapy ± radiotherapy. Preoperative chemotherapy is only given where masses are bilateral, unresectable or have vascular extension.
- Staging is carried out during laparotomy and resection.
  - Stage I: limited to kidney, completely resected (~45%).
  - Stage II: extra renal extension, completely resected (~25%).
  - Stage III: residual non-haematogenous tumour, confined to abdomen (or stage II with intraoperative capsule rupture or tumour spillage) (~25%).
  - Stage IV: haematogenous metastasis (~10%).
  - Stage V: bilateral tumours (~5%).
- Staging and histology determines the chemotherapy regimen.
  - Stages I and II with favourable histology: 18 weeks of vincristine and actinomycin D.
  - Stage II unfavourable (anaplastic) histology and stage III: 24 weeks of vincristine, actinomycin D, and doxorubicin (cardiotoxic).

- Stage IV: chemotherapy + radiotherapy to abdomen ± chest.
  - Stages II to IV (with poorest histology): 24 weeks vincristine, doxorubicin, cyclophosphamide and etoposide + radiotherapy.
- Cure rate in stage I disease is >85%. For other stages outcome is dependent on staging and histology.
- 5% are bilateral (each is staged independently). After initial staging and 6–8 weeks of chemotherapy to shrink tumours (one side may disappear completely), a definitive operation is performed aiming for resection of the tumour with minimal loss of function. 5-year survival is 70% (and there is an incidence of renal failure).

Preoperative assessment

Preoperative evaluation includes chemotherapy history (if any), sites of previous vascular access, renal function, FBC, coagulation screen (up to 10% have an acquired von Willebrand's disease with platelet dysfunction and coagulopathy) and cross match. Polycythaemia is occasionally seen due to ↑ erythropoietin. ACE inhibitors (captopril), and the angiotensin II antagonist, saralasin may be used preoperatively to treat hypertension. If coagulopathy from acquired von Willebrand's disease is present preoperatively then cryoprecipitate and/or FFP are given according to haematological advice. The results of CT and, in the case of IVC or atrial extension, angiography and an echocardiogram are reviewed. Discuss postoperative care and analgesia with the parents. Sedative premedication if the child is anxious.

Anaesthetic technique

- In most cases an IV induction is possible. Some anaesthetists perform a rapid sequence induction because of the large upper abdominal mass.
- Endotracheal intubation and IPPV are necessary. A nasogastric tube is passed.
- Maintenance is with volatile in oxygen an air. An infusion of remifentanil 0.1–0.25 mcg/kg/min reduces volatile requirements and helps maintain cardiovascular stability.
- Two wide bore peripheral IV cannulae are required, in the upper limbs if possible. IVC compression from the tumour mass or surgical manipulation may reduce venous return. In most cases an arterial line and central venous line are inserted. Blood pressure is often labile during surgery due to contracted intravascular volume, left ventricular hypertrophy (LVH) and IVC compression (acute hypertension during handling of the tumour is not common).
- Blood loss is usually replaced with colloid and blood transfused if necessary.
- This may be lengthy abdominal (retroperitoneal) surgery. Meticulous thermoregulation and fluid balance is essential. A warming mattress, warming blanket, and fluid warmer should be used and central temperature monitored.

- Analgesia is best provided, in the absence of contraindications, by a thoracic epidural. The incision is transverse across the upper abdomen so the contralateral kidney can be examined). Epidural veins are often dilated by IVC compression but the benefits of an epidural are usually considered to outweigh the risks. Alternatively, a bolus of morphine sulphate 100–150 mcg/kg should be given before the end of surgery and, if necessary, more given in the recovery area until the child is pain free. NSAIDs are not used in view of the significant blood loss and potential renal impairment.
- Intravascular extension (renal vein, IVC, right atrium) has no effect on survival but may require cardiopulmonary bypass for resection. Assessment is by preoperative CT, angiography and echocardiogram. Preoperative chemotherapy will shrink the tumour and reduces operative complications.
- Hypertension that is labile or severe (similar situation to phaeochromocytoma and neuroblastoma with contraction of intravascular volume and LVH) may require intraoperative phenoxybenzamine, phentolamine or sodium nitroprusside to control.

Postoperative care

Patient usually nursed in HDU. Oxygen may be required because of splinting of the diaphragm. FBC and U&E are checked. Maintenance fluids plus colloid or blood (depending on haemoglobin) if required to maintain fluid balance and urine output. An epidural infusion of LA plus opioid or an IV infusion of morphine sulphate (📖 Chapter 6) is usually required for 48 hours. Regular paracetamol can be prescribed but NSAIDs are avoided. Blood pressure may take several weeks to return to normal.

Neuroblastoma

- Malignancy of primitive neural crest cells from the adrenal medulla and sympathetic ganglia.
- Most common malignant neoplasm in children <1 year old.
- Accounts for 7% of all paediatric cancers, 15% of cancer deaths in children.
- Over >70% are abdominal, 20% thoracic, 5% cervical. Of the abdominal tumours, one-third arise from the retroperitoneal sympathetic chain and two-thirds from the adrenal medulla.
- 50% are diagnosed at <2 years of age and 75% <4 years.

Aetiology

- Usually caused by a sporadic gene mutation.
- 1 to 2% are familial.

Presentation

- Abdominal mass with CT evidence of calcification and necrosis in 85%, abdominal pain.
- Hypertension (compression of renal vasculature or direct secretion of catecholamines).
- Diarrhoea (secretion of vasoactive intestinal peptide).
- Respiratory distress (5% of posterior mediastinal masses cause tracheal compression or deviation).
- Thoracic or abdominal tumours may invade the epidural space causing back pain or spinal cord compression.
- Metastases are present in >50% at diagnosis. Tend to invade surrounding structures (nephroblastoma and hepatoblastoma tend to grow without local invasion, compressing neighbouring tissue).
- Associated with von-Recklinghausen's neurofibromatosis, Hirschsprung's disease, and Ondine's curse (central failure of ventilation).

Investigations

- MRI.
- Neuroblastomas produce catecholamines in 85% of cases. Detected in urine (24-hour collection) as vanillylmandelic acid (VMA) and homovanillic acid HVA.
- mIBG (meta-iodo-benzyl guanidine) scan.
- Excess catecholamine exposure may induce cardiomyopathy, LVH and cardiac failure. Full cardiac assessment is required including echocardiography.

Treatment

- Surgery is for localized tumours without distant metastases. Postoperative chemotherapy if unfavourable histology.
- For tumours that have spread resection is delayed until after chemotherapy to shrink the tumour. Common chemotherapeutic agents include: doxorubicin (cardiac dysrhythmias, acute cardiomyopathy), cisplatin, cyclophosphamide, and etopside.
- Radiotherapy for disseminated disease.

- Staging
  - Stage I: localized tumour, completely excised.
  - Stage IIA: localized tumour, incompletely excised.
  - Stage IIB: localized tumour, incompletely excised, local lymph nodes.
  - Stage III: tumour crosses midline, regional bilateral nodes.
  - Stage IV: distant metastases.
  - Stage IVS: <1 year old, localized tumour, metastasized to liver, skin, or marrow.
- Cure rate >80–90% for localized tumours which are fully resected. Much lower for metastatic disease unless age <1year.

Preoperative assessment

Preoperative evaluation includes chemotherapy history, sites of previous vascular access, renal function, FBC, U&E, cross match. There may be airway compression with posterior mediastinal masses. Preoperative blood pressure control and plasma expansion as indicated. Preoperative control of blood pressure allows re-expansion of the intravascular compartment, can reverse catecholamine induced myocardial dysfunction; and reduces the incidence and severity of intraoperative hypertensive events (see 📖 phaeochromocytoma, p.341 for blood pressure management).

Although hypertension is common at presentation, intraoperative hypertensive crises during tumour manipulation are rare when compared to phaeochromocytoma (relatively fewer intracellular catecholamine storage granules, a mix of cholinergic and adrenergic cells in the tumour and a relative lack of the enzymes necessary to convert dopamine to noradrenaline and noradrenaline to adrenaline in neuroblastoma cells). However, surges in blood pressure can occur. Discussion of postoperative care and analgesia.

Anaesthetic technique
- Similar to nephroblastoma and phaeochromocytoma.
- Endotracheal intubation and IPPV. Nasogastric tube.
- Maintenance is with volatile in oxygen an air. An infusion of remifentanil 0.1–0.25 mcg/kg/min reduces volatile requirements and helps maintain cardiovascular stability.
- Two wide bore peripheral IV cannulae.
- In most cases an arterial line and central venous line are inserted. Blood pressure is sometimes labile during surgery (similar situation to phaeochromocytoma and nephroblastoma with contraction of intravascular volume and LVH). May require intraoperative phenoxybenzamine, phentolamine or sodium nitroprusside to control.
- Meticulous thermoregulation and fluid balance. Measure central temperature. Use a warming mattress, warming blanket, and fluid warmer.
- For abdominal tumours, analgesia is best provided by a thoracic epidural unless there are contraindications. Alternatively, a bolus of morphine sulphate 100–150 mcg/kg should be given before the end of surgery and, if necessary, more given in the recovery area until the child is pain free. NSAIDs if no contraindications.

Postoperative care

Patient usually nursed in HDU. Oxygen may be required because of splinting of the diaphragm. FBC and U&E are checked. Maintenance fluids plus colloid or blood (depending on haemoglobin) if required to maintain fluid balance and urine output. An epidural infusion of LA plus opioid or an IV infusion of morphine sulphate (📖 Chapter 6) is usually required for 48 hours. Regular paracetamol can be prescribed. NSAIDs if no contraindications.

Phaeochromocytoma

- These tumours arise from chromaffin tissue of the adrenal medulla and the sympathetic ganglia (around aortic bifurcation, GI tract, bladder, and in the chest).
  - If functional, they can secrete large amounts of noradrenaline, adrenaline, and dopamine.
  - Rare: 2–8 cases per million population per annum.
  - 5–10% occur in children. Most cases in children occur in teenagers, very rare under 8 years of age.
  - ♂:♀ ratio 2:1.
- In children, compared with adults:
  - Malignancy is less common.
  - Bilateral and extra-renal or multiple sites are more common.
  - Noradrenaline is the predominant catecholamine in most cases.
  - There is an increased incidence of MEN (multiple endocrine neoplasia). MEN includes hyperparathyroidism, medullary carcinoma of thyroid and phaeochromocytoma.
  - Associated with neurofibromatosis and tuberous sclerosis.

Presentation

Presentation is essentially with symptoms of sympathetic overdrive:
- Nausea, vomiting.
- Fatigue.
- Abdominal pain.
- Sweating.
- Headaches.
- Palpitations.
- A hypertensive crisis may occur with possible cerebrovascular haemorrhage, pulmonary oedema or cardiac failure.

Investigations

- 24 hour urine collection for the metabolites of catecholamines– vanillylmandelic acid (VMA) and homovanillic acid (HVA). Collection and analysis must conform to strict protocols. False negatives can occur.
- CT (95% accuracy) and/or MRI (99% accuracy) are used to locate tumours and plan resection.
- mIBG scan can also be used (radiolabelled isotope taken up into neural cells – 80% sensitivity).

Treatment

- Treatment is surgical removal. Laparoscopic phaeochromocytoma excision is becoming common and is associated with less surgical stimulation and better postoperative recovery than open surgery.

Preoperative management

Assessment of the extent of end-organ hypertensive damage. Cardiac effects include LVH, cardiomyopathy (dilated or obstructive), dysrhythmias, ischaemia, and heart failure. ECG and echocardiogram required. Cardiac dysfunction precludes the use of perioperative beta blockers (negative inotropic effects—pulmonary oedema, hypotension). Cardiac dysfunction is usually reversible and treatment reduces intraoperative morbidity and overall mortality. There may also be pulmonary oedema, renal impairment, biochemical changes ($\uparrow$ Ca^{2+} (hyperparathyroidism), $\downarrow$ K^+ ($\uparrow$ renin $\rightarrow$ secondary hyperaldosteronism), hyperglycaemia (alpha receptor stimulation in pancreas $\rightarrow$ $\downarrow$ insulin).

Preoperative preparation for surgery requires alpha receptor blockade to reverse the effects of excess catecholamines. Phenoxybenzamine, a selective alpha$_1$ antagonist (some alpha$_2$ blockade), forms a non-competitive alkylated bond with the receptor. It is long acting and so can act into the postoperative period resulting in resistant hypotension (until new alpha receptors are produced). Children are started at 0.25–1.0 mg/kg/day orally and this is increased until control is achieved (may take weeks). Criteria for adequate blockade include normal blood pressure, orthostatic hypotension and a fall in haematocrit of around 5% due to plasma expansion. Beta blockers to treat reflex tachycardia from unopposed alpha blockade are rarely needed in children. Preoperative alpha receptor blockade has reduced mortality from phaeochromocytoma from 50% to 3%.

Anaesthetic technique

- Should minimize adrenergic responses and catecholamine release.
- Sedative premedication e.g. midazolam 0.5 mg/kg oral maximum 20 mg.
- IV induction in older children.
- Endotracheal intubation and IPPV. The larynx is often sprayed with lidocaine 1% and a bolus of remifentanil (0.1–1 mcg/kg) or fentanyl (1–2 mcg/kg) given to attenuate the pressor response to laryngoscopy.
- Two wide gauge IV cannulae.
- Maintenance with volatile in oxygen and air or nitrous oxide. Ensure adequate depth of anaesthesia prior to patient positioning, incision etc. Remifentanil 0.1–0.25 mcg/kg/min helps provide cardiovascular stability.
- Standard monitoring plus arterial line, central venous line, urine output, and temperature.
- For open procedures a thoracic epidural provides good analgesia but will not prevent release of catecholamines during handling of the tumour. For laparoscopic procedures a bolus of opioid is given towards the end of surgery if an infusion of remifentanil is used or at the start if not.

- Intraoperatively unpredictable swings in blood pressure may occur. Volatile anaesthetics provide a rapidly titratable vasodilator effect. Short acting vasodilators and pressors (once the adrenal vein is ligated, there may be a precipitous fall in blood pressure) should be available. Most commonly used are:
  - Sodium nitroprusside: 0.5–4 mcg/kg/minute is a direct vasodilator with quick onset and offset. Tachyphylaxis and cyanide toxicity (only if rate >10 mcg/kg/min) are possible problems.
  - Phentolamine: 5–50 mcg/kg/min is a short acting alpha antagonist. Tachycardia and tachyphylaxis occur.
  - Esmolol: 0.5 mg/kg over 1 min or 25–200 mcg/kg/min is a short acting beta-blocker.
  - Magnesium sulphate: up to 50 mg/kg reduces catecholamine release from the adrenal medulla and sympathetic nerve endings, blocks adrenergic receptors, has direct vasodilator effect, and is an antidysrhythmic.
  - Hypotension after tumour removal should be treated with fluid boluses initially. If required
  - Phenylephrine: 2–10 mcg/kg is an alpha agonist.
  - Noradrenaline: 0.02–0.1 mcg/kg/min or 20–100 nanograms/kg/min.
- Measure glucose hourly until the adrenal vein is ligated then more often.

Postoperative care

Patient nursed in HDU. FBC and U&E are checked. Maintenance fluids plus colloid if required to maintain fluid balance and urine output. Hypotension may be due to bleeding or residual alpha blockade from the preoperative period. May be transient hypoglycaemia so glucose is monitored regularly and 10% dextrose infused if necessary. An epidural infusion of LA plus opioid or an IV infusion of morphine sulphate (📖 Chapter 6) is usually required for 48 hours after open surgery. Morphine infusion or PCA overnight for laparoscopic procedures. Regular paracetamol can be prescribed and a NSAID if no contraindication. Patients may remain hypertensive for several weeks. Laparoscopic procedures are associated with faster resumption of feeding and discharge.

Radiotherapy

- Anaesthesia for radiotherapy is usually requested for children up to 5 or 6 years of age who will be unable to lie still and tolerate the planning preparation and execution of radiotherapy.
- Indications:
  - Leukaemia: ALL and AML
  - Wilms' tumour, neuroblastoma, retinoblastoma.
  - CNS tumours.
  - Others.
- Usually daily treatments for several weeks (6 weeks is not uncommon).
- The child's clinical condition may change during the course of treatment. Side effects of radiotherapy will develop—hair loss, skin damage, nausea, fatigue. There may be intercurrent problems, especially respiratory infections or psychological effects of daily fasting and anaesthesia.
- Takes place in a remote site, often in another hospital, almost always with limited facilities for induction, maintenance, and recovery from anaesthesia.
- Issues of patients and staff transport.
- Usually a logistical problem and a drain on the anaesthetic department.
- Patient must be left alone in radiotherapy room while being treated—cameras to observe patient and monitor.
- Anaesthesia is required for planning and simulation and then treatments.
  - Actual treatments are usually fairly short—each field to be irradiated may only be exposed for 30–90 sec.
  - Prior to therapy, the fields are marked after plotting. The usual sequence involves constructing a unique plastic 'shell' from a plaster cast of the region of the body to be treated, upon which marks are made to guide the focused radiation beam. This can be used repeatedly, and can also be used in conjunction with imaging to simulate the radiotherapy prior to actual exposure.
  - Simulation: numerous images of the tumour and surrounding tissue are used to form a 3D 'model' of the patient's anatomy (usually computer based). This can be used to ascertain the best approach to the tumour, with minimal injury to surrounding organs and tissue. Different approaches can be tried, until a plan is constructed for actual radiotherapy.

Anaesthetic technique

- Preferably done as first case in morning to minimize disruption to the child caused by fasting, disruption to radiotherapy suite activity, and disruption to anaesthetic activity.
- Anaesthetic machine usually uses cylinders rather than piped gases and because it is in a remote location there may be limited stocks of drugs and equipment. Appropriate checks are performed.
- Patients have a Hickman line or portacath with Gripper® needle in place.

- May arrive from home once the routine is established. Alternatively, transported from the oncology ward.
- Induction is usually IV. Inhalational if preferred.
- Almost always a LMA is used with SV and maintenance in oxygen and volatile. 100% oxygen preferred in case of an airway or ventilation problem during treatment while the anesthetist is remote from the child. TIVA is an alternative technique.
- Analgesia not required.
- Once recovered, the child eats and is often discharged straight home.

Radiology

- Anaesthesia for imaging often takes place in a suite where anaesthesia was 'designed in' with piped gases, induction and recovery areas, integrated monitors, and modern anaesthetic machines designed for use in a radiology setting e.g. elective MR lists.
- Many elective scans are performed in sedated patients (📖 Chapter 16) without the involvement of an anaesthetist.
- Occasionally an unusual investigation is required in an unfamiliar setting with less ideal equipment and radiology staff who do not normally work with anaesthetized children. This combines the challenges of working in a site remote from theatre (unfamiliar equipment, personnel, and room layout) and a complex patient population. In these situations good communication with radiology staff is essential.
    - Planned procedure.
    - Duration.
    - Patient position—supine/prone/lateral?
    - Is the patient anaesthetized in one location then transferred to another room?
    - Will the patient be moved during procedure?
    - Is the patient airway and IV cannula accessible while scanning?
    - Head first or feet first into scanner?
    - What is being done? Risks and complications? Stimulating or non-invasive? Will contrast or heparin be used? Will you be asked to administer it?
    - What are the likely sequelae of the procedure—PONV, pain, bleeding from puncture or biopsy site, CVS, or respiratory complications, anaphylactoid or anaphylactic reactions to contrast solutions.
    - Oxygen is often supplied from a cylinder—have a spare.
    - Suction is dedicated for anaesthetic use.
    - A resuscitation trolley and defibrillator is present and that the drill for extricating the child in an emergency is known.
    - In the event of a cardiac arrest removing the patient to the induction room is usually preferable—be familiar with protocol.
    - Do not let the resuscitation team into the MRI room.

Staff

Require anaesthetic assistance and recovery nurse as for all other general anaesthetics. Radiology staff may need to help to move larger children on and off scan table.

Equipment

For induction, maintenance and recovery must meet appropriate standards and be familiar to the anaesthetist and assistants.

Patients

- Assessment and examination should be as for any general anaesthetic, paying special attention to syndromes and concomitant illnesses.
- Patients for investigation of CNS pathology are common and frequently have associated CVS or respiratory conditions. Assess the airway with care.

Radiation

- With most modern equipment (shielded and coned) there is negligible radiation exposure >2 m from the source.
- However, all personnel should take precautions to minimize total exposure, wearing a lead apron, thyroid shield, and an exposure badge if exposure is frequent. Take advice from the radiographers.
- If possible (and the patient is appropriately monitored) leave the immediate vicinity and observe from behind leaded glass screen. Protect the patient from unnecessary exposure (testis, ovaries, thyroid and eyes).

Patient access

- Limited space, immovable tables and equipment, dark rooms, and numerous staff can make it impossible to position anaesthetic equipment close to the patient.
- Long ventilation tubing and IV lines are easily caught or dislodged.
- Ask the radiographer to do a trial run with the table into the scanner so that the extra 'slack' required can be ascertained.

Temperature

- Radiology suites often contain superconductors (MRI), which require cooling. Measure patient temperature for all but the briefest scans.
- Warming blankets can interfere with imaging.

Contrast media

Iodinated contrast media are frequently administered during a scan to enhance the images obtained. Occasional side effects:

- Dose dependent reactions. Due to the physicochemical properties of the agent and include heat, pain, vasodilatation, cardiac depression and hypotension.
- Dose independent reactions. Nausea and vomiting, hypersensitivity reactions—minor (flushing, nausea and vomiting, pruritis, urticaria, arm pain); moderate (severe urticaria, facial oedema, hypotension, bronchospasm); severe (shock, laryngeal oedema, convulsions, cardiac arrest). Most reactions are minor. Moderate reactions are seen in 1% of contrast administrations and severe reactions occur in 0.1% (history of atopy doubles the incidence). Most reactions are anaphylactoid and true anaphylaxis with contrast media is rare. Mortality rate is 1:75000. Adverse reactions may be less common with low osmolar media, which should also be used in all intra-arterial injections (less pain).

Computed tomography (CT)

- A rotating X-ray emitter and detector provide images taken at numerous different angles such that a 2D image of a thin cross-sectional slice of the body is produced.
- Structures of differing densities (bone and muscle) within the body are clearly separated, while those of similar densities are less well differentiated.
- Quick—head scans are often produced in <30 sec. Modern 'spiral' CT machines are very quick, but so is the table movement. Check the full extent of movement that the patient will experience during the scan and ensure that the anaesthetic circuit and IV extensions are long enough.
- No restriction on type of anaesthetic and monitoring equipment.
- Relatively large doses of radiation are used. If possible monitor from the control room.
- Patients for CT under general anaesthesia range from well infants with a congenital cystic adenoidal malformation of the lungs who are fasted and scanned electively to trauma patients who are undergoing resuscitation during the scan.
- Access to the head and airway is limited, especially for head scans. Ensure a secure airway prior to scanning.
- Keep IV sites visible and accessible.
- Keep metallic leads (ECG cables etc) away from the site of the scan since they cause interference
- Ensure adequate staff for a controlled transfer from trolley to scan table.
- Discuss positioning and use of contrast before scan, so that the dose can be decided, method of administration, note allergies to iodine.

Anaesthetic technique

- Many elective CT cases are infants and inhalational induction is often easier than IV.
- A LMA is sometimes appropriate for airway management. In many cases an ETT is preferable either because the child is small and access is limited or because they are undergoing a CT of the thorax and the radiographers will request that the child is rendered apnoeic in inspiration for short periods of time. This is easier with an ETT in a paralysed patient.
- Maintenance either with volatile in oxygen and air or nitrous oxide or with a propofol infusion. Syringe pumps are small, lightweight, and can usually be placed on the scan table with the patient and monitor if required.
- Emergency cases with a head injury and reduced level of consciousness require an IV rapid sequence induction.

Postoperative care

Elective cases usually recover rapidly, feed and are discharged within 1–2 hours. Emergency cases go to theatre, ITU, or HDU depending on the result of the scan and clinical situation.

Magnetic resonance imaging (MRI)

Hydrogen atoms contained in water molecules within the body, are arranged in a random fashion, but when placed in a strong magnetic field, a few of these atoms align in the direction of the field. At the same time, the atoms spin on their axis. This is called resonance. Radio waves of the same frequency as the spin of the hydrogen atoms transfer energy to them. The transferred radiofrequency energy enables the spinning hydrogen atoms to spin out wider until they are spinning at 90° to the magnetic field. At this point the radiofrequency is turned off; the magnet starts to influence the atoms again and drags them back in line with the field. The hydrogen atoms must give up energy so they can 'relax' back to the lower energy state, in line with the magnetic field. An antenna (coil) will detect this emitted energy. The entire process is repeated over and over again and each time the coil receives a signal. These signals are assembled to create a digital image. Different tissues relax at different rates (and therefore have different energy signals) and so appear different on the resulting image.

In order to generate the large magnetic (static—always on) field required, a superconductor is used (electrical current passing along wire surrounded by liquid helium at −269°C resulting in no resistance and allowing a massive current).

Field strength: 0.5 to 1.5 Tesla (T) (1 Tesla = 10000 Gauss).
- Earth's magnetic field: 0.3–0.7 Gauss i.e. the magnet is 10000 times stronger.
- Any ferromagnetic material will be influenced by this field.
- Below 0.5 mT (5 Gauss) this influence is considered minimal. This boundary should be noted within the scan room. No magnetic material (including syringe pumps) should be any closer than 0.5 mT.

Equipment:
- All equipment must be MR 'safe' or MR 'compatible' and labelled. Includes patient trolleys, oxygen cylinders for transfer to wards, and laryngoscopes.
- MR safe: must present no risk to patients or staff in the MR environment (may still malfunction or interfere with quality of MR image).
- MR compatible: MR safe and functions normally and does not interfere with image quality.

Monitoring. The usual minimum standards apply. Cables should be padded or directed away from the skin and should not be coiled (may burn skin). MR compatible fibreoptic pulse oximeter cables, temperature probes, and carbon fibre ECG electrodes are available. Capnography tubing is long, increasing the interval between sampling and recording. ECG may be inaccurate—currents generated in the large vessels and heart by the magnetic field may be displayed as artefact on the ECG trace. Audible alarms may not be noticed above the MR noise especially if ear defenders are worn. Many anaesthetists prefer to remain outside the scanning room with a slave monitor and observe the patient through a window.

- Noise: the average noise produced is around 85–90 decibels. Ear defenders should be placed on the child once anaesthetized (and worn by staff in the scanning room).
- Temperature: the cooling system required by the large electromagnet results in a cold room temperature and the potential for significant heat loss. Forced air warming blankets can interfere with the radiofrequency signal and degrade the image quality. The radiofrequency energy itself can result in heating of the tissues (short wave diathermy), such that small infants may actually gain heat. Neonates, infants, or children undergoing a long scan should have body temperature monitored.
- Contrast: paramagnetic contrast media are used (the most common is gadolinium DTPA). The incidence of adverse reactions is low (nausea and vomiting, pain on injection). Although rare, anaphylaxis has been reported.
- Magnetism: ferromagnetic material close to the magnetic field will accelerate towards the most powerful point. Radiology staff use a checklist for patients, parents, and staff to ensure they have no metallic implants (clips on vessels, coils, stents, pacemakers, implants). Care is required to ensure that magnetic material is not taken near the magnet inadvertently. Conventional laryngoscopes and ferromagnetic oxygen cylinders are a particular risk.
- Quenching: sudden release of large quantities of helium from the superconductor and may be due to a deliberate shutdown or fault. Increasing helium concentration in the room produces a hypoxic environment.
- The MRI unit must be self-sufficient in dealing with emergencies including CPR, anaphylaxis, and anaesthetic complications.

Preoperative assessment

Patients may have conditions or syndromes that present specific anaesthetic concerns. Apart from noise and the enclosed environment, MRI is not stimulating. Most older and cooperative children are scanned awake while listening to music with a parent present. Anaesthesia (or sedation) is reserved for those who are too young to lie still for the duration of the scan or have a medical condition which limits cooperation.

Anaesthetic technique

- Induction can be inhalational or IV.
- ETT or LMA depending on patient—age, risk of reflux, respiratory function, ICP.
- Usually SV but IPPV for neonates, if poor respiratory function or raised ICP.
- Maintenance with volatile in oxygen and air or nitrous oxide. Alternatively, an infusion of propofol with or without formal airway management is easy to titrate, wears off rapidly, and may reduce nausea.

Postoperative care

Elective cases usually recover rapidly, feed and are discharged within 1–2 hours.

Thoracotomy and thoracoscopy

- Indications:
  - Closed cardiac procedures e.g. ligation of patent ductus arteriosus, repair of coarctation, modified Blalock–Taussig shunt (📖 Chapter 11).
  - Repair of tracheo-oesophageal fistula (📖 Chapter 12).
  - Resection of congenital cystic adenomatoid malformations. Incidence 1:5000 births, size may compromise surrounding lung, low risk of malignant change).
  - Congenital lobar emphysema is resected when size compresses adjacent lung (IPPV pressure worsens).
  - Bronchiectasis.
  - Mediastinal masses—biopsy or resection.
  - Drainage of empyema.
  - Decortication.
  - Anterior approach in scoliosis (📖 Chapter 9).
  - Lung sequestrations. Large blood supply can cause left to right shunt to the IVC. May result in high output cardiac failure. Association with diaphragmatic hernia.
- Morbidity—stump leak, hypoventilation, hypoxia, intrapulmonary bleeding and haemothorax.
- Many diagnostic and operative procedures are now done thoracoscopically after production of a CO_2 capnothorax.
- General considerations:
  - Oxygen consumption in neonates and infants is double that in adults (7 mL/kg/min compared with 3 mL/kg/min).
  - Closing volume is greater than FRC (up to age 6–8 years).
  - Due to immature hypoxic pulmonary vasoconstriction, ↑ chest wall compliance and volatile anaesthetics the nondependent (operated) lung may receive greater perfusion than the dependent lung, leading to shunting.
  - Avoid heat loss in open procedures—↑ ambient temperature, warm fluids, gases, warming mattress. Hypothermia is rarely a problem during thoracoscopic procedures.
  - Assessment for associated cardiac disease.
- A number of techniques are used for lung isolation depending on patient age, equipment available, and local expertise.
  - Open thoracic surgery can be performed with a conventional ETT in the trachea and the operated lung collapsed by the surgeon using swabs and retractors to expose the operative site.
  - Selective endobronchial intubation. A single lumen ETT is used for intentional endobronchial intubation of the main bronchus of the non-operated ventilated lung. If possible, cuffed tubes are used to achieve a satisfactory seal and the position should be confirmed by fibreoptic bronchoscopy (proximal protrusion of the cuff above the carina may occlude the contralateral bronchus). There may be obstruction of the right upper lobe if the right main bronchus is intubated, inability to suction operative lung and an inadequate seal (if an uncuffed ETT is used) leading to soiling of the healthy lung.

- Double lumen tube (DLT). Currently the smallest conventional DLT manufactured is a size 26FG (Rusch®) that can be used in children >8–10 years old. A bilumen DLT consisting of two uncuffed single lumen tubes of different lengths attached longitudinally has been described for use in neonates and infants (Marrano).
- Bronchial blockers. These are either improvised from embolectomy or atrioseptostomy catheters or designed for the purpose and incorporate a bronchial blocker and ETT together (Univent® and Arndt® equipment). The end result is an ETT in the trachea that ventilates one or both lungs depending on whether or not the balloon of the bronchial blocker is inflated or deflated. Placed in accordance with the manufacturers instructions.
- In all cases of lung isolation, the use of a bronchoscope to ensure correct placement and to assess the airway in the event of changes during the procedure is very useful.

Table 10.1 Airway equipment: sizes for thoracic surgery

Age	Weight kg	ETT ID mm	DLT FG	Univent	Bronchial blocker FG
Newborn	>3.5	3.5			5
6/12	7	3.5			5
1	10	4			5
2	15	4.5–5.0			5
4	17	5.0–5.5			5
6	21	5.5–6.0		3.5	6
8	25	6.0–6.5	26	3.5	6
10	31	6.5–7.0	26–28	4.5	6
12	40	7.0–7.5	32	4.5	6
14	50	7.5–8.0	35	6.0	7

Preoperative assessment

Likely pathology. Relevant previous treatment e.g. chemotherapy or radiotherapy. Review imaging—CXR, CT, or MRI. Assess risks of lung soiling, haemorrhage, and impaired postoperative respiratory function. Potential requirement for postoperative IPPV. FBC, U&E, and cross match. Arterial blood gas or capillary gas if hypoxic. Formal respiratory function tests are difficult <8–10 years of age. Avoid sedative premedication if there is hypoxia and/or hypercarbia.

Anaesthetic technique

- Induction is usually as requested by parent/child. Occasionally an inhalational induction is necessary as in anaesthesia for resection or biopsy of a mediastinal mass.
- Endotracheal intubation, DLT, or bronchial blocker technique with fibreoptic confirmation of correct positioning.
- IPPV.
- Maintenance of anaesthesia is with volatile in oxygen and air. A remifentanil infusion (0.1–0.25 mcg/kg/min) reduces volatile requirements and helps provide cardiovascular stability. As well as routine monitoring, there is a low threshold for insertion of an arterial line, central line, and urinary catheter depending on age, size, pathology, and the likely course of surgery.
- Lateral position with the operative side uppermost.
- Depending on circumstances, hand ventilation with a T-piece circuit may be preferred for all or part of the procedure if there are changes in compliance, episodes of hypoxia, or hypercarbia.
- A high F_IO_2 is often required during one lung anaesthesia.
- It may be necessary to use intervals during the surgical procedure to expand the collapsed lung and ventilate both lungs to allow expiration of CO_2 or to improve oxygenation.
- Hypercarbia occurs during thoracoscopic procedures in neonates. A capnothorax may cause hypotension that requires a fluid bolus and/or an inotrope infusion to treat.
- Analgesia for thoracotomy is usually provided by a bolus of opioid (morphine sulphate 100–150 mg/kg IV or fentanyl citrate 1–5 mcg/kg) plus a regional technique of some kind. Options for a regional technique are:
  - Thoracic epidural
  - Intercostal nerve blocks placed by the surgeon at the end of surgery—at least two nerves above and below the incision must be blocked.
  - Paravertebral block.
  - Interpleural block using an epidural catheter placed by the surgeon at the end of the procedure and tunnelled externally.
  - For thoracoscopy opioid is given and infiltration of the port sites with LA and adrenaline is performed.
  - In both cases a NSAID can be given if there are no contraindications.

Postoperative care

HDU care. Oxygen if required and early chest physiotherapy. Maintenance fluids until feeding. Chest drains may cause as much pain as the incision. Options for analgesia include a combined epidural infusion of LA and opioid or a regional technique instituted in theatre (intercostal blocks, paravertebral block, interpleural block.) combined with an IV infusion of morphine sulphate, PCA or NCA (Chapter 6). In most cases a regular NSAID can be prescribed and is very useful.

Dental and oral surgery

- Comprises:
  - Extractions of decayed deciduous or permanent teeth.
  - Restorative work.
  - Surgical exposure of impacted or unerupted teeth.
  - Extraction of undecayed permanent teeth to facilitate orthodontic treatment.
- 56% of 5-year-olds have signs of dental disease. In 5-year-olds only 8% of tooth decay has been restored, 20% extracted, and 70% remains untreated.
- In the UK, anaesthesia for dental surgery in children is provided in hospitals or in clinics equipped and staffed to the same standard as a hospital.
- Simple extractions of deciduous teeth may only take few minutes. Complex extractions, restorations oral surgery may take 1–2 hours.
- The majority of straightforward extractions are performed under local anaesthesia.
- General anaesthesia is used in children:
  - Too young to cooperate with local anaesthesia only.
  - Too anxious to cooperate.
  - With developmental delay.
  - With complex medical conditions where treatment under LA alone will not be tolerated.
  - For complex or prolonged procedures.
  - After previous failed treatment under local anaesthesia.
  - With allergy to LA.

Preoperative assessment

The majority of children undergoing dental extractions under general anaesthesia are between 3–8 years old. They (and their parents) are often anxious and may have had a previous unpleasant dental experience. Sedative premedication is commonly required e.g. midazolam (0.5 mg/kg oral or 100–150 mcg/kg nasal; maximum 20 mg).

Respiratory tract infections are common and cause an ↑ in adverse anaesthetic respiratory events, especially where the airway is shared, and consideration should be given to postponing surgery. Patients with learning difficulties and CNS or neuromuscular disease often present for dental care under general anaesthesia. The medical condition often has implications for the conduct of anaesthesia e.g. reflux in severe cerebral palsy, cardiomyopathy in muscular dystrophy. Antibiotic prophylaxis is usually required if there is congenital cardiac disease (even if it has been surgically corrected or palliated). A full anaesthetic history (congenital heart disease, fasting, respiratory tract infection, experience of previous dental treatment) and examination as appropriate with special attention to the airway, tonsils, and any loose teeth is required.

Anaesthetic technique

- Induction: IV or inhalational with IV cannula placed after induction.
- Airway management depends on the procedure, the patient, and the preferences of anaesthetist and dental surgeon.
- Nasal mask (McKesson or Goldman). This must be held at the same time as applying jaw thrust to maintain the airway. They provide no protection from blood or debris entering the pharynx. Largely superseded by the LMA.
- LMA (usually armoured or flexible LMA) provides 'hands free' airway maintenance and protection from debris, but its bulk can restrict surgical access within the mouth. It is easily displaced in small children as bite blocks are placed and repositioned. The LMA is usually suitable for extractions but not for oral surgery procedures.
- ETT: south facing preformed RAE or north facing nasal ETT. Used when there are multiple extractions or restorations in a small child, a risk of reflux or a requirement for IPPV. Provides a secure protected airway, more space in mouth for surgical manoeuvres. Preferred for oral surgery.
- Throat packs are used with LMAs and ETTs to protect against aspiration of blood or debris.
- Usually SV but IPPV for longer restorative cases or in compromised children.
- Maintenance is usually with volatile in oxygen and air or nitrous oxide. Alternatively, for longer cases TIVA with propofol with or without remifentanil 0.05–0.3 mcg/kg/min.
- The dental surgeon usually inserts a bite block taking care not to displace the LMA or ETT.
- Analgesia is provided by one or more of LA, NSAID and opioid depending on the procedure performed and dental and anaesthetic preference.
  - LA infiltration or nerve block. Lidocaine 2% with 1:80000 adrenaline is the most commonly used. Maximum dose 7 mg/kg (one cartridge contains 2.2 mL = 44 mg lidocaine; maximum = one cartridge per 7 kg body weight. Prilocaine 3% with felypressin 0.03 IU/mL ((felypressin is a synthetic hormone with properties similar to vasopressin, it does not cause local or distal ischaemia at injection site) is useful if adrenaline is contraindicated. Maximum dose is 6 mg/kg. Articaine 4% with adrenaline 1:100000 is also available for infiltration only. Maximum dose 7 mg/kg.
  - NSAID. Ibuprofen 10 mg/kg oral preoperatively or diclofenac sodium 1 mg/kg rectal while anaesthetized.
  - Opioid. Fentanyl 1–2 mcg/kg IV or codeine phosphate 0.5–1 mg/kg IM.
- An antiemetic is usually given especially to children undergoing longer cases or receiving opioids—ondansetron 100 mcg/kg (max 4mg) IV or dexamethasone 100–200 mcg/kg.
- Remove throat pack.
- Patients are recovered and the LMA or ETT is removed in the left lateral head down (tonsil position) especially if bleeding from extractions.

Postoperative care

Oral fluids are encouraged. Paracetamol, a NSAID and an oral opioid e.g. codeine phosphate 1 mg/kg 4-hourly are prescribed. Postoperative stay depends on the patient and type of procedure performed. Healthy children after a few extractions of deciduous teeth may be discharged after 1 hour. Medically compromised children or an oral surgical procedure may require several hours before discharge or overnight admission.

Congenital heart disease

Anne Goldie

Overview and classification of congenital heart disease

- Incidence of congenital heart disease (CHD) is 5–10:1000 live births.
- Reported incidence figures generally exclude mitral valve prolapse, bicuspid aortic valve, and patent ductus arteriosus in premature infants.
- More than 80% of children with CHD survive beyond the first year of life and approximately 80% of these survive to adulthood. Complex disease is increasingly represented among survivors.
- Currently more than half of surgery for CHD is done in children under one year old with an ongoing trend towards early complete repair rather than staged repairs.

Classification of CHD

- The anatomical classification of CHD studies the morphology of the cardiac chambers and takes a segmental, sequential approach, examining each element (atrium, ventricle, great artery or vein) and their relation. This classification method continues to be developed and refined.
- As far as anaesthesia is concerned, the important consideration is the effect of the anatomical lesion on cardiovascular and respiratory physiology. Therefore defects may also be classified on a physiological basis to provide a starting point in planning anaesthetic management.
- Defects are often grouped depending on shunting, oxygenation, pulmonary blood flow, and volume or pressure loading of cardiac chambers. However, there is overlap between categories and the physiological effects of a defect may change with time.
- For each patient, one should visualize the path of blood flow, the shunts, the changes in pressures within chambers and vessels, and the likely effects of manipulation of systemic and pulmonary vascular resistances. The effects of drugs, ventilation, and fluid administration may then be anticipated.

Table 11.1 Incidence of lesions observed in infancy

VSD	25–30%
ASD (ostium secundum type)	6–8%
PDA	6–8%
Coarctation of the aorta	5–7%
Tetralogy of Fallot	5–7%
d-Transposition of the great arteries	3–5%
Complete AVSD	1–2%

VSD ventricular septal defect, ASD atrial septal defect, PDA patent
ductus arteriosus, AVSD atrioventricular septal defect.

Table 11.2 Physiological classification of CHD

Left–right shunt	↑ pulmonary blood flow, volume overload	VSD ASD AVSD PDA
Right–left shunt	↓ pulmonary blood flow, hypoxia	Tetralogy of Fallot Pulmonary atresia
Mixed shunt	Hypoxia, variable volume and pressure overload	Transposition of the great arteries Hypoplastic left heart
Obstruction	Pressure overload	Coarctation of aorta Valvular stenosis

Fetal circulation

- The fundamental difference in the fetal circulation compared to the postnatal is that the placenta is responsible for gas exchange. The lungs receive little blood flow and there is high pulmonary vascular resistance (PVR).
- Three vascular structures are unique to the fetal circulation—the ductus venosus, the foramen ovale, and the ductus arteriosus.
- Blood returns from the placenta with a pO_2 of 4.0–4.7 kPa. Approximately 50% passes via the ductus venosus to mix with deoxygenated blood from the lower body and enter the inferior vena cava (IVC).
- In the right atrium, blood from the IVC is preferentially directed across the foramen ovale to the left atrium. This more highly oxygenated blood is pumped by the left ventricle to supply the coronary circulation, the brain and upper extremities.
- Deoxygenated blood returning via the superior vena cava (SVC) enters the right ventricle. The majority of its output is directed via the ductus arteriosus to the lower body, umbilical arteries and placenta.

Changes to the fetal circulation at birth

- The placenta is disconnected, increasing SVR and reducing IVC flow.
- The lungs are expanded, reducing PVR and increasing pulmonary blood flow.
- Blood flow in the ductus venosus reduces greatly and it closes to become the ligamentum venosum.
- ↑ pulmonary blood flow leads to an ↑ in left atrial volume. At the same time there is a reduction in IVC flow to the right atrium, such that left atrial pressure exceeds right atrial pressure and there is functional closure of the foramen ovale.
- ↑ pulmonary blood flow also results in reduced flow in the ductus arteriosus. This and other factors including ↑ oxygen levels and prostaglandins result in its closure. Functional closure of the ductus occurs hours after birth, with anatomical closure by 2–3 weeks of age.

Abnormalities of transition from fetal to neonatal circulation

- PVR may remain high giving rise to persistent fetal circulation (PFC) or primary pulmonary hypertension of the newborn.
  - Management is supportive until the condition resolves spontaneously.
  - Ventilatory strategies include high frequency oscillation and inhaled nitric oxide. Inotropic support may also be required.
  - PFC may be encountered by the anaesthetist during some neonatal surgical procedures e.g. repair of congenital diaphragmatic hernia.
- The ductus arteriosus may not close.
  - This causes volume overload of the left ventricle and ↑ pulmonary blood flow.
  - This is more common in premature infants, can prevent weaning from mechanical ventilation and may require surgical ligation of the duct.

- In some forms of CHD, persistence of the ductus arteriosus is a prerequisite for survival. Patients with such duct-dependent lesions may present with cardiovascular collapse if the duct closes.
  - Examples include neonatal coarctation of the aorta, pulmonary atresia, and transposition of the great arteries.
  - As part of the immediate management of these conditions, ductal patency can be maintained using an infusion of alprostadil 5–50 nanograms/kg/min. Alprostadil may cause apnoea so respiration must be monitored and occasionally IPPV instituted. It is also a potent vasodilator and volume or inotropic support may be needed after it is started.

Assessment of patients with CHD

- Diagnosis of CHD is generally made in three circumstances:
  - Routine checks (including preoperative assessment).
  - Prenatal.
  - Presentation in infancy with cardiovascular compromise.
- Clinical aspects of diagnosis remain important but the definitive diagnosis is likely to be made by echocardiography and now less frequently cardiac catheterization.
- Magnetic resonance imaging is used increasingly in the diagnosis of CHD as software development allows delineation of the anatomy of small, rapidly beating hearts.

Preoperative assessment should follow the standard approach (📖 Chapter 3), paying attention to:
- Cardiac function:
  - Review cardiac investigations to gain as complete an understanding as possible of the patient's anatomy and physiology to aid anticipation of problems.
  - Check for evidence of limited cardiac reserve or cardiac failure indicated by poor exercise tolerance, poor growth, and recurrent respiratory infections. In neonates and infants, cardiac failure is associated with poor feeding, failure to thrive, tachypnoea at rest, pallor, and hepatomegaly.
  - Consider the effects of medication e.g. diuretics may result in borderline preload and electrolyte abnormalities.
  - Check ECG for conduction abnormalities and dysrhythmias due to the cardiac lesion or previous surgery.
  - Can cardiac function be improved preoperatively in the time available?
- Hypoxia:
  - Check severity and whether episodic i.e. hypercyanotic spells.
  - Polycythaemia develops in response to hypoxia and causes hyperviscosity and abnormal coagulation. There may be a persistent metabolic acidosis in severe hypoxia.
  - Avoid prolonged preoperative fasting in polycythaemic patients (2 hours for clear fluids). Preoperative IV fluids may be required.
  - Consider need for intraoperative coagulation factor replacement.
- Respiratory abnormalities:
  - Airway abnormalities are not uncommon, including difficult intubation, shortened trachea, compression of the airways by cardiovascular structures, and tracheobronchomalacia.
  - ↑ or ↓ pulmonary blood flow, pulmonary hypertension.
  - Concurrent respiratory infections are associated with an ↑ incidence of intraoperative and postoperative complications and prolonged intensive care stay. It is prudent to postpone non-emergency surgery. However it can sometimes be difficult to separate the symptoms and signs of respiratory infection from those of the underlying CHD.
  - Review CXR.

- Associated abnormalities and syndromes:
  - Non-cardiac anomalies are found in approximately 25% of infants with CHD.
  - Check for other organ dysfunction.

Table 11.3 Commonly encountered abnormalities and some of their associated lesions

Trisomy 21	AVSD, Tetralogy of Fallot, VSD
DiGeorge sequence	Aortic arch anomalies, truncus arteriosus
VATER association	VSD
CHARGE association	Tetralogy of Fallot, septal defects
Turner syndrome	Coarctation of aorta, septal defects
Noonan syndrome	Pulmonary stenosis, septal defects

Previously undiagnosed murmur

- A common finding in children (📖 Chapter 3).
- The majority are innocent.
- A normal history and otherwise normal cardiac examination make the diagnosis of an innocent murmur more likely. ECG to check for ventricular hypertrophy may be useful. CXR is generally unhelpful.
- Innocent murmurs are early to mid systolic (except venous hum—continuous murmur), soft, and may alter with changes in patient position. There are normal femoral pulses and there is no parasternal impulse or heave.
- Paediatric (ideally paediatric cardiology) opinion should be sought preoperatively if the child is younger than 1 year, the murmur is diastolic, pansystolic, late systolic, continuous, loud, or there are associated cardiac symptoms or signs.
- If the nature of the murmur is in question, cardiology opinion unavailable, and surgery urgent, the decision as to how to proceed is based on the patient's clinical status. Antibiotic prophylaxis should be given in this situation.

Conduct of anaesthesia in CHD

In order to safely manage anaesthesia for a patient with CHD, one should understand the anatomy of the defect and that of the planned surgical procedure. Then the effects of the defect on physiology and likely effects of anaesthetic manipulations can be determined. The complexity of anaesthesia depends on the nature of the cardiac defect and on the proposed surgery. Many CHD patients for non-cardiac surgery can be managed conventionally. Others with more complex lesions require the expertise of a paediatric cardiac centre.

Premedication

- The usual indications and contraindications apply (📖 Chapter 3).
- Commonly used prior to major surgery including bypass, but avoided in younger infants and neonates.
- Reducing anxiety may be helpful in maintaining cardiovascular stability.
- Examples include midazolam 0.5 mg/kg (maximum 20 mg) oral 30 min before induction and alimemazine (trimeprazine) 2 mg/kg (maximum 60 mg) oral 1 hour before induction.

Monitoring

- Full routine monitoring is standard with the addition of arterial and central venous lines as required by the patient's cardiovascular status and the procedure.
- Unlike adult practice, invasive monitoring lines are generally inserted following induction of anaesthesia and endotracheal intubation.
- Sites of intravascular line insertion are chosen depending on the patient's cardiac anatomy and previous and proposed surgery e.g. right radial arterial line for repair of coarctation of the aorta, left radial arterial line for creation of a right Blalock–Taussig shunt. Typically a 22G cannula is used for arterial cannulation (24G in small neonates).
- Percutaneous central lines are often inserted into the right internal jugular vein. Ultrasound guidance may be used (📖 Chapter 5). Diameter and length are chosen depending on patient size.
- For cardiopulmonary bypass (CPB) surgery:
  - Core and peripheral temperature are monitored.
  - A urinary catheter is inserted.
  - For repeat bypass surgery, defibrillation pads should be applied and the surgeon may wish to have access to femoral vessels to allow partial bypass in the event of damage to the right ventricle or great vessels during sternotomy or dissection.
  - The surgeon may insert lines directly into the right or left atria or the pulmonary artery. Directly placed atrial lines are an alternative to percutaneous central lines.
  - The use of intraoperative echocardiography (epicardial or transoesophageal) is becoming standard practice.
  - Neurological monitoring is employed in some centres and is of particular interest in deep hypothermia and circulatory arrest. Techniques include the processed electroencephalogram, transcranial Doppler, and near infra-red spectroscopy.

Induction and maintenance of anaesthesia

- The cardiovascular profile should be considered when selecting anaesthetic agents. The effect on cardiac output, heart rate, peripheral and pulmonary vascular resistance may influence the choice of drug. Cardiovascular effects can be ameliorated to some extent by careful titration to effect. Onset will be delayed by the prolonged circulation time in cardiac failure.
- Sevoflurane is cardiovascularly stable and well tolerated for induction. Ketamine is a useful agent in neonates and when there is cardiac compromise. Etomidate is a useful alternative in older children. Propofol may be used, but with caution in cardiac impairment. An opioid may also be given at induction especially if there is cardiac failure.
- For neuromuscular blockade, pancuronium (100 mcg/kg) is often used for its relatively long duration of action and vagolytic effect. Vecuronium and rocuronium have stable cardiovascular profiles and a shorter duration of action.
- Nasal endotracheal intubation is performed when postoperative IPPV is planned i.e. most CPB cases. Nasal intubation is suitable up to 8–10 years of age and allows more stable fixation of the ETT than oral intubation.
- Anaesthesia is maintained using a volatile agent e.g. isoflurane in oxygen and air or a propofol infusion which may be target controlled. Opioids are given to those with cardiac compromise and as dictated by the procedure.
- Nitrous oxide may also be used if desired, but in CPB cases is limited to the induction period to minimize the risk of significant air embolism.
- In cases undergoing CPB, moderate to high dose opioids are given to maintain anaesthesia. Fentanyl, alfentanil, morphine, and remifentanil have all been used. There is a trend towards using more moderate doses of opioids combined with a volatile agent.
- While on CPB, anaesthesia is usually maintained intravenously. Volatile agents may be administered in the gas supply to the bypass pump membrane and may contribute to myocardial preconditioning and neuronal protection.
- Endocarditis prophylaxis may be required. CHD lesions can be stratified according to risk of developing infective endocarditis. Those at high or moderate risk should receive antibiotic prophylaxis when undergoing procedures likely to produce bacteraemia e.g. dental extractions, tonsillectomy. The highest risk is associated with previous infective endocarditis, valve replacements, and surgically created systemic–pulmonary shunts or conduits. Local or national guidelines should be consulted.
- Care should be taken to avoid injection of air bubbles particularly in those with a right–left shunt.
- Resuscitation drugs should be readily available.

Examples of anaesthetic recipes for a 3-year-old cardiovascularly stable child scheduled for secundum ASD repair on bypass.

- Premedication: midazolam 0.5 mg/kg oral.
- Induction: propofol 3–4 mg/kg, fentanyl 2–3 mcg/kg, pancuronium 100 mcg/kg.
- Maintenance: isoflurane (including in bypass gases), fentanyl 30 mcg/kg in divided doses (aim to have given 10 mcg/kg by the time of sternotomy). Pancuronium 100 mcg/kg as required and midazolam 100–200 mcg/kg on initiation of CPB. Morphine sulphate 250–500 mcg/kg while rewarming on bypass.
- Minimal or no inotropic requirement expected.
- Plan for early extubation in intensive care.

- Premedication midazolam 0.5 mg/kg oral.
- Induction and maintenance with propofol by target controlled infusion (2–5 mcg/ml, but taking care to limit dose infused).
- Alfentanil 10–20 mcg/kg at induction and in further increments to 50 mcg/kg by time of sternotomy, followed by infusion of 1–5 mcg/kg/min. Pancuronium 100 mcg/kg at induction with further doses as required. Morphine 250 mcg/kg towards the end of surgery.
- Minimal or no inotropic requirement expected.
- Plan for early extubation in intensive care.

Regional anaesthesia

- Insertion of a thoracic epidural catheter can be considered for postoperative analgesia in patients undergoing thoracotomy and will be particularly useful in providing postoperative analgesia when early extubation is planned.
- Neuraxial blockade for CPB procedures remains controversial because of the use of anticoagulants and the low but catastrophic risk of epidural haematoma.

Non-cardiac surgery

- CHD patients may be encountered on any surgical list. They frequently appear on dental lists in particular.
- The anaesthetic technique chosen will depend on the nature and severity of the CHD and on the surgical procedure. Equally this will influence where and by whom the anaesthetic is given.
- Remember antibiotic prophylaxis for patients at risk of endocarditis.
- The anaesthetic techniques used for the various types of cardiac procedures can be modified to apply to non-cardiac procedures.
- Provision of good postoperative analgesia including regional and peripheral blocks is important, but the impact of the method used on cardiovascular and respiratory function should be taken into consideration.

Cardiac catheterization

- Diagnostic cardiac catheterization is now performed less commonly than previously but includes post-repair identification of residual and undiagnosed defects in potentially severely compromised patients.
- Interventional cardiac catheterization is increasing and includes ballooning of stenosed vessels and valves, stent placement, device closure of defects (e.g. PDA, ASD) and aberrant pathway ablation.
- Carried out in the catheter laboratory rather than in an operating theatre. A balanced anaesthetic technique with intubation and ventilation, low dose opioids, and limited volatile agent is suitable. Procedures can be prolonged. Take care to maintain patient temperature and protect pressure points.
- Be prepared for dysrhythmias, sudden loss of cardiac output, and significant blood loss.

Closed cardiac procedures

- These are cardiac surgical procedures carried out without the need for bypass.
- Endotracheal intubation and ventilation are required.
- Neonates and infants are likely to require ventilation postoperatively.
- Arterial access is usual, central venous access is used in the major procedures.
- Surgical approach is either via a thoracotomy or median sternotomy. During thoracotomy the lung is retracted by the surgeon in order to gain access to cardiovascular structures.

Systemic arterial–pulmonary arterial shunt

- Intended to improve pulmonary perfusion and improve oxygenation in conditions with restricted pulmonary blood flow and cyanosis e.g. tetralogy of Fallot, pulmonary atresia, tricuspid atresia.
- Usually a modified Blalock–Taussig shunt using a 3.5–5 mm graft to provide a connection between the subclavian artery and ipsilateral pulmonary artery.
- Approached via thoracotomy. Collapse of one lung to achieve surgical access can worsen oxygenation in an already hypoxic patient.
- The aim is to produce sufficient reliable pulmonary blood flow to give acceptable oxygenation without volume overloading the left ventricle to the point of cardiac failure. Postoperative SpO_2 is usually in the 80s.
- Management of patients with a pre-existing systemic arterial–pulmonary arterial shunt should avoid dehydration and include antibiotic prophylaxis.

Coarctation of the aorta

- Causes pressure overload of the left ventricle and reduced volume femoral pulses.
- May be diagnosed at any age.
- Neonates can present with cardiac failure or collapse. Immediate management is resuscitation and an IV infusion of prostaglandin E_1 (5–50 mg/kg/min) in an attempt to re-open the ductus arteriosus. Ventilation and inotropic support may be required.
- Surgical repair is via a left thoracotomy with excision of the coarctation. Any residual gradient may require future balloon dilatation at cardiac catheterization.

Patent ductus arteriosus

- ↑ pulmonary blood flow and volume overload of the left ventricle.
- May require surgical ligation in premature neonates to facilitate weaning from mechanical ventilation. May be suitable for transcatheter closure in older patients.

Epicardial pacemaker insertion

- Used to provide pacing in infants and younger children, most commonly for atrioventricular block.
- Surgical approach is via median sternotomy and effective placement of pacing leads may take some time.
- Consider siting an arterial line, and be prepared for significant and/or sudden blood loss if the patient has had previous cardiac surgery.

Pulmonary artery banding
- Intended to restrict pulmonary blood flow and prevent development of heart failure and pulmonary hypertension.
- Originally used in conditions with large left–right shunts where definitive repair was delayed e.g. AVSD, large VSD. Most of these conditions are now repaired early in life.
- Current indications include:
  - Multiple VSDs where early repair is not feasible.
  - Single or multiple VSDs with coarctation of the aorta or interrupted aortic arch.
  - Preparation of the left ventricle for an arterial switch procedure by ↑ afterload.
- Median sternotomy or left thoracotomy.
- A Dacron or PTFE band is placed around the pulmonary artery and tightened while pulmonary artery pressure is monitored until pulmonary pressure is less than 50% of systolic or the lowest pulmonary pressure with an acceptable SpO_2 is achieved.
- The band is removed at the time of definitive surgery.
- If the band is too loose, heart failure and pulmonary hypertension result. If too tight, right–left shunt and profound hypoxia are possible.

Cardiopulmonary bypass

A team approach is essential—involve surgeon, anaesthetist, perfusionist, and cardiology staff. Communication is key.

Pre-cardiopulmonary bypass

- Maintain stable cardiac and respiratory status. Anticipate haemodynamic instability during siting of the CPB cannulae particularly in neonates and small infants. Precise placement of these cannulae is crucial in maintaining global systemic perfusion and good venous drainage. Periods of relative hypotension and dysrhythmias caused by surgical manipulation may have to be tolerated up to a point. Communication with the surgeon is important in interpreting and managing haemodynamic changes.
- Greatest stimulation occurs at the time of skin incision and at sternotomy. Anaesthesia and analgesia should be titrated appropriately.
- Check arterial blood gases and baseline activated clotting time (ACT). In-theatre testing of electrolytes, haematocrit, glucose, and lactate is also done.
- Heparin (300 units/kg) is given when requested by the surgeon. Some surgeons prefer to inject heparin directly into the heart. Aim for a post-heparin ACT of greater than 400 secs before CPB is initiated.
- Consider the use of anti-fibrinolytic agents. Aprotinin may be used in re-do operations and complex neonatal procedures. A test dose is given after induction. Dosing regimens vary, but usually consist of a loading dose, followed by an infusion, with a further dose added to the bypass circuit prime.
- Pre-bypass time will vary considerably depending on previous surgery and the need to identify and ligate any extra-cardiac shunts.

Cardiopulmonary bypass

- The standard components of a bypass circuit are used—size appropriate arterial and venous cannulae, circuit tubing, a venous reservoir, cardiotomy suction, a roller pump, a membrane oxygenator and gas supply, and a blood warmer.
- Circuit priming volume is reduced compared to an adult circuit, but is still high compared to patient blood volumes (up to 100% compared to 25–30% in adults). Blood is added if necessary so that the desired haematocrit is achieved while on CPB (usually 24–28%).
- Blood flow is calculated depending on the patient's body surface area. Perfusion pressure varies depending on patient age. Vasopressors e.g. phenylephrine, vasodilators e.g. phentolamine, glyceryltrinitrate, and anaesthetic drugs are used to alter perfusion pressure as required. Continuous monitoring of mixed venous saturation will help to confirm adequate CPB. Continuous monitoring of some electrolytes and haematocrit may also be available.
- Ventilation is discontinued once full bypass flow is established. Anaesthesia is maintained intravenously using opioids, with the addition of benzodiazepines, propofol, and volatile agents (added to bypass gases) as desired.

- Hypothermia is generally used, and to a greater degree than in adult surgery. Commonly 25–32°C and for some procedures 18–20°C with circulatory arrest (see below).
- During hypothermia, blood gas management uses alpha stat and/or pH stat methods depending on local protocols. Blood gas samples are warmed to 37°C before measurement (temperature uncorrected), then a nomogram is used to convert results to the patient's temperature (temperature corrected). Alpha stat (using temperature uncorrected values) has become the more generally used method. It maintains electrochemical neutrality and preserves cerebral autoregulation during moderate hypothermia. pH stat management (using temperature corrected values) maintains pH and pCO_2 at normal values for 37°C, which is done by the addition of CO_2 to bypass gases. There has been a recent ↑ in interest in the pH stat strategy for circulatory arrest (see below).
- Many procedures require the aorta to be cross-clamped and the heart arrested in order to facilitate surgical access. Myocardial preservation is provided by hypothermia and by perfusion of a cardioplegia solution into the aortic root and thence the coronary arteries. Cardioplegia may be a crystalloid or, now more commonly, a blood-based solution. The main effective component is potassium.
- Ultrafiltration helps reduce the adverse effects of CPB and haemodilution. Various methods are used either during or immediately following bypass.

Separation from cardiopulmonary bypass

- Before weaning from CPB, ensure adequate rewarming, normal electrolytes and neutral acid–base status. Confirm adequate ventilation. Anticipate the need for inotropic drugs. Mild hypothermia may confer neuroprotection and certainly hyperthermia should be avoided. A core temperature of 36–36.5°C at separation from CPB is appropriate.
- Cardiac filling can be assessed by direct visualization of the heart and by measured central venous or atrial pressures.
- Pacing may be required if the heart rate is slow or there is atrioventricular dissociation. As it is difficult to anticipate the need for postoperative pacing, the surgeon will place atrial and ventricular epicardial pacing wires in all but the simplest of cases.
- Epicardial (surface) echocardiography following separation from bypass is usually performed to assess the repair and exclude residual lesions. It also provides an indication of ventricular filling and function. The availability of small transoesophageal echo probes is making the use of this technique a more realistic option. Appropriate expertise is required in order to interpret complex echocardiography images and data.

- Protamine (2–5 mg/kg) is given slowly once off CPB and stable to reverse the effects of heparin. It should not be given until requested by the surgeon. Cardiotomy suction to the CPB pump is stopped immediately. Adverse effects due to protamine occur less commonly than in adults.
- Coagulation defects may require administration of blood components, most commonly in neonates and cyanosed patients. In particular, reduced platelet numbers and function can be expected.

Problems post-cardiopulmonary bypass

Residual defects
- Diagnosed by echocardiography or if necessary cardiac catheterization.
- Significant residual defects should be corrected and this may require a further period of CPB.

Ventricular dysfunction
- Can affect left and/or right ventricle.
- Manage by optimizing preload, heart rate and rhythm, correcting ionized calcium levels, and starting inotropic drugs.
- Dopamine remains the most commonly used first line inotrope (3–10 mcg/kg/min) producing a favourable response across the paediatric age range.
- Adrenaline (0.02–0.5 mcg/kg/min) is useful if systemic hypotension is persistent despite adequate preload.
- Milrinone (0.35–0.75 mcg/kg/min) has inotropic, lusitropic (diastolic relaxation) and vasodilator actions and is therefore an attractive drug for paediatric patients, particularly neonates, after CPB. A loading dose (25–50 mcg/kg) may be given, usually while on CPB.
- Right ventricular dysfunction can also be managed in selected cases by creating a right–left shunt at atrial level. The patient becomes cyanosed but systemic perfusion is maintained.
- The chest may be left open for 24–48 hours in some cases of ventricular dysfunction to allow recovery from the effects of surgery and CPB. This benefits right ventricular function in particular.
- Mechanical support with extracorporeal membrane oxygenation or a ventricular assist device is used in less than 5% of CPB cases. Outcome is best for those with right ventricular failure, who have undergone reparative rather than palliative surgery and where there has been an initial period of successful weaning from CPB.

Pulmonary hypertension
- More likely to occur following surgery for large left–right shunts e.g. AVSD, large VSD, in pulmonary venous obstruction or in neonates.
- Causes right ventricular failure.
- Managed in the early post-bypass period by careful attention to ventilation, ↑ inspired oxygen concentration and inhaled nitric oxide. Mechanical support may be required in some cases.

Postoperative care

- Requires a team approach and specialized staff in a paediatric intensive care unit.
- Analgesia is usually provided by an IV opioid infusion. Morphine is used frequently, but fentanyl or alfentanil are useful if there is cardiovascular instability. Additional sedation can be provided by benzodiazepines, triclofos and alimemazine (trimeprazine). IV or oral clonidine is a useful adjunct. Propofol infusion in this setting is contraindicated in children because of adverse effects.
- Selected patients may be suitable for rapid weaning and extubation, possibly in theatre. Those with a passive pulmonary circulation may benefit from early spontaneous ventilation. Some will require mechanical ventilation for longer periods of time.
- Inotropes are used to maintain cardiac function. Fluid input is restricted if possible and diuretics are used to avoid fluid overload.
- Goals prior to extubation include, cardiac stability with minimal inotrope requirement, minimal ongoing blood loss, adequate respiratory function and oxygenation, and adequate conscious level.
- Renal and neurological dysfunction can complicate the postoperative course.

Deep hypothermic circulatory arrest (DHCA)

- Employed in cases where surgical access requires removal of the CPB cannulae, mainly complex neonatal procedures e.g. transposition of the great arteries, interrupted aortic arch, total anomalous pulmonary venous connections.
- The patient is cooled on bypass for at least 20 mins to 18–20°C, after which blood is drained into the bypass circuit and the cannulae removed.
- Neurological impairment is reported to be minimal if DHCA lasts for less than 40 mins.
- Cerebral protection is provided by rapid and even cooling on bypass. Vasodilators may be used to aid even cooling e.g. phenoxybenzamine or phentolamine.
- The choice of blood gas management strategy is debated. The pH stat method may offer better neurological protection during extreme hypothermia. Cerebral blood flow is higher with pH stat management because of vasodilatation due to a higher pCO_2. This is believed to provide faster brain cooling. However, the clinical data available does not provide firm evidence of benefit.
- Pharmacological agents used to provide neuroprotection include steroids and barbiturates, but none have been demonstrated to improve neurological outcome.
- An alternative to DHCA involves regional low flow perfusion via the right innominate artery, but despite the theoretical advantages there is as yet no clear evidence for improved neurological outcome over DHCA.

Open cardiac procedures—notes on specific lesions

Atrial septal defect

- ↑ pulmonary blood flow and volume overload of the right atrium and right ventricle.
- Closed either using a transcatheter technique (secundum ASD) or on CPB depending on size, location and associated cardiac defects. Usually done at age 3–5 years of age unless the defect is large with signs of cardiac failure necessitating earlier closure.
- In stable patients, conventional anaesthetic management is usually suitable for non-cardiac procedures.

Ventricular septal defect

- ↑ pulmonary blood flow and volume overload of the left ventricle.
- 30–40% close spontaneously depending on site and size. Muscular defects are most likely to close spontaneously. VSDs can be single or multiple.
- Restrictive defects i.e. diameter less than that of the aortic root tend to be asymptomatic and then standard anaesthetic management is suitable for these patients.
- Non-restrictive defects are more likely to have cardiac failure and early development of pulmonary vascular disease. Repair may be required at 3–6 months of age.

Atrio-ventricular septal defect

- The anatomy varies from a primum ASD with cleft mitral valve and minimal cardiovascular disturbance to a complete AVSD with volume overload of both ventricles and atria and common atrio-ventricular valve regurgitation. The latter patients develop pulmonary vascular disease early and may have cardiac failure. They require repair at 3–6 months of age.
- Associated with trisomy 21 (30% of complete AVSDs). Also with other congenital abnormalities including other cardiac anomalies.

Tetralogy of Fallot

- Tetralogy of Fallot has four elements—infundibular stenosis, aortic override, ventricular septal defect, and right ventricular hypertrophy. The degree of cyanosis depends on the severity of right ventricular outflow tract obstruction.
- Surgical management is either a primary complete repair in infancy or less commonly now a two-stage repair with an initial systemic arterial–pulmonary arterial shunt (usually a modified Blalock–Taussig shunt—tube graft from subclavian artery to pulmonary artery) in the neonatal period followed by definitive repair around 1 year of age.
- Tetralogy spells are episodes of hypercyanosis and rapid, deep breathing with a peak incidence at 2–4 months of age. Their aetiology is unclear, but they are associated with ↑ oxygen demand, acidosis, and hypercapnoea. Treatment may include abdominal compression, flexion of the legs, oxygen, morphine (or other opioid), IV fluid administration, beta-blockers (esmolol, propranolol), vasoconstrictors (noradrenaline, phenylephrine).

- Patients should not be fasted for prolonged periods as this results in worsening hyperviscosity. There is a risk of clotting a surgical shunt if dehydration is allowed to occur.
- Anticipate coagulation defects if there is significant polycythaemia.
- Despite reduced pulmonary blood flow, sevoflurane is a useful induction agent.
- There may be conduction defects and pulmonary regurgitation after repair.

Transposition of the great arteries

- In this condition, the pulmonary artery arises from the left ventricle and the aorta from the right ventricle. Approximately 25% also have a significant VSD.
- Systemic to pulmonary artery shunts are necessary to maintain life. In the fetus, the ductus arteriosus and foramen ovale provide such shunts, but as these close in the neonate the patient is compromised. Initial treatment is with alprostadil by IV infusion. In addition, an atrial septostomy may be performed.
- In the first 14 days of life the neonate undergoes an arterial switch procedure. The great arteries are divided and reattached to the correct ventricle and the coronary arteries are re-implanted above the neo-aortic valve. Operation may be delayed if a VSD is present.
- Deep hypothermia and DHCA or low-flow CPB are used during the arterial switch procedure.
- The left ventricle requires afterload reduction post-CPB. Milrinone may be useful for this.
- Consider using aprotinin as this is a complex neonatal procedure.
- Atrial switch (physiological but not anatomical repair) was performed previously with reasonable outcomes. This is now performed rarely, but older patients who have had this procedure may be encountered. Careful attention to haemodynamic management is required when anaesthetizing these patients.

Section 5

Neonatal and emergency procedures

Emergency surgery: neonatal, general, and airway

Emma Dickson

Rapid sequence induction

- Rapid sequence induction (RSI) is considered in cases associated with an ↑ risk of aspiration. As in adults, it involves:
  - Preoxygenation.
  - Near simultaneous administration of an induction dose of a rapidly acting IV anaesthetic agent (thiopentone or propofol are the commonest) and suxamethonium.
  - Application of cricoid pressure from the period immediately prior to induction until confirmation of correct placement of the ETT.
  - Avoiding ventilation by face mask before endotracheal intubation because of concern that this may inflate the stomach.
- In children, the indications for RSI are the same as those in adults:
  - Any concern about an ↑ risk of aspiration.
  - Abdominal pathology.
  - Emergency surgery with no time for appropriate fasting.
  - Recent preoperative opioids.
- An RSI requires a reasonable amount of cooperation and understanding from the child and so this presents a number of challenges to the anaesthetist, their assistant, and the parents. There is no ideal solution to these problems and a degree of adaptability is necessary. Good communication with all these parties beforehand can help. Factors which limit its usefulness in children include:
  - Difficulty in securing IV access.
  - Application of monitoring pre-induction.
  - Difficulty in preoxygenation and denitrogenation. Neonates and infants have a high oxygen consumption relative to FRC and rapidly become hypoxic when apnoeic (📖 Chapter 1). This problem is compounded if preoxygenation has been incomplete because the child is struggling and distressed.
  - Discomfort associated with cricoid pressure.
  - Distortion of the view of the laryngeal inlet by cricoid pressure.
  - Parental presence and anxiety.

In small children, it is possible to end up in a situation where the first attempt at endotracheal intubation is unsuccessful because of the anterior larynx and cricoid pressure, the child is becoming hypoxic because of high oxygen consumption, the suxamethonium is wearing off, and attempts at ventilation by facemask cause gastric distension. In practice, RSI is usually limited to older (>5 years) cooperative children whose anatomy and physiology are virtually adult. In younger children, many paediatric anaesthetists prefer an inhalational or IV induction followed by administration of a depolarizing relaxant and IPPV by face mask to provide optimal conditions for endotracheal intubation in a fully oxygenated patient.

Following the discontinuation of anaesthesia after a rapid sequence induction, the child should be extubated awake with intact airway reflexes.

Principles of neonatal anaesthesia

A neonate is defined as a newborn up to 44 weeks postconceptual age. Anaesthetizing neonates requires special consideration and attention. They have developing physiological systems and handle drugs differently to infants and older children. Preoperative and postoperative care of neonates should take place in units with experienced staff trained in neonatal care.

Specific physiological and pharmacological considerations in neonates are covered in Chapters 1 and 2. Some features of neonatal anaesthetic care require specific attention. These include temperature measurement and its control, fluid balance and pharmacokinetics.

Preoperative assessment

- Surgical pathology: intended procedure and possible variations on this, likely duration, likely blood loss, options for postoperative analgesia.
- Gestation: determines to some extent the likely surgical pathology, respiratory reserve, likelihood of postoperative IPPV.
- Congenital anomalies: may be the surgical problem or can affect anaesthetic management as with the big tongue of Beckwith–Wiedemann or congenital heart disease often seen in Down's syndrome.
- Cardiovascular status: if there is associated CHD does the child have heart failure, are they shunt (ductus arteriosus) dependent, what is the direction and flow through any shunts which are present, presence of pulmonary hypertension, drugs such as diuretics or digoxin?
- Respiratory status: partly determines degree of monitoring required postoperatively and the need for postoperative IPPV, prematurity (bronchopulmonary dysplasia and risk of postoperative apnoeas), previous IPPV, baseline oxygenation, oxygen requirement if any.
- Volume status: consider hypovolaemia, hypervolaemia, capillary refill, skin turgor, core-peripheral temperature gradient, wet nappies, nasogastric losses, abdominal distension, and extravascular sequestration.
- Discussion with parents. If possible, meet the parents (not always possible if the child has been transferred from another hospital immediately after birth), take a history and examine the baby. Discuss the anaesthetic, analgesia, and likely postoperative scenarios with the parents and give them an opportunity to ask questions.

Investigations

- Full blood count, U&E and blood glucose are routine.
- Others investigations are indicated by surgical pathology and associated anomalies—clotting screen (sepsis or jaundice), chest film (respiratory disease, cardiac disease, diaphragmatic hernia, oesophageal atresia and tracheo-oesophageal fistula), ECG and cardiac echo (congenital heart disease), abdominal film (bowel obstruction, enterocolitis), MRI (↑ ICP, fits).

Premedication

- Sedative premedication is rarely used in neonates because of their sensitivity to them and the risk of airway obstruction and respiratory depression.
- An anticholinergic is commonly given. This may be atropine 20 mcg/kg IM. More commonly this is given IV around the time of induction.
- Vitamin K is usually given to all newborns in the UK (as prophylaxis against haemorrhagic disease of the newborn) and this should be verified from the notes before surgery. Neonates are relatively deficient in clotting factors II, VII, IX, and X and at risk of excessive bleeding during surgery.

Preoperative preparation

- Set the ambient temperature of the operating theatre.
- Calculate drug doses, including emergency ones, beforehand.
- Check anaesthetic machine, circuits, masks, airways, laryngoscope blades and ETTs.

Induction

- Neonates are usually anaesthetized in the operating theatre where ambient temperature can be kept high and monitoring need not be disconnected for transfer from the anaesthetic room.
- The child is at risk of hypothermia during induction and associated activity such as obtaining venous access. The ambient temperature is set at about 26–28°C, unnecessary exposure is avoided, and an overhead radiant heater used.
- ECG electrodes and an oximeter probe are applied prior to induction.
- The choice between IV and inhalational induction depends on the clinical situation and the preference of the anaesthetist.
- If an IV cannula is in situ then an IV induction is appealing. Smaller doses of induction agents are used than in older children (thiopental 2–3 mg/kg, ketamine 1–2 mg/kg). Neonates rapidly become hypoxic when apnoeic and it is important to attempt preoxygenation and to ensure effective ventilation by face mask between induction and endotracheal intubation.
- An inhalational induction is common if there is no IV access and avoids the need to attempt this in the struggling child. It also has the advantage of ensuring oxygenation as the child is anaesthetized and gives the anaesthetist the chance to obtain a clear airway as the child relaxes. Using a T-piece circuit makes handling of the airway easier.
- Intramuscular induction with ketamine 5 mg/kg is occasionally used if venous access is difficult, the child is cardiovascularly unstable or has significant CHD and is dependent on a left to right shunt.
- Endotracheal intubation is almost always used in neonates during general anaesthesia. Once the child is adequately anaesthetized and effective ventilation by face mask is ensured, a neuromuscular blocker is given to facilitate endotracheal intubation. These drugs have a higher volume of distribution in neonates than in older children. If suxamethonium is used, a larger dose than normal (3 mg/kg) is given while non-depolarizers are given in the same doses as normal while the increased sensitivity of the neonatal muscles offsets the large volume of distribution (📕 Chapter 2). It is also possible to intubate on deep inhalational anaesthesia.

Maintenance
- Is usually with volatile in oxygen and air or nitrous oxide Nitrous oxide reduces the requirement for volatile agent and has the same contra-indications as in older children. Very premature neonates are at risk of retrolental fibroplasia (retinopathy of prematurity) from high concentrations of oxygen (and several other factors) and the inspired oxygen concentration in these patients is titrated to maintain an S_pO_2 of 92–95%
- Patients are almost always ventilated during anesthesia and this can be done mechanically if the ventilator is sophisticated enough or, very commonly, by hand used a T-piece circuit (although this cannot be scavenged effectively).

Temperature maintenance
- Humans are homeothermic and control body temperature within a narrow range. This is required for optimal enzyme activity and metabolic processes.
- Neonates are at a considerable disadvantage for this type of system. They have numerous ways to lose heat and have inefficient methods to generate heat. General anaesthesia and opiates abolish non-shivering thermogenesis.
- Maintaining temperature: ↑ ambient temperature, heat and moisture exchanger for inspired gases, use of active warming devices (heated water mattress and convective warm air blanket), avoid unnecessary exposure of the child, cover the head with a hat, warmed solutions for surgical skin preparation, warmed IV fluids, monitor core and peripheral temperatures during surgery.

Fluids
- Maintenance fluids are required for all but the briefest of procedures.
- These should usually contain 4% or 5% glucose e.g. 4% glucose with 0.18% saline.
- Blood glucose is monitored during longer procedures.
- Fluids are warmed before administration.
- Fluids are administered through a pump or syringe to ensure accuracy.
- Volume replacement (blood volume calculated as 90 mL/kg) is with crystalloid (0.9% saline or Ringer's lactate) or colloid. Blood and blood products as indicated depending on ongoing losses and preoperative haemoglobin concentration. Haemoglobin can be measured intra-operatively if there is adequate access.

Analgesia
- If extubation is planned then, when possible, a regional technique is used to avoid opioid administration This can be infiltration for superficial procedures such as inguinal herniotomy or pyloromyotomy, peripheral nerve blocks for penile or groin surgery, or a central block especially caudal epidural for more extensive surgery below the umbilicus such as a colostomy for imperforate anus.
- When opioids are used they are usually given in smaller doses at longer intervals than in older children—morphine sulphate 25–50 mcg/kg IV or fentanyl citrate 1–2 mcg/kg IV. If the child is to be ventilated postoperatively then larger doses of opioids can be given.

- NSAIDs are often relatively contraindicated in neonates because of renal immaturity, hypovolaemia, or potential sepsis.
- Paracetamol by rectum has a very variable absorption and the IV route (15 mg/kg) is preferable.

Reversal and extubation
- Carried out when the child is normothermic, normovolaemic and has a minimal concentration of expired volatile agent.
- Neuromuscular blockade is reversed with neostigmine 50 mcg/kg and atropine 20 mcg/kg or glycopyrronium bromide 10 mcg/kg.
- Gentle suction to pharnx and nostrils (nasal breathing).
- Nasogastric tube aspirated if present.
- Child is extubated 'awake' when breathing adequately and moving vigorously.
- CPAP by face mask may be required for laryngospasm.

Postoperative care

- Requires appropriate area with relevant nursing and medical expertise.
- Pulse oximetry, ECG and temperature. Other monitors—apnoea monitor, urine output, CVP as indicated.
- Blood glucose measured at regular intervals until feeding.
- Bloods if indicated.
- Maintenance fluids until feeding. Other fluids as required—replace nasogastric losses, volume replacement, blood transfusion.
- Paracetamol 15 mg/kg oral or nasogastric 6-hourly. If child is nil by mouth then prescribe 15 mg/kg 6-hourly IV.
- Weak opioid such as codeine phosphate 0.5 mg/kg oral or nasogastric 4-hourly if required.
- If required IV infusion of morphine sulphate 5–10 mcg/kg/hour (📖 Chapter 6). Occasionally 20 mcg/kg/hour is required.

Pyloromyotomy

- Indicated for congenital hypertrophic pyloric stenosis. This occurs in about 1:300–1:400 children (80% are boys). The pathology is thickening of the smooth muscle of the pylorus, which obstructs gastric outflow. Pyloromyotomy requires incision of the 'tumour' down to but not through the mucosa and is curative.
- Infants generally aged <12 weeks present with non-bilious projectile vomiting following a feed.
  - Vomiting causes loss of fluid, hydrogen ions, and chloride ions.
  - A secondary hyperaldosteronism develops due to the hypovolaemia. The high aldosterone levels causes the kidneys to avidly retain sodium (to correct the intravascular volume depletion) and excrete ↑ amounts of potassium into the urine (resulting in hypokalaemia) as the kidneys retain sodium and hydrogen ions.
  - Infants may be dehydrated and exhibit a hypochloraemic, hypo-kalaemic metabolic alkalosis.
  - More often in the UK nowadays medical care is sought quickly and many infants have only a mild metabolic derangement. Some have none at all.
- Diagnosis is made from the history and examination, which reveals the pyloric 'olive' on palpation. Ultrasound scanning shows hypertrophy of the muscle of the pyloric wall (thickness >4 mm or length of pylorus >16 mm).
- Surgery is not an emergency. The dehydration and biochemical abnormality are corrected before theatre. If necessary, a bolus of 20 mL/kg of 0.9% saline or colloid is given for resuscitation. More often, children receive 0.45% saline with 5% glucose as 150% of calculated maintenance requirements with added potassium chloride (15 mmol per 500 mL bag) once urine output is confirmed. A nasogastric tube is passed and regular gastric lavage performed to ensure that the stomach is as empty as possible prior to surgery and anaesthesia. Significant naso-gastric losses are replaced with 0.9% saline or Hartmann's solution.
- The procedure can be carried out in the traditional 'open' style via an incision in the left upper quadrant or around the umbilicus or laparo-scopically.

Preoperative assessment

A general history with details of pregnancy, birth, and progress since birth is taken. The presence of a nasogastric tube is confirmed and the results of gastric lavages noted. The child's state of hydration is assessed—skin turgor, capillary refill, wet nappies. Details of the fluid regimen are noted. Laboratory results and capillary blood gas results are checked. Once the child is rehydrated, serum chloride is >100 mmol/L, pH <7.5, base excess <6 mmol/L, and bicarbonate <30 mmol/L the infant is ready for theatre.

Anaesthetic technique

- Pyloromyotomy is a short surgical procedure not associated with blood loss or fluid shifts. Patients have an IV cannula in situ and IV fluids running.
- Anticholinergic premedication is given if desired—atropine 20 mcg/kg IV just prior to induction.
- The nasogastric tube is aspirated.
- Options for induction include:
  - Rapid sequence induction (📖 p.388).
  - IV induction followed by face mask ventilation, administration of a non-depolarizing neuromuscular blocker, and endotracheal intubation.
  - Inhalational induction followed by administration of a non-depolarizing neuromuscular blocker and endotracheal intubation.
  - Inhalational induction followed by endotracheal intubation under deep volatile anaesthesia.
- IPPV is the norm and maintenance is with volatile in oxygen and air or nitrous oxide.
- The surgeon may ask for the stomach to be distended with 40–60 mL of air injected through the nasogastric tube to look for a mucosal perforation. This air is aspirated prior to wound closure.
- The incision or laparoscopic port sites are infiltrated with LA by the surgeon.
- At then end of surgery, the nasogastric tube is aspirated and the child extubated 'awake'.

Postoperative care

Maintenance fluids are continued until feeding is established (clear fluids initially followed by milk if tolerated). Some surgeons feed the child after 4 hours, other wait for up to 16 hours. The nasogastric tube is often removed at the end of the surgical procedure. Paracetamol 15 mg/kg oral 6-hourly (maximum 60 mg/kg/day) is prescribed for analgesia. Neonates are usually monitored with an oximeter and ECG. Older infants can return to a general ward.

Oesophageal atresia (tracheo-oesophageal fistula) repair

- Oesophageal atresia has an incidence of 1:3000 live births.
  - Survival is of the order of 90% and is determined largely by the presence of associated anomalies.
  - It is associated with maternal polyhydramnios and premature birth. Diagnosis is usually made antenatally. If not it presents in the neonatal period with choking episodes, production of frothy mucous from the mouth, and repeated chest infections.
  - There is a risk of aspiration and subsequent pneumonitis.
  - After repair, many children suffer one or more of gastro-oesophageal reflux, oesophageal stricture, and tracheomalacia later in life.
- Associated conditions occur in 30–50%:
  - Prematurity.
  - CHD.
  - Additional gastrointestinal abnormalities.
  - Renal and genitourinary conditions.
  - VATER (vertebral, anal, tracheo-oesophageal, radial or renal anomalies).
  - VACTERL (vertebral defects, anorectal malformation, cardiovascular anomalies, tracheo-esophageal, renal (genitourinary), and limb malformations).
  - Tracheomalacia and other associated conditions of the trachea.
- A variety of forms of atresia and fistula exist:
  - Type 1 (85%). Proximal oesophageal atresia, distal oesophageal fistula into the trachea usually about 1 cm above the carina. Unable to pass an orogastric tube into the stomach. A CXR reveals the tube curled in the proximal oesophageal pouch. There is a gastric air bubble.
  - Type 2 (8–10%). Pure oesophageal atresia with no fistula. There may be a large gap between the upper and lower segments of the oesophagus. CXR reveals the nasogastric tube curled in the upper segment of the oesophagus and there is no gastric air bubble.
  - Type 3 (2–4%). H-type tracheo-oesophageal fistula without oesophageal atresia. This is often a late and difficult diagnosis.
  - Type 4 (1%). Proximal pouch tracheo-oesophageal fistula.
  - Type 5 (1%). Double tracheo-oesophageal fistula.
- Preoperative management:
  - A double lumen 'Replogle' suction catheter is inserted in to the upper pouch and connected to constant low suction to aspirate swallowed secretions and prevent aspiration in to the lungs.
  - The child is nursed head up, kept nil by mouth, and given IV maintenance fluids.
  - Assessment for associated anomalies—examination, echocardiogram, and renal ultrasound.
  - FBC, U&E, glucose, and cross match.

- Surgery usually involves a right thoracotomy in the lateral position, identification and ligation of a tracheo-oesophageal fistula, and anastomosis of the two ends of the oesophagus. A thoracoscopic technique is possible. A fistula may not be present. In some cases, the oesophagus cannot be made continuous and a gastrostomy is performed.
- A bronchoscopy may be performed prior to the thoracotomy to help identify the position of the tracheo-oesophageal fistula.
- Postoperative morbidity:
  - Anastomotic leak—10–20%.
  - Oesophageal stricture requiring dilatation—20–40%
  - Oesophageal reflux.
  - Aspiration, atelectasis and recurrent pneumonia.
  - Stridor and tracheomalacia—20%.

Preoperative assessment

The degree of prematurity, episodes of aspiration, and associated CHD are most relevant to anaesthetic management. A premature child with previous aspiration will be difficult to ventilate and postoperative IPPV will be obligatory. Limb anomalies may make venous access and arterial cannulation difficult. If there is no tracheo-oesophageal fistula present then gastric distension during induction of anaesthesia will not occur.

Anaesthetic technique

- Premature babies or those who have aspirated may already be intubated. In this case, the positioning and length of the ETT are checked. Ideally, the distal end will be distal to the tracheo-oesophageal fistula so that distension of the stomach by ventilation through the fistula is avoided.
- The Replogle tube is aspirated.
- The main concern during induction is gastric distension by ventilation through the tracheo-oesophageal fistula. Whatever the induction technique used ventilation by face mask is performed gently at low inflation pressures.
- Options for induction include:
  - IV induction followed by neuromuscular blockade and endotracheal intubation.
  - Inhalational induction followed by neuromuscular blockade and endotracheal intubation.
  - Inhalational induction and endotracheal intubation under deep volatile anaesthesia to avoid the need for IPPV by face mask.
- Ideally, the tip of the ETT should lie distal to the fistula to prevent inflation of the stomach during ventilation. Occasionally, the ETT is inserted into the fistula inadvertently. Some anaesthetists deliberately intubate a bronchus then withdraw the ETT until bilateral lung ventilation is noted and then secure the ETT in this position in the expectation that the distal end of the ETT is distal to the tracheo-oesophageal fistula.

- In most cases, nasotracheal intubation is performed since postoperative IPPV is required in many cases.
- Rarely, a needle gastrostomy may be necessary to deflate the stomach before the fistula is tied off.
- An arterial line is often sited to help assess cardiac output during surgery and to aid postoperative management.
- Maintenance is with volatile in oxygen and air. Nitrous oxide is avoided to prevent gastric distension.
- IPPV is necessary and this is usually done by hand using a T-piece circuit at a high frequency of 30–40 minute and low tidal volumes. Surgery often involves episodes where ventilation is difficult because of reduced lung compliance, lung compression, or obstruction/kinking of major airways. Inspired oxygen may need to be ↑, ventilation ↑ or occasionally surgery stopped for a period to allow adequate ventilation and removal of carbon dioxide. Cardiac output can fall dramatically if surgical manoeuvres compress major vessels. Good communication and cooperation with the surgeon are essential.
- In many cases postoperative IPPV is planned and a generous bolus of opioid (morphine sulphate 100–150 mcg/kg; fentanyl citrate 5–10 mcg/kg) is given or an infusion started (fentanyl 2–4 mcg/kg/hour; remifentanil 0.25–0.5 mcg/kg/min).
- If extubation is planned a small bolus of opioid is given (morphine sulphate 25–50 mcg/kg; fentanyl citrate 1–2 mcg/kg) and a regional technique performed—a thoracic epidural catheter inserted directly or via the sacral hiatus or intercostal nerve blocks by the surgeon prior to wound closure.
- The anaesthetist may be asked to help identify the distal end of the proximal pouch within the thorax by manipulating the Replogle tube from above.
- Once the two ends of the oesophagus are approximated the anesthetist usually passes a fine transanastomotic nasogastric tube before the anastomosis is fashioned to allow enteral feeding in the postoperative period.

Postoperative care

In many cases the child is returned to ITU for a period of IPPV. This may be because of the condition of the child or in order to protect the anastomosis by keeping the child still. Traditionally, patients are nursed with the head in the midline and the neck slightly flexed for 3–5 days to minimize tension on the anastomosis. If the anastomosis is not tight and the condition of the child allows, extubation is performed. Analgesia may be provided by a thoracic epidural infusion of LA (often without opioid in neonates) or an IV infusion of morphine sulphate (📖 Chapter 6) plus paracetamol by nasogastric tube or IV. A chest film is required. The child is fed by nasogastric tube or parenterally for 5–7 days until a contrast study confirms anastomotic integrity.

Necrotizing enterocolitis

- This condition develops almost exclusively in premature infants (5–15% of those with birth weight <1500 g) and is characterized by intestinal mucosal injury secondary to ischaemia of the bowel. It can progress to intestinal perforation and sepsis.
- Clinically it presents with increasing gastric aspirates, abdominal distension, bloody diarrhoea, temperature instability, and apnoeas. As the disease progresses evidence of sepsis becomes apparent—thrombocytopenia, anaemia, coagulopathy, and metabolic acidosis.
- Initial medical treatment involves fluid resuscitation, stopping enteral nutrition, decompressing the stomach with a nasogastric tube, and antibiotics.
- Around 50% of cases require surgical intervention.
- Surgical options include insertion of a peritoneal drain or drains and laparotomy to remove necrotic bowel with stoma formation. A tunnelled central line is often inserted for sampling and parenteral nutrition during the postoperative period.

Preoperative assessment

These babies are often extremely unwell. They are usually intubated and ventilated in the SCBU before transfer to theatre. Discussion with the neonatologist is informative and helpful. Details of the ETT, ventilator settings, and increasing ventilation are important. The type and volume of fluid administered are noted. Circulating volume is assessed. Patients are frequently hypovolaemic, as third space losses are considerable. May be receiving an inotrope preoperatively. Recent blood results—FBC, clotting, electrolytes, and arterial blood gas—and trends in these give an indication of the state of the patient. Blood must be cross matched before surgery. Both platelet and red cell transfusion may be required before surgery. The vascular access is noted. An arterial line is very useful (if it can be placed without delaying surgery) to provide serial assessments of acid–base status, clotting parameters, electrolytes, haemoglobin, and platelet values.

Anaesthetic technique

- The patient is often transferred to theatre by neonatal staff. A thorough handover of recent events is required.
- Patients are unstable and require careful handling and continuous monitoring—they often deteriorate when lifted and transferred from the incubator to the operating table.
- Maintenance fluids, analgesia and sedation instituted in the SCBU are continued. A further bolus of analgesia is given and a neuromuscular blocker if necessary.
- Maintenance is with volatile in oxygen and air. Nitrous oxide is contraindicated.
- IPPV is continued and it may be preferable to do this by hand with a T-piece circuit rather than using a ventilator.

- Inspired oxygen concentration is titrated against S_pO_2 to ensure an adequate arterial oxygen saturation of 92–95% but avoiding hyperoxia and possibly contributing to the risk of developing retinopathy of prematurity.
- Ventilatory requirements often ↑ during surgery as handling of the bowel reduces lung compliance.
- Patients may become more cardiovascularly unstable during surgery as ischaemic bowel is handled and bleeding occurs. Significant volume replacement is often required and is titrated in aliquots of 10 mL/kg against clinical response. Blood is sequestered in the ischaemic bowel and a (further) blood transfusion is often required. It is common to replace a circulating volume or more with a mixture of colloid, red cells, platelets, and fresh frozen plasma during an extensive bowel resection. It is often difficult to weigh up the need for volume against inotrope (or ↑ inotrope). A CVP measurement is rarely available and blood loss is difficult to measure accurately.
- Despite all precautions—↑ ambient temperature, warmed fluids, warming mattress, and warm air blanket—patients often become hypothermic during this type of surgery.
- Urine output is monitored if possible.
- Arterial blood gases, FBC, and electrolytes are checked at intervals if it is possible to sample.

Postoperative care

Patients are returned to the neonatal intensive care unit, usually for a prolonged period of IPPV and parenteral nutrition.

Abdominal wall defects: gastroschisis and exomphalos

- These are congenital abdominal wall defects. Exomphalos is a herniation into the umbilical cord and gastroschisis is a defect in the abdominal wall lateral to the umbilicus. Together they have an incidence of 1:3000 live births. They are usually detected antenatally and are apparent at birth.
- Exomphalos (also known as omphalocele):
  - Occurs following failure of gut migration from the yolk sac to the abdomen with incomplete closure of the rectus muscles in the abdominal wall and herniation of the midgut within the umbilical cord.
  - In about 50% of cases there is liver, spleen, or gonads in the hernia.
  - The extruded viscera are contained in a translucent sac (unless it ruptures during birth) and the umbilical vessels radiate on to the wall of this sac. The bowel is usually morphologically and functionally normal.
  - Babies with this condition often have a low birth weight and in around 40% there are other associated malformations including imperforate anus, bowel atresias, Beckwith–Wiedemann syndrome, CHD, and bladder exstrophy. Mortality is determined largely by the associated anomalies.
- Gastroschisis:
  - There is a congenital defect in the abdominal wall lateral to the umbilical cord (right side is more common) causing herniation of the abdominal contents through the anterior abdominal wall.
  - The herniated bowel is exposed to amniotic fluid in utero and air after delivery and becomes inflamed, oedematous, shortened, and functionally abnormal.
  - Lower incidence of associated congenital anomalies than exomphalos.
- In both cases the immediate management following delivery is to cover the contents with a sterile dressing or plastic bag to prevent heat loss, fluid loss, and infection. A nasogastric tube should be passed to decompress the bowel. The child is transferred to a neonatal surgical unit.
- Surgical repair involves excision of a sac if present, stretching of the abdominal wall and placement of the bowel in the abdomen followed by primary closure.
- Gastroschisis is usually reduced urgently. If primary closure is not possible the bowel is placed in a silastic silo taped to the edges of the defect that covers the bowel until closure is possible. In many centres application of a silo without general anaesthesia is now the initial method of treatment. The extra-abdominal bowel is reduced gradually over several days followed by definitive closure of the defects under general anaesthesia.
- Exomphalos surgery may be delayed to allow investigation for other anomalies. Surgical repair follows the same principles as gastroschisis.
- A feeding line may be inserted.

Preoperative assessment

Volume status is assessed. Fluid resuscitation is often required. FBC, electrolytes, and acid–base status are checked. Regular blood glucose checks. Blood is cross matched. Examination for associated anomalies and echocardiogram.

Anaesthetic technique

The child may be transferred from ITU intubated and ventilated. If not anaesthetized then:

- Aspirate nasogastric tube.
- IV or inhalational induction as preferred. Many anaesthetists prefer a RSI for these patients.
- Endotracheal intubation (nasal tube since IPPV will probably be required postoperatively) and IPPV are required.
- Maintenance with volatile in oxygen and air.
- Unless the child is to be extubated at the end of surgery a bolus of opioid—morphine sulphate 50–100 mcg/kg IV or fentanyl citrate 2–4 mcg/kg—is given for analgesia. If there is a small exomphalos the child may be extubated postoperatively. In this case less opioid is given or a caudal epidural block performed.
- During surgery intra-abdominal pressure ↑, lung compliance falls, and ventilation usually becomes more difficult. Ventilatory rate and pressure along with the F_IO_2 usually need to be ↑. A slight degree of head up may be helpful.
- IVC compression may reduce cardiac output and organ perfusion.
- An arterial line is useful in addition to standard monitoring.
- All the available measures to prevent hypothermia in a neonate are required since a large volume of bowel is often exposed.

Postoperative care

Unless there is a very small exomphalos, patients are usually ventilated postoperatively. In addition to the usual aspects of intensive care, ventilation may be difficult because of high intra-abdominal pressure. Cardiac output may be reduced because of compression of the IVC and this is most commonly manifested as oliguria and metabolic acidosis. An infusion of inotrope e.g. dopamine 3–5 mcg/kg/min may be necessary to improve renal and mesenteric perfusion. There may be congestion and cyanosis of the lower body that will affect NIBP and oximetry readings from the legs. In gastroschisis a prolonged period of parenteral nutrition is usually required.

Imperforate anus

- One of the congenital anorectal anomalies.
  - Incidence is 1:5000 births.
  - More common in ♂ than ♀.
  - Presents during the initial physical examination after birth or as failure to pass meconium.
- Lesions are described as 'high' or 'low'. In high lesions, the end of the rectum is above the levator ani muscle while in low lesions it is below this muscle. High lesions are usually more complex and long term faecal continence is less likely. This differentiation determines the type of surgery required:
  - High lesions commonly communicate with the urethra in males while in females the fistula is to the vagina.
  - Low lesions usually open on to the skin in the perineum, the median raphe of the scrotum, or in to the vaginal vestibule.
  - Surgery for a high-type defect involves a colostomy prior to a more complex anal repair when the child is older. Surgery for the low-type imperforate anus involves some form of perineal anoplasty with closure of the fistula, creation of an anal opening, and reposi tioning the rectal pouch into the anal opening.
- Patients may have abdominal distension with impairment of ventilation, apnoeas, or be at risk of bowel ischaemia.
- This are often other congenital anomalies associated with imperforate anus. It may be part of the VACTERL spectrum and in about 25% there is tethering of the spinal cord.

Preoperative assessment

Assess for other anomalies—ultrasound of renal system, CXR, ECG, echocardiogram, X-rays of lumbar and sacral spine. The degree of abdominal distension and any effects of respiration are noted—S_pO_2 in air, oxygen requirement, occurrence of apnoeas. Patients have IV access and maintenance fluids. Blood is cross matched for high lesions requiring a colostomy. If a regional technique is planned, this is discussed with the parents.

Anaesthetic technique

- Atropine 20 mcg/kg IV if desired.
- Induction can be IV or inhalational.
- Endotracheal intubation and IPPV.
- Maintenance is with volatile in oxygen and air.
- Patients are positioned supine for colostomy. For anoplasty or EUA of the perineum the lithotomy position (or as near to it as possible in a neonate) is used with the hips and knees flexed and then taped in this position. The child is usually positioned at the far end of the operating table.

- Options for analgesia include:
  - Anoplasty: a caudal epidural block (📖 Chapter 8) as a single injection to block sacral dermatomes— 0.3–0.5 mL/kg 0.25% levobupivacaine or similar.
  - Colostomy: requires blockade of thoracic dermatomes. A single caudal epidural injection—1.25 mL/kg 0.125% levobupivacaine or similar—or insertion of a caudal epidural catheter. The catheter can be used for a postoperative infusion.
  - The sacrum is occasionally anatomically abnormal in anorectal anomalies and a caudal technique may not be possible.
  - An intervertebral epidural to block thoracic dermatomes.
  - IV opioid: morphine sulphate 25–50 mcg/kg IV; fentanyl citrate 1–2 mcg/kg IV.
  - All of these techniques can be supplemented by IV paracetamol 15 mg/kg.
- Occasionally during a colostomy some volume replacement is required.

Postoperative care

Patients are usually extubated. Maintenance fluids are required until feeding is established. After anoplasty oral analgesia is adequate—paracetamol 15 mg/kg oral 6-hourly (maximum 60 mg/kg/day) and a weak opioid such as codeine phosphate 0.5 mg/kg oral 4-hourly. After formation of a colostomy the options are an IV infusion of morphine sulphate or an epidural infusion of LA (📖 Chapter 6) usually for 24 hours.

Congenital diaphragmatic hernia

- Babies with this condition generally present early in the neonatal period (if not already picked up antenatally) with cyanosis and respiratory distress in the presence of a scaphoid abdomen.
- It results from failure of the pleuro-peritoneal membrane to develop adequately and close to separate thorax and abdomen before the intestines return to the abdomen during the 10th week of gestation. The intestines then enter the pleural cavity.
- The incidence is 1:4000 live births.
- Left sided herniae via the postero-lateral foramen of Bockdalek are the most frequent (85%). In this location there is herniation of both small and large bowel as well as solid organs into the thoracic cavity. Right sided herniae generally only involve the liver and large bowel. Rarely bilateral hernias occur but they are usually fatal.
- On the affected side there is lung hypoplasia along with surfactant dysfunction, pulmonary hypertension, and right-to-left shunting. The hypoplasia is often bilateral even though the hernia is unilateral. These respiratory consequences rather than the anatomical hernia are the fundamental problem in this condition. These babies should be cared for in a specialist unit and their medical management optimized prior to surgical treatment.
- Surgical repair is achieved via an abdominal, thoraco-abdominal, or trans-thoracic incision. A patch of artificial material is sometimes required.
- Prognosis is related to the degree of pulmonary hyperplasia and pulmonary hypertension and the presence of other congenital anomalies. Mortality is 30–50%.
- Occasionally a congenital diaphragmatic hernia may present later in infancy or adulthood with respiratory distress or bowel obstruction. In this situation there is normally a good outcome.

Preoperative assessment

Respiratory support with endotracheal intubation and IPPV is usually required. Face mask ventilation should be performed with low pressures and tidal volumes to avoid distension of the intrathoracic intestine. A nasogastric tube is passed to decompress the intrathoracic intestine. Respiratory acidosis and metabolic acidosis need to be treated. Limiting inflation pressures and permissive hypercapnia is a common ventilatory strategy to minimize barotrauma. Specific treatment for pulmonary hypertension is often required. This may include nitric oxide, high frequency ventilation, oscillation, and extracorporeal membrane oxygenation (ECMO). Vasodilators (prostaglandin E1, nitroglycerin, nitroprusside) can be used but cause systemic hypotension and an inotrope may be needed to counter this. The arterial line should be preductal i.e. right radial. If a central venous line is inserted this should be a femoral line or a neck line on the side of the hernia since a pneumothorax on the side of the good lung may be fatal. The child is assessed for associated anomalies especially CHD. FBC, U&E, cross match and a CXR are required if not already done.

Anaesthetic technique

- Most patients are transferred to theatre from ITU intubated and ventilated.
- Anaesthesia is essentially a continuation of intensive care with the addition of volatile agent and supplementary opioid (morphine 100–200 mcg/kg, fentanyl 5–10 mcg/kg, an infusion of fentanyl 2–4 mcg/kg/hour, or remifentanil 0.25–0.5 mcg/kg/min).
- Positioned supine. Usually a sub costal incision.
- Pressure limited ventilation is the preferred mode. If hand ventilation is used great care should be taken to avoid high inflation pressures and pneumothorax. An airway pressure gauge is sometime used with the T-piece circuit to help avoid this.
- Frequent arterial line sampling is performed.

Postoperative care

Patients return to ITU. Respiratory function is usually worse after surgery and treatment of pulmonary hypertension and right to left shunting through the ductus arteriosus is continued.

Myelomeningocele

- Myelomeningocele occurs secondary to a failure of fusion of the embryonic neural tube during the 4th week of gestation. It is associated with varying degrees of neurological dysfunction below the level of the lesion. There may or may not be a covering of skin.
- 75% of lesions occur in the lumbo-sacral region.
- Myelomeningocele refers to a lesion containing neural tissue; if the bulge contains CSF without neural tissue it is a meningocele.
- Myelomeningocele is associated with an Arnold–Chiari type II lesion and hydrocephalus is present in 70–85% of neonates with myeloeningocele.
- The Arnold–Chiari type II lesion comprises a bony abnormality of the posterior fossa and upper cervical spine with caudal displacement of the cerebellar vermis, fourth ventricle, and lower brainstem below the plane of the foramen magnum. Medullary cervical cord compression can occur with abnormal ventilatory responses to hypoxia and hyper-carbia and occasionally lower cranial nerve lesions resulting in problems with swallowing and upper airway reflexes.
- The condition is usually diagnosed antenatally by ultrasound.
- There is a high risk of infection and the rate of ventriculitis is related to how quickly the surgical correction is performed. Ideally, defects are closed within 24 hours to avoid infection.
- A ventriculo-peritoneal shunt is usually inserted at the time of primary repair or shortly afterwards.

Preoperative management

The level and extent of the lesion will affect positioning during induc-tion, duration of surgery, and potential blood loss. The child will have undergone a neurological examination and the neurological findings are noted for comparison with the postoperative situation. The lesion is covered with a damp dressing to stop tissues drying out. The presence of other congenital anomalies especially CHD may affect the anaes-thetic management. Patients have blood cross matched.

Anaesthetic technique

- The child usually has an IV cannula in place with maintenance fluids.
- Premedication—atropine 20 mcg/kg IV prior to induction if desired.
- Induction is IV or inhalational as preferred. The child may need to be supported on a cushion or jelly ring to avoid pressure on the lesion or placed in the lateral or semi-lateral position depending on the exact anatomy.
- Endotracheal intubation with an armoured ETT and IPPV are required.
- Maintenance is with volatile in oxygen and air or nitrous oxide.
- Consider arterial and central line depending on the size of the lesion.
- The patient is positioned prone for surgery. Rolls of soft material or jelly bolsters are placed under the shoulders and pelvis to allow free abdominal movement during ventilation.

- The extremities are padded.
- The surgeon may wish to stimulate nerves during the procedure. Discuss this before giving a long acting neuromuscular blocker.
- Blood loss is not usually a problem but some large lesions require extensive undermining of skin to fashion a flap or flaps when bleeding does become an issue.
- The surgical site is usually infiltrated with LA and adrenaline to ensure haemostasis. Additional opioid analgesia (morphine sulphate 25–50 mcg/kg or fentanyl citrate 1–2 mcg/kg) can be given if this is inadequate. The sensory level is usually unclear at this point so analgesic requirements are variable.
- IV antibiotics are given according to surgical request or local protocol.
- If stable, extubate at the end of procedure.

Postoperative care

A tight closure of an extensive lesion may impair ventilation. A co-existing Chiari malformation may also affect postoperative respiratory function. The child is nursed in a neonatal surgical unit with ECG monitoring and pulse oximetry. Maintenance fluids are continued until feeding is established. Paracetamol 15 mg/kg oral 6-hourly (maximum 60 mg/kg/day) and a weak opioid such as codeine phosphate 0.5 mg/kg oral 4-hourly are prescribed for analgesia. If the lesion is extensive, an IV infusion of morphine sulphate can be used (Chapter 6).

Appendicectomy

- Appendicitis is the commonest reason for non-elective general surgical procedures in children.
- It is usually seen in school age children but does occur in younger children including infants and rarely neonates.
- Appendicitis classically presents with a history of central colicky abdominal pain which migrates to right iliac fossa, low grade fever, and vomiting.
- Abdominal ultrasound is frequently used to aid diagnosis and has a sensitivity and specificity of >80%. CT is less frequently used but has a sensitivity and specificity of >90%.
- The diagnosis is often made relatively late in younger children where, the presentation may be atypical and diagnosis difficult. There is a higher rate of perforation, abscess formation, and peritonitis in preschool children. Their ability to compensate for hypovolaemia and sepsis means that they may be quite sick by the time of surgery.
- Appendicectomy is performed through a traditional muscle splitting open approach or laparoscopically (which can also be of use in diagnosis).

Preoperative assessment

General assessment of intercurrent illness, past medical history, previous anaesthetics, allergies, and drugs. Most patients are normal healthy children. Children have often not been drinking for a day or two and may have been vomiting. They are frequently febrile. Assessment of fluid balance and IV fluids is important. Analgesia is given as required. FBC and U&E.

Anaesthetic technique

- Patients usually have IV access.
- A rapid sequence induction is normally performed.
- Endotracheal intubation and IPPV is the norm.
- Maintenance is with volatile in oxygen and air or oxygen and nitrous oxide.
- The need for analgesia is variable and depends on preoperative analgesia, whether the procedure is open or laparoscopic and whether there is a perforation with an abscess or peritonitis. Options include a bolus of opioid—morphine sulphate 100–150 mcg/kg IV or fentanyl citrate 2–4 mcg/kg IV. This can be supplemented by wound infiltration with LA and a NSAID if there are no contraindications. Some people prefer to give less opioid initially until the nature and extent of the surgical pathology and the procedure are clear.
- An antiemetic is given e.g. ondansetron 100 mcg/kg IV.
- Young children and those with a late diagnosis may decompensate when anaesthetized and need a couple of boluses of 20 mL/kg of fluid for resuscitation. Their management is along the lines of a more major abdominal procedure such as intussusception.

Postoperative care

In most cases patients return to the surgical ward. Maintenance fluids and antibiotics are continued. For analgesia options include an IV infusion of morphine sulphate or PCA plus paracetamol and a NSAID or an oral opioid such as codeine phosphate 1 mg/kg 4-hourly plus paracetamol and a NSAID. The choice depends on the state of the patient, the presence of peritonism and the extent of the surgical procedure.

Some younger children with a late diagnosis may require HDU care with oxygen, further fluid resuscitation, and monitoring of urine output.

Intussusception

- Intussusception is the result of invagination of one segment of small bowel into another.
  - Most commonly it involves the segment of bowel just proximal to the ileocaecal valve.
  - The affected bowel is compressed and there is traction on the mesentery. Local lymphatic and venous obstruction develops and the bowel becomes swollen and oedematous.
  - The arterial supply is compromised and, without urgent reduction of the intussusception, the bowel will become gangrenous.
- Incidence is 2–4:1000 and there is ♂:♀ ratio of 3:2. It is seen most frequently in the age range 5–18 months.
- Most cases are 'idiopathic' i.e. of unknown cause. Features which may be identified as the lead point of the intussusception include a Meckel's diverticulum, lymph nodes, polyps, and intestinal duplications.
- Classically infants present with intermittent colicky abdominal pain and blood and mucous in the stool ('red currant jelly stool').
- Diagnosis is confirmed by ultrasound or CT.
- Treatment initially involves an air or barium enema performed in the radiology department. If reduction is unsuccessful or the child is septic and there is concern about gangrenous bowel an urgent laparotomy is performed. Laparoscopy is also a surgical option.

Preoperative assessment

Significant fluid resuscitation may be required (20 mL/kg repeated once or twice is not unusual). Analgesia e.g. morphine sulphate 100–200 mcg/kg IV may be needed. Bloods for FBC, U&E, and group and save.

Anaesthetic technique

- The child usually has IV access.
- A RSI is usually performed although many younger children will not cooperate with preoxygenation and a period of IPPV with a face mask after induction and before endotracheal intubation may be needed to avoid hypoxia.
- A second IV cannula is inserted. Nasogastric tube. Appropriate antibiotics, if not already given, are needed.
- Neuromuscular blockade and IPPV are the norm.
- Maintenance is with volatile in oxygen and air. An infusion of remifentanil 0.25–0.5 mcg/kg/min reduces volatile requirements and promotes cardiovascular stability.
- Regional analgesic techniques other than wound infiltration are usually relatively contraindicated. In most cases, morphine sulphate 100–150 mcg/kg IV or fentanyl citrate 2–4 mcg/kg is given (depending on preoperative opioid administration and the use of remifentanil).
- Several boluses of 20 mL/kg of fluid for resuscitation may be required during surgery especially if there is resection of necrotic bowel. Blood transfusion is a possibility.

- A warming mattress and a warming blanket should be used. IV fluids are warmed. Central and peripheral temperature should be monitored.
- If bowel is resected and the child will be admitted to HDU or ITU postoperatively then a central venous line and arterial line can be inserted while the child is still anaesthetized at the end of surgery. A urinary catheter should also be inserted at this stage.

Postoperative care

If well, i.e. no bowel resection, cardiovascularly stable, and no oxygen requirement, then return to a surgical ward is appropriate. Maintenance fluids and IV antibiotics are continued. An IV infusion of morphine sulphate (Chapter 6) is run for 24–48 hours. Children are nil by mouth but IV or rectal paracetamol are useful adjuncts. The use of a NSAID requires careful assessment in the light of recent hypovolaemia and potential sepsis. They are usually withheld for 12–24 hours until the child is clearly recovering.

If the child requires oxygen to maintain saturations, is cardiovascularly unstable, has ongoing fluid requirements or is oliguric then admission to HDU or ITU is necessary.

Very similar principles of anaesthetic care apply to children undergoing laparotomy for any reason.

Acute scrotum

- This presents with a short history of acute scrotal pain. Depending on the age, the differential diagnosis includes epididymo-orchitis, trauma, incarcerated hernia, appendicitis, and tumour.
- Neonates:
  - May present with trauma or torsion from the birth often due to a breech delivery.
  - A neonatal testicular torsion involves twisting of the whole spermatic cord that occurs because of the unfixed nature of the newly descended testis.
  - Almost all neonatal torsions present late with testicular necrosis.
- Infants and toddlers:
  - The commonest cause is an acute epididymo-orchitis.
  - This is caused by bacterial or viral infection and there is no definitive way to exclude torsion.
  - Diagnosis is, therefore, usually made after surgical exploration.
  - In infants, an irreducible inguinal hernia can mimic an acute scrotal condition.
- School age boys have the highest prevalence of acute scrotal problems. The important diagnoses to consider are torsion of the testis, torsion of a testicular appendages (hydatids of Morgagni) and acute epididymo-orchitis.
  - In testicular torsion the spermatic cord is twisted, cutting off the testicular blood supply. Prolonged testicular torsion results in necrosis of the testicle. In most boys, the testicles are attached to the inner lining of the scrotum. Boys who do not have this natural attachment are at risk of testicular torsion. This anomaly is known as 'bell clapper testis' and is a common cause of testicular torsion. Torsion is commonest in adolescents and epididymo-orchitis in younger boys.
  - The testicular hydatids of Morgagni are embryological remnants of the mullerian duct on the upper pole of the epididymis or the testis itself. Torsion of these appendages is most common near the onset of puberty.
  - Rarely, testicular tumours present as an acute scrotum.
- No sign or investigation can exclude testicular torsion and so urgent surgical exploration of the acute scrotum is required, ideally within 6 hours of the onset of pain in order to salvage the testicle.
  - Testicular salvage is dependent on the time between onset of symptoms and surgery (80% within 6 hours, <25% after 18 hours).
  - The testis is derotated and sutured to the scrotal lining with non-absorbable sutures. Because the anatomical abnormality predisposing to torsion (the bell clapper testis) is commonly bilateral, the contralateral testis is fixed at the same time.
  - There is an incidence of late testicular atrophy.

Preoperative assessment

Neonatal anaesthesia is discussed on 🕮 p.390. Younger boys with epididymo-orchitis are frequently febrile, toxic, and occasionally dehydrated. They have often had a systemic illness for several days. There is not usually time for preoperative fluid administration and this is done during surgery. Older boys may be quiet and frightened. Patients are rarely fasted and even if they have not eaten for 6 hours the pain and distress of the condition and urgent admission to hospital probably mean that adequate emptying of the stomach cannot be assumed.

Anaesthetic technique

- In older boys a RSI is performed. This may not be possible or appropriate in neonates and infants. An inhalational induction may have to be done for these patients.
- The younger boys with a febrile illness are at ↑ risk of laryngospasm.
- The commonest technique involves endotracheal intubation with spontaneous ventilation or IPPV as preferred. A LMA is an option only if the anaesthetist is confident that there is no ↑ risk of regurgitation.
- Maintenance is with volatile in oxygen and air or nitrous oxide.
- IV fluids are given to patients who have been febrile and unwell preoperatively.
- Options for analgesia include:
  - Infiltration of the incision with LA plus a NSAID.
  - As above plus a bolus of intraoperative opioid—morphine sulphate 100–150 mcg/kg IV or fentanyl citrate 2–4 mcg/kg IV.
  - Caudal epidural blockade. This is useful in older boys if the incision is scrotal (sacral dermatomes) but less useful for inguinal incisions (lumbar dermatomes). In neonates and infants a caudal epidural block is useful for both scrotal and inguinal incisions. It is usually regarded as contraindicated if the child is toxic.
- An antiemetic is given other than to neonates and infants e.g. ondansetron 100 mcg/kg IV.
- Manipulation of the testis may cause a vagal response and atropine or glycopyrronium bromide should be at hand.

Postoperative care

Patients usually recover rapidly from anaesthesia and surgery. Oral intake is usually resumed rapidly. Febrile infants should have maintenance IV fluids until drinking. A combination of paracetamol 15 mg/kg oral 4-hourly, ibuprofen 10 mg/kg oral 6-hourly, and codeine phosphate 1 mg/kg oral 4-hourly is prescribed.

Bleeding tonsil or adenoids

- This presents either within the first 6 hours (primary) or about a week following surgery (secondary) and is potentially life threatening.
- Children present with fresh blood in the mouth, frequent swallowing, pallor, sweating, and haematemesis. Significant blood loss may have been swallowed and gone unnoticed. Hypotension is a late and serious sign that indicates gross hypovolaemia with decompensation.

Preoperative assessment

The child is assessed for hypovolaemia, cannulated, and IV fluids started (20 mL/kg 0.9% saline, Hartmann's or colloid repeated if necessary). Assessment of blood loss may be difficult as it is not possible to assess the volume of swallowed blood. Check pulse, BP, capillary refill time. Healthy children have a large physiological reserve and will mask signs of hypovolaemia. Blood is sent for FBC, U&E, and group and save. The child is regarded as having a full stomach and being at ↑ risk of regurgitation and aspiration. The chart for the recent anaesthetic is read for information on any airway difficulties (especially if the indication for surgery was obstructive sleep apnoea) and the ease or otherwise of endotracheal intubation. Consultant anaesthetist involved.

Anaesthetic technique

- The child usually comes to theatre with an IV cannula.
- A RSI is the norm. An inhalational induction may be performed for a particular indication or if venous access is very difficult.
- The stomach is emptied with a large bore orogastric tube.
- Spontaneous ventilation or IPPV as preferred.
- Maintenance is with volatile in oxygen and air or oxygen and nitrous oxide.
- Ongoing fluid resuscitation may be required during surgery.
- Analgesia may not be required if the child is immediately postoperative and has received analgesia in theatre and on the ward.
- If analgesia is needed, a dose of opioid—codeine phosphate 1 mg/kg IM, morphine sulphate 100–150 mcg/kg IV, fentanyl citrate 1–2 mcg/kg IV—is given. Ondansetron 100 mcg/kg IV is also given. IM codeine is not used if the patient is hypovolaemic. NSAIDs are not given.
- The child is extubated awake in a head down left lateral position.

Postoperative care

Patients usually recover rapidly. Maintenance fluids are required until drinking resumes. Analgesia is restricted to oral opioid and paracetamol without a NSAID. If there has been adenoidal bleeding, and a pack is left in the post-nasal space, the child is admitted to HDU in case the pack dislodges and causes airway obstruction.

Foreign body removal

- Inhalation or swallowing of a foreign body is most common between 1–3 years of age and can be life threatening.
- Inhaled foreign bodies are usually organic with peanuts being common. Few are radio opaque. All organic material but especially peanuts can cause airway hyper reactivity. Coins usually end up in the upper oesophagus
- Large (>20 mm) objects are held up in the oropharynx. Medium-sized (8–15 mm) or irregularly shaped objects are held up in the larynx. Small, smooth, and linear objects tend to enter the trachea and bronchi. If a foreign body is small enough to pass through the cords it rarely occludes the trachea. Most end up in a main bronchus (right 50%, left 45%, and trachea 5%). A foreign body in the oesophagus can produce respiratory distress by compressing the trachea.
- A foreign body in the airways may cause hyperinflation of the lung by allowing air entry during inspiration but preventing expiration.
- Presentation is usually with one or more of cough, cyanosis, choking, wheezing, or dyspnoea. Sometimes the aspiration goes unnoticed and the child presents with fever and a chest infection some days later (or months later with atypical respiratory symptoms).
- Signs may be of airway obstruction, wheeze, and ↓ breath sounds.
- CXR may be normal. A radio opaque foreign body will be seen. Other common features include collapse of a lobe or lung, mediastinal shift, and pneumothorax. An end expiratory film may show unilateral emphysema or hyperinflation on the side of the foreign body.
- Examination and removal under general anaesthesia are required. This may involve laryngoscopy, rigid oesophagoscopy and/or rigid bronchoscopy. See 📖 Chapter 9.
- Following removal of the foreign body there may be laryngeal, subglottic or tracheal mucosal oedema.

Preoperative assessment

The degree of respiratory distress varies. Many children are calm and not distressed. The degree of urgency varies depending on symptoms and the extent of respiratory distress. It is usually possible to fast the child before anaesthesia. If the child is partially obstructed, hypoxic, or very distressed, anaesthesia and surgery proceed even if the child is not fasted since the risks of delay outweigh the risk of regurgitation and aspiration.

Anaesthetic technique

- Sedative premedication is avoided.
- The aim is to maintain a patent airway while keeping the patient breathing spontaneously throughout the procedure
- An inhalational induction with halothane or sevoflurane in 100% oxygen is performed.

- In a child with upper airway obstruction induction may be slower than normal. Gentle application of CPAP helps to overcome upper airway obstruction.
- Once adequately anaesthetized, an IV cannula is inserted and atropine (20 mcg/kg) or glycopyrronium bromide (5–10 mcg/kg) given (to dry secretions and protect against bradycardia from airway instrumentation or high concentrations of halothane).
- If the foreign body is thought to be in the oropharynx or near the laryngeal inlet, the surgeon will perform a direct laryngoscopy.
- If the child is to undergo bronchoscopy, the vocal cords are sprayed with lidocaine (up to 4 mg/kg) to provide topical analgesia to the larynx before the bronchoscope is introduced. Dense topical anaesthesia of the larynx is vital to help avoid coughing and breath-holding during the procedure.
- The patient is positioned supine with a support beneath the scapulae to extend the neck and push the trachea anteriorly.
- A T-piece circuit is attached to the side arm of the Storz bronchoscope.
- Maintenance is with volatile in 100% oxygen. Spontaneous ventilation is preferred but if the child hypoventilates, is not adequately anaesthetized or is hypoxic then gentle assisted ventilation is needed.
- When the telescope is introduced, the cross sectional area of the bronchoscope is reduced and the work of breathing may be significantly ↑. This is a significant problem in infants. Adequate gas exchange may require intermittent removal of the telescope from the bronchoscope to allow a period of uninterrupted ventilation.
- Once the foreign body has been removed, the trachea is intubated with a conventional endotracheal tube (0.5–1 mm smaller than calculated by age) to maintain the airway until the child emerges from anaesthesia and is extubated awake. Dexamethasone 250 mcg/kg IV is often given to reduce oedema and swelling.
- If there is evidence of significant oedema and swelling of the airway (stridor, use of accessory muscles, hypoxia requiring oxygen) then the child should remain intubated and ventilated in the ITU.
- For oesophagoscopy the child is paralysed and the trachea intubated. Extubate awake.

Postoperative care

Most patients return to a general ward. Admission to ITU if ventilated or HDU for observation if there is stridor. Nebulized adrenaline 400 mcg/kg of 1:1000 will relieve stridor caused by mucosal oedema but the effect is short lived (2–3 hours) and it needs to be repeated regularly. Dexamethasone can be continued (100 mcg/kg IV 6-hourly) for 24 hours. IV maintenance fluids until oral intake resumes. Paracetamol and a NSAID for analgesia. Antibiotics if indicated for infection with a late presentation. A CXR is required. There is a risk of oesophageal perforation after rigid oesophagoscopy. Indicators are pain, tachycardia, and pneumomediastinum on the CXR.

Stridor

- Stridor is a high pitched sound that occurs as a result of partial obstruction in the upper airways.
    - Inspiratory stridor suggests obstruction at or above the larynx e.g. croup, laryngomalacia.
    - Expiratory stridor suggests obstruction below the larynx in the lower trachea or bronchi e.g. asthma, bronchiolitis.
    - Biphasic stridor (inspiratory and expiratory) suggests a midtracheal lesion e.g. vascular ring, foreign body.
    - Hoarseness suggests involvement of the vocal cords e.g. croup.
- Stridor is often accompanied by:
    - Dyspnoea.
    - Use of accessory muscles, tracheal tug, supraclavicular and intercostal recession.
    - Tachypnoea.
    - Tachycardia.
    - Hypoxia.
    - Hypercapnia.

Causes

Acute

- Infection:
    - Laryngotracheitis.
    - Laryngotracheobronchitis (croup).
    - Epiglottitis (now rare in UK).
    - Infectious mononucleosis.
    - Retropharyngeal abscess.
- Allergy:
    - Angioneurotic oedema.
- Trauma:
    - Inhaled foreign body.
    - Inhalation of hot gases.
    - Post-extubation laryngospasm.

Chronic:

- Laryngomalacia.
- Tracheobronchomalacia.
- Laryngeal web or stenosis.
- Laryngeal papillomatosis.
- Subglottic haemangioma.
- Tumour.
- Foreign body.
- Vascular ring.

For anaesthesia for diagnosis and treatment of chronic conditions requiring bronchoscopy see 📖 Chapter 9.

Table 12.1 Features of epiglottitis and croup

	Epiglottitis	Croup
Age	2–5 years	6 months–2 years
Cause	Haemophilus influenzae B	Parainfluenza
		Respiratory syncytial virus
		Influenza
Features	Short onset	Gradual onset
	Fever and systemic upset	Barking cough
	Adoption of tripod position and drooling	
Treatment	Endotracheal intubation	Supportive
	Antibiotic therapy	Humidified oxygen
		IV fluids
		May require endotracheal intubation

Anaesthesia for the child with acute severe stridor

Preoperative assessment

Assess airway, breathing, and degree of obstruction. Agitation may indicate severe hypoxia. Avoid interventions that will distress the child such as venous cannulation or CXR. S_pO_2 monitoring and high flow oxygen. In cases of severe croup, nebulized adrenaline (400 mcg/kg of 1:1000) will improve the child while waiting for theatre. Accompany child to theatre from A&E or ward with appropriate airway equipment. Consultant ENT surgeon and anaesthetist involved.

Anaesthetic technique

- Similar technique as for diagnostic bronchoscopy and removal of inhaled foreign body.
- Principles of a safe technique are inhalational induction, maintenance of spontaneous ventilation and avoidance of neuromuscular blockade until the airway is secured with an ETT.
- Sedative premedication is avoided.
- The child is induced in the position they prefer. This is often sitting. They must not be forced to lie flat if unwilling.
- An inhalational induction with halothane or sevoflurane in 100% oxygen is performed.
- Induction is slower than normal. Gentle application of CPAP helps to overcome upper airway obstruction. Total airway obstruction is a risk as the child is anaesthetized and loses muscle tone.
- An IV cannula is inserted and atropine (20 mcg/kg) or glycopyrronium bromide (5–10 mcg/kg) given (to dry secretions and protect against bradycardia from airway instrumentation or high concentrations of halothane).

- Once adequately anaesthetized, laryngoscopy and endotracheal intubation are performed under deep inhalational anaesthesia.
- In epiglottitis, gentle compression of the chest may produce bubbles that give an indication of the position of the laryngeal inlet.
- Once the child is intubated, the ETT is assessed for correct length and diameter. It may be appropriate to change it for a nasal ETT if the intubation was not difficult to make care in ITU easier. Before transfer to ITU the child is sedated and paralysed. A nasogastric tube, second IV cannula, and an arterial line are inserted.
- Occasionally, endotracheal intubation is not possible and a tracheostomy is required with the child maintained on oxygen and volatile breathing spontaneously through the face mask. If a 'can't intubate, can't ventilate' situation develops, this is managed as described in 📖 Chapter 14.

Postoperative care

Admit to ITU. CXR. Specific treatment for the underlying cause.

Tracheostomy

- Indications:
  - Congenital or acquired upper airway obstruction e.g. Pierre Robin syndrome, severe laryngomalacia.
  - Long term respiratory support as in Ondine's curse (congenital central hypoventilation syndrome).
- Anaesthetic considerations:
  - Shared airway.
  - Potentially difficult endotracheal intubation.

Preoperative assessment

The indication for tracheostomy largely determines the anaesthetic technique. The aetiology of airway obstruction and the ease of endotracheal intubation, if known, are extremely important. Respiratory function in the second group is determined from the notes. Examination of the airway and prediction, in so far as possible, of the anticipated degree of difficulty in airway maintenance and endotracheal intubation. Consultation between surgeon and anaesthetist is important. An ITU bed may need to be booked.

Anaesthetic technique

- When possible, endotracheal intubation, neuromuscular blockade and IPPV are preferred.
- The child may come to theatre from ITU already intubated.
- If indicated, the child is treated as a difficult endotracheal intubation with a gaseous induction and endotracheal intubation under deep inhalational anaesthesia.
- If necessary, tracheostomy can be performed with the child breathing spontaneously through a face mask or LMA.
- Maintenance is with volatile in oxygen and air or 100% oxygen. Nitrous oxide is usually avoided in case of pneumothorax.
- Patient is positioned with a roll or bolster under the shoulders to extend the neck fully and bring the trachea anteriorly.
- The surgical field is infiltrated with LA and adrenaline to provide haemostasis and analgesia. A bolus of opioid can also be given in most cases to provide a degree of postoperative sedation and avoid the child being agitated and potentially dislodging the tracheostomy.
- In children a tracheostomy is performed between the second and third tracheal rings. It is important to operate below the first tracheal ring to reduce the risk of tracheal stenosis. If the tracheostomy is too low there is a risk of endobronchial intubation. The size of the tracheostomy tube is normally 0.5 mm bigger than the ETT it replaces.
- Prior to the incision in the trachea, the child is ventilated with 100% oxygen for a few minutes to provide a reserve in the event of difficulty during the transition from ETT to tracheostomy tube.

- As the tracheostomy tube is inserted the ETT is pulled back but is not removed (so it can be pushed back in to the trachea if necessary) until there is adequate ventilation via the tracheostomy.
- Two stay sutures are inserted on either side of the tracheal incision and taped to the chest wall. These can be used to hold the tracheal incision open if the tracheostomy tube is dislodged and needs to be replaced during the first few days.
- A fibrescope is often passed through the ETT to visualize the insertion of the tracheostomy tube. When this is seen in a good position the ETT is withdrawn. A fibrescope can also be passed through the tracheostomy tube to check the distal end is proximal to the carina.
- Before the tracheostomy tube is taped in place, the shoulder roll is removed to flex the neck so the tapes are not too loose.

Postoperative care

Usually nursed in HDU. ITU and IPPV occasionally depending on the circumstances. The natural mechanism for warming and humidifying inspired air has now been bypassed and patients require humidified oxygen and frequent suctioning of the tracheostomy tube. A CXR should be carried out in the early postoperative period to confirm correct placement and length and exclude a pneumothorax.

Common problems encountered following the procedure include bleeding, surgical emphysema, decannulation, blockage, pneumothorax, and pneumomediastinum.

If the tracheostomy tube comes out the airway and ventilation should be managed from above i.e. face mask or LMA and oral endotracheal intubation if required. The tracheostomy tube is then replaced under controlled circumstances to minimize morbidity. Replacement should not be the initial method of airway management. There is a significant risk of trauma to the trachea and creation of a false passage if this is attempted as an emergency procedure by unskilled personnel.

It takes 7–9 days for the tracheostomy track to mature and during this time the child must be under constant nursing supervision.

Choanal atresia

- This is a congenital anomaly of the anterior skull base with closure of one or both nasal cavities. The obstruction can be membranous or bony.
- The incidence is 1:7000 live births. There is a unilateral to bilateral ratio of 2:1. It is more commonly seen in girls and in up to 50% there are associated congenital abnormalities.
- Bilateral atresia presents early in the neonatal period with respiratory distress. The condition is suspected if a fine suction catheter cannot be passed through the nostrils to the pharynx. CT usually confirms the diagnosis. Unilateral atresia may remain undiagnosed for years before presenting with unilateral nasal discharge.
- Most neonates are obligate nasal breathers for the first few months of life. During quiet inspiration the tongue is pulled up to the palate and obstructs the oral airway. When the child cries this obstruction is relieved.
- Immediate management involves inserting an oropharyngeal airway or a McGovern nipple (rubber teat with a hole at the end which holds the oral airway open and allows the child to breath through it). An orogastric tube can be placed to facilitate feeding. If respiratory distress continues then the baby may require oral endotracheal intubation until definitive surgical correction. This is usually performed within the first week.

Preoperative assessment

Bilateral atresia may be part of the CHARGE syndrome (**C**oloboma, **H**eart defects, choanal **A**tresia, **R**etarded growth, **G**enitourinary and **E**ar anomalies. The child is assessed to exclude other congenital anomalies.

See neonatal anaesthesia 📖 p.390.

Anaesthetic technique

- The child usually comes to theatre with IV access, an oropharyngeal airway in place, and an orogastric tube.
- Atropine or glycopyrronium bromide are given if desired.
- The orogastric tube is aspirated and removed.
- An inhalational induction is performed with the oropharyngeal airway in place.
- The ability to perform IPPV with the face mask is confirmed, the child is paralysed and an oral endotracheal tube inserted. This is usually a south facing preformed RAE type.
- If the child is already intubated it is important to check with the surgeon the practicality of the endotracheal tube in place. This may need to be changed to a south facing preformed RAE type.
- IPPV and maintenance with volatile in oxygen and air or nitrous oxide.

- Surgery is carried out via an endonasal or oral transpalatal approach. The aim is to open up the choanae and insert stents from the nostrils to the nasopharynx. These are left in place for 6–12 weeks so that the choanae heal around them and remain patent (there is a 25–30% restenosis rate for bilateral choanal atresia).
- Analgesia—morphine sulphate 25–50 mcg/kg IV or fentanyl citrate 1–2 mcg/kg IV. IV paracetamol 15 mg/kg is beneficial because of its lack of airway and respiratory effects

Postoperative care

Most patients are extubated and returned to a neonatal intensive care unit. Maintenance fluids are required until feeding is established. An orogastric tube can be passed to ensure enteral feeding if the child is slow to feed by mouth. Analgesia is usually a combination of paracetamol 15 mg/kg and a weak opioid e.g. codeine phosphate 0.5 mg/kg oral 4-hourly both given orally or by orogastric tube. The stents require suction every few hours to maintain patency especially before feeding during which the child will need to breath through them. Eventually the parents are taught to do this so they can care for the child at home.

Emergency anaesthesia: orthopaedics, plastics, neurosurgery, ophthalmology, maxillofacial

Alison Carlyle

Orthopaedics

Considerations in emergency orthopaedic surgery

- The provision of anaesthesia for urgent orthopaedic surgery comprises a significant proportion of the non-elective workload in paediatric anaesthesia.
- Many cases are deferred to the next daytime non-elective theatre session but some require surgery 'out of hours' for clinical or organizational reasons.
- Other than in the case of pathological fractures, most patients are healthy and there is little in the way of intercurrent illness to consider.
- The main safety consideration is the risk of regurgitation and aspiration. The fact that children have suffered trauma and have often received opioid analgesia means that they are often at risk regardless of the time since last oral intake.
- Children are often upset and fretful and accompanied by worried and shocked parents.
- Any number of straightforward and complex conditions will be seen but the common ones are fractures of the forearm, supracondylar humerus and distal tibia.
- Fractures of the femur and septic arthritis provide a small but significant workload.
- The classic paediatric condition associated with pathological fractures is osteogenesis imperfecta. Others include fibrous dysplasia or Ollier's disease, severe cerebral palsy, and the metabolic bone disease associated with renal and hepatic impairment.

Forearm fractures

- These are the commonest orthopaedic condition requiring non-elective paediatric anaesthesia and one of the commonest indications overall.
- 70% of children's fractures involve the upper limb and 50% the forearm and hand.
- Most occur in older, independent children over the age of 5 years and are the result of falls during play or sport.
- Greenstick fractures are more common in younger children and complete fractures in older children.
- They usually heal rapidly with active remodelling and little or no overgrowth. These factors allow conservative management of most forearm fractures with casting alone or manipulation under anaesthesia (MUA) followed by casting.
- Some require fixation with a percutaneous Kirschner wire or wires while a small number require formal open reduction and internal fixation with plating.

Preoperative assessment

Many of these fractures are deferred until the child is fasted and done on the next planned trauma list. These patients are usually treated as elective cases. In some cases, the child may be technically fasted but is pale and frightened. They may be in pain and have received opioid analgesia. Under these circumstances, the stomach is unlikely to have emptied and the child should be regarded as a regurgitation risk. Some fractures require urgent surgery irrespective of fasting status. Communication with the orthopaedic staff is necessary to determine the nature of the fracture and the type of surgical management planned since this may affect the anaesthetic technique. The recent administration of analgesia should be noted as this may influence what is given during anaesthesia. Regional techniques such as brachial plexus block rather than a general anaesthetic are poorly tolerated by children and are not usually considered.

Anaesthetic technique

- IV or gaseous induction may be used as appropriate in a fasted patient.
- A rapid sequence induction is required if the child is regarded as a regurgitation risk.
- Airway management depends, to a certain extent, on what surgery is planned. For an MUA spontaneous ventilation with an LMA is a suitable technique. For longer cases or in young children endotracheal intubation with or without IPPV may be preferable.
- Laryngospasm may occur due to surgical stimulation during manipulation of the fracture. Ideally, this should be anticipated and prevented by deepening anaesthesia or by giving a bolus of short acting opioid such as fentanyl 1–2 mcg/kg IV or alfentanil 10–20 mcg/kg IV.

- An unstable fracture may require percutaneous K wires across the fracture to maintain the reduction or an open reduction and internal fixation. These slightly longer procedures (30 and 90 minutes) require temperature monitoring and a warming mattress. Maintenance IV fluids should be given if the child has fasted for a long time.
- A tourniquet is used during open reduction and internal fixation so blood loss is minimal.
- Opioid analgesia is required for operative procedures. It should also be considered for a simple manipulation. Although the pain of fracture manipulation is not usually regarded as severe most children are not comfortable postoperatively unless they receive an opioid of some kind. The surgical technique of manipulation is usually to ↑ the deformity of the fracture before trying to reduce it and a child who was pain free in a back slab preoperatively may emerge from anaesthesia in pain if analgesia is not given. Options include morphine 100–150 mcg/kg IV, fentanyl 2–4 mcg/kg IV or a weaker opioid such as codeine phosphate 1–1.5 mg/kg IM unless the child received opioid analgesia shortly before surgery. In this case, they are titrated to comfort in the recovery area if necessary. Adjuncts such as a NSAID or paracetamol and an antiemetic may also be given.
- Regional analgesic techniques such as brachial plexus block are usually avoided for these cases. Neurological function is monitored postoperatively and this is complicated by the residual numbness and motor block produced by a regional technique. Local anaesthetic can be infiltrated around the incision by the surgeon if an open reduction and internal fixation is performed.

Postoperative care

Patients usually eat and drink early in the postoperative period. A combination of paracetamol 15 mg/kg oral 4-hourly, a NSAID e.g. ibuprofen 10 mg/kg oral 6-hourly and an oral opioid e.g. codeine phosphate 1 mg/kg oral 4-hourly is prescribed. Following manipulation under anaesthesia, it is common to discharge patients on the day of operation, provided that they fulfil the discharge criteria in the local day-surgery protocol. After more prolonged anaesthetics or complex surgery performed 'out of hours', patients may be kept overnight and discharged the following day.

Supracondylar fracture

- This is the commonest elbow fracture in children and accounts for about 75% of fractures in this area.
- Caused by trauma with the elbow in hyperextension (95%) or hyperflexion (5%).
- May be an indicator of significant force and the presence of other less obvious injuries on presentation should be excluded during preoperative assessment.
- Management may include closed reduction and casting, closed reduction and internal fixation with K-wires or, commonly, open reduction and internal fixation.
- There is a significant incidence of neurological and vascular complications associated with supracondylar fractures.
- Neurological injury most commonly involves the anterior interosseus branch of the median nerve, followed by the radial and ulnar nerves.
- There is a risk of iatrogenic damage, particularly to the ulnar nerve, during operative reduction. Most nerve lesions due to the fracture comprise a neuropraxia and resolve spontaneously over 6–18 months.
- It is relatively common for ischaemia (evidenced by a weak radial pulse or slow capillary refill) to develop distal to the fracture due to impingement of the brachial artery on or between fragments of the fracture. This usually resolves with reduction of the fracture.
- Rarely an arterial laceration occurs which requires exploration and repair during the procedure.

Preoperative assessment

These fractures are usually reduced urgently because of concerns about neurological and vascular damage. They are extremely painful and ideally an IV cannula is sited in the emergency department and IV morphine administered. Patients have usually suffered considerable force and should be regarded as at risk of regurgitation. Other injuries should be considered and excluded.

Anaesthetic technique

- A rapid sequence induction is usually performed with preoxygenation and cricoid pressure performed by a trained assistant.
- The surgical procedure may be prolonged. The airway is secured with an ETT and a standard anaesthetic technique of volatile agent in oxygen and air or nitrous oxide used. It is common to ventilate the patient for the duration of the case.
- The patient is usually positioned supine but may occasionally be in the lateral position to facilitate a posterior approach to the elbow.
- Upper limb nerve blocks are not usually performed. They delay reduction of the fracture and postoperative motor block and numbness confuses the assessment of distal neurological function.

- Intraoperative analgesia depends on the circumstances. If IV morphine was given just prior to surgery then analgesia may be withheld and the child assessed in the recovery area. Otherwise morphine sulphate 100–150 mcg/kg IV or fentanyl citrate 2–4 mcg/kg IV can be given. Paracetamol 15 mg/kg IV or 40 mg/kg rectal and a NSAID may also be used and have an opioid sparing effect.
- Analgesia should not be withheld because of concerns about a compartment syndrome. If this is a concern, a pressure monitor may be inserted at the time of operation.
- A tourniquet is used and operative blood loss is usually minor.
- Maintenance fluids are given as crystalloid.
- Patients are extubated awake.
- The patient may require further IV morphine in the recovery room to achieve adequate analgesia.

Postoperative care

IV maintenance fluids are prescribed until oral intake is established. A combination of paracetamol 15 mg/kg oral 4-hourly, a NSAID e.g. ibuprofen 10 mg/kg oral 6-hourly and an oral opioid e.g. codeine phosphate 1 mg/kg oral 4-hourly is prescribed. Patients are not discharged on the day of surgery. They are nursed with the affected arm in an elevated sling to help reduce the swelling and allow careful observation of neurological function and vascular sufficiency distal to the operation site.

Femoral shaft fractures

- These account for 1.6% of paediatric fractures in the developed world. The male: female ratio is 2.3:1.
- There is a bimodal distribution with one peak between 4–7 years of age and another in teenagers.
- In young children, relatively weak bone may fracture with little force. In older children when bone is mature high velocity trauma is needed to fracture the femur. Resuscitation and treatment of other injuries may take initial priority over the femoral fracture.
- Treatment depends on age. Below 4 years of age, traction or application of a hip spica plaster cast are the usual treatments. Older children can also be put in traction but are candidates for external fixation (compound fractures), intramedullary nailing or plating. Children over 10 years of age usually undergo external fixation, intramedullary nailing or plating.
- Pain is severe. Acute pain management is required on presentation and later to allow traction. This should comprise morphine sulphate 200 mcg/kg IV with further boluses of 50 mcg IV titrated every 5–10 min until the child is comfortable. This may be supplemented by a femoral nerve block (📖 Chapter 7). The nerve block is usually done blind without the aid of a nerve stimulator and may not be successful so IV morphine should be the first analgesic measure.
- Ongoing pain management is required for 7–14 days. A combination of oral paracetamol 15 mg/kg oral 4-hourly, NSAID e.g. ibuprofen 10 mg/kg oral 6-hourly and an opioid e.g. codeine phosphate 1 mg/kg oral 6-hourly is prescribed.
- Anaesthesia may be required for fitting of a splint and adjustment of traction or manipulation with or without open reduction and internal fixation.

Preoperative assessment

For an urgent procedure the relevant concerns are the presence of other injuries, volume status, fasting status and analgesia administered. More often there is a planned procedure a day or two after the injury to adjust traction. In this case, the child is fasted and treated as an elective case.

Anaesthetic technique

- Urgent cases, even if technically fasted, are regarded as having a full stomach and undergo a rapid sequence induction and endotracheal intubation.
- Maintenance is with a volatile agent in oxygen and air or oxygen and nitrous oxide.
- Additional morphine may be given if several hours have elapsed since the last dose. Alternatively, the child can be titrated to comfort postoperatively with boluses of morphine sulphate 50 mcg/kg IV in the recovery room.

- It is difficult to position the child for an epidural or caudal even if this is an option and most anaesthetists would leave the child supine and perform a femoral nerve block using a nerve stimulator or a fascia iliaca compartment block (📖 Chapter 7).
- For a planned case, induction can be gaseous or inhalational depending on circumstances. An LMA may be appropriate for airway management. Again, central blocks are very difficult to perform if the child is in traction and one of the anterior blocks—femoral nerve or fascia iliaca compartment are usually preferred.

Postoperative care

Once the fracture has been immobilized in a splint or internally fixed, pain ↓ markedly. After an operative procedure, an IV morphine infusion or PCA (📖 Chapter 6) is appropriate for 24 hours followed by a combination of paracetamol, NSAID, and oral opioid.

Septic arthritis

- Infection of a joint by pyogenic bacteria. An indication for urgent surgery.
- Incidence in children (5–10/10000 per year).
- Over half of affected children are under 2 years of age.
- Any joint may be involved but the hip, knee, shoulder and elbow are most commonly affected. Only one joint is affected in over 90% of cases.
- Infection is usually haematogenous but direct infection from trauma or surgery and local spread from infected tissues also occur.
- In neonates and infants, the hip is most commonly affected while in older children it is the knee.
- A febrile illness may precede symptoms and signs localized to the infected joint.
- Diagnosis may be difficult because of the subtle and non-specific presentation of a child who is generally unwell before localizing signs are identified. The child may appear septicaemic. Signs include abnormal posture, pain on passive movement, and a reduction in spontaneous movement of the joint.
- Differential diagnosis includes osteomyelitis, acute arthritis, post-traumatic joint effusion, Perthe's disease, and cellulitis. Anaesthetic involvement may start with a request for venous access in a septic infant.
- The commonest organisms involved are *Staphylococcus aureus*, *Staphylococcus epidermidis*, and *Streptococcus pyogenes*.
- Treatment requires rapid evacuation of the pus and aggressive treatment with appropriate antibiotics. Articular cartilage is particularly susceptible to the lytic effects of pus and a delay in treatment may damage the joint and result in long-term deformity and disability. Aspiration of the joint may be performed but in most cases, arthrotomy and generous irrigation of the joint are preferred. An arthroscope is usually used for the knee.

Preoperative assessment

Some anaesthetists are prepared to anaesthetize the child as soon as possible, irrespective of fasting status, to reduce the chances of damage to the joint. Anaesthesia can be delayed until the child is fasted but in a septic infant oral intake will often have been poor for some time. Older children may be systemically well with symptoms and signs limited to the infected joint. Infants may be systemically unwell, febrile, tachycardic, and dehydrated. Respiratory symptoms are common in this situation. Venous access may be present already for antibiotic treatment. Preoperative IV fluids may be needed. Recent administration of paracetamol or a NSAID is noted since this prevents their administration during anaesthesia.

Anaesthetic technique

- IV or inhalational induction is appropriate depending on the circumstances.
- In an older child who is systemically well an LMA and spontaneous ventilation with volatile agent in oxygen and nitrous oxide or air is a suitable technique. In infants and children who are 'toxic' or systemically unwell then endotracheal intubation and IPPV are preferable.
- Arthrotomy and irrigation is usually a short procedure but large volumes of irrigation fluid may be used, some of which soaks into the drapes and sheets. Temperature monitoring is required, particularly in infants as the patient can cool rapidly in this environment. A warming mattress should be in place but may not need to be switched on in the febrile child.
- Blood loss is minimal. Crystalloid fluids are given to replace the calculated fasting deficit and maintenance needs. Pyrexia ↑ insensible losses and maintenance fluids are ↑ by 10% per °C ↑ in temperature.
- The child is likely to have received paracetamol and a NSAID preoperatively. During surgery, a short acting opioid such as fentanyl 1–2 mcg/kg IV may be given.

Postoperative care

IV maintenance fluids until drinking. Paracetamol 15 mg/kg oral 4-hourly and a NSAID e.g. ibuprofen 10 mg/kg oral 6-hourly are continued for postoperative analgesia and can be supplemented with a weak opioid such as codeine phosphate 1 mg/kg oral 4-hourly if necessary. It is important to leave secure venous access for the postoperative administration of IV antibiotics. Occasionally in infants, this may require some form of central venous access.

Plastic surgery

- The majority of non-elective plastic surgery in children comprises peripheral lacerations and finger injuries.
- Most children are fit and well.
- Emergency procedures are rare and most children are operated on during the day or early evening.
- Burns and scalds require anaesthetic involvement in initial resuscitation, intensive care, surgical procedures, and acute and chronic pain management.

Lacerations

- Traumatic lacerations to the head and peripheries and fingertip injuries are very common and form a substantial part of the 'on call' paediatric anaesthetic workload.
- Surgery usually involves exploration to exclude damage to underlying structures, debridement of dead and dirty tissue, cleaning and suturing of the wound.
- Many of these procedures can be performed with LA only but this is often poorly tolerated especially in younger children and when general anaesthesia is available many surgeons prefer this option.

Preoperative assessment

Most children are fit and healthy. Surgery is delayed until the child is fasted and is often done on a planned trauma list. Occasionally, these cases are done in the evening more because of organizational than clinical reasons. An IV cannula may have been placed already for administration of antibiotics or analgesia.

Anaesthetic management

- IV or gaseous induction are both appropriate.
- Anaesthetic maintenance usually involves spontaneous ventilation through an LMA with volatile agent in oxygen and air or nitrous oxide.
- A digital nerve block or ring block provides very effective analgesia for digits. Some surgeons prefer to perform these blocks themselves. Otherwise, the surgeon usually performs wound infiltration with LA. A NSAID and or paracetamol may also be given.
- A tourniquet is often used and blood loss is usually minimal.
- This procedure may turn into a prolonged and complex nerve or tendon repair if underlying damage is found during the surgical exploration.

Postoperative care

The requirement for postoperative analgesia is usually low. Paracetamol and NSAID with or without a weak opioid are prescribed. Unless lacerations are surgically complex or require continued IV antibiotics, patients are usually discharged later on the day of surgery or early next morning.

Nerve and tendon repairs

- These procedures are classically required in children after injuries to the hands involving broken glass.

Preoperative assessment

Patients are usually normal healthy children. Surgery is delayed until the child is technically fasted. If opioid analgesia has been given in the emergency department, the child is often regarded as a regurgitation risk.

Anaesthetic technique

- A rapid sequence induction is performed if there is concern about regurgitation.
- IPPV may be preferable to spontaneous ventilation for prolonged procedures and in younger children.
- Surgery may be prolonged and pressure area care, temperature monitoring, and maintenance IV fluids should be considered.
- A tourniquet is usually used and blood loss is minimal.
- An opioid (morphine sulphate 100–150 mcg/kg IV or fentanyl citrate 2–4 mcg/kg IV) is usually given and the wound infiltrated with LA solution by the surgeon.
- Nerve blocks are usually relatively contraindicated in nerve repair procedures as they can make postoperative assessment of neurological function difficult.

Postoperative care

The main concern is the recovery of function and frequent assessments of motor and neurological function are required. IV maintenance fluids are prescribed until oral intake resumes. A combination of paracetamol 15 mg/kg oral 4-hourly, a NSAID e.g. ibuprofen 10 mg/kg oral 6-hourly and an opioid e.g. codeine phosphate 1 mg/kg oral 4-hourly is prescribed for analgesia.

Burns and scalds

- Approximately 50000 children each year in the UK attend emergency departments following a burn or scald. Between 5000–6000 require admission.
- Burns and scalds account for 6% of paediatric injuries.
- The majority involve pre-school children, burns being most common between 1–2 years. Between 5–18 years, flame burns are the commonest cause of injury.
- House fires are the cause of most fatal burns (approximately 80%), with smoke inhalation being the immediate cause of death in many cases.
- Non-fatal burns generally involve flammable clothing and liquids.
- Scalds are most commonly associated with hot drinks in toddlers but can also occur with over-heated bath water and hot cooking oil.
- Children have nearly three times the body surface area:body mass ratio of adults. Fluid losses are proportionately higher in children than in adults. Consequently, children have relatively greater fluid resuscitation requirements and more evaporative water loss than adults.
- Children younger than 2 years have thinner layers of skin and insulating subcutaneous tissue than older children and adults. Because of disproportionately thin skin, a burn that may initially appear to be partial thickness in a child may instead be full thickness in depth. Thus, the child's thin skin may make initial burn depth assessment difficult.
- Severity of a burn or scald is related to the temperature and the duration of contact. The time needed to cause tissue damage ↓ exponentially with temperature. At 44°C contact with a heat source would require 6 hours for tissue damage to occur; at 70°C epidermal injury occurs in 1 second.
- Burns are categorized by the percentage of body surface area (BSA) involved and the depth of the burn. For children there are three age related assessment charts (Fig 13.1), and for assessment of smaller areas, the child's hand is used as an indicator of 1% of BSA.
- Superficial burns:
  - Involve the outer epidermal tissues, are erythematous and painful but cause minimal tissue damage.
  - The protective function of the skin remains intact.
- Partial thickness burns:
  - Involve the entire epidermis and variable portions of the dermis. There is blistering of the skin, weeping transudates, and they are extremely painful.
  - Superficial partial thickness burns heal quickly with re-epithelialization of hair follicles and sweat glands and minimal scarring.
  - In deep partial thickness burns there are few viable epithelial cells. Re-epithelialization is very slow and scarring occurs if skin grafting is not performed.

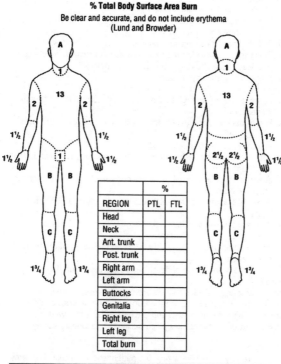

% Total Body Surface Area Burn
Be clear and accurate, and do not include erythema
(Lund and Browder)

	%	
REGION	PTL	FTL
Head		
Neck		
Ant. trunk		
Post. trunk		
Right arm		
Left arm		
Buttocks		
Genitalia		
Right leg		
Left leg		
Total burn		

AREA	Age 0	1	5	10	15	Adult
A = ½ OF HEAD	9½	8½	6½	5½	4½	3½
B = ½ OF ONE THIGH	2¾	3¼	4	4½	4½	4¾
C = ½ OF ONE LOWER LEG	2½	2½	2¾	3	3¼	3½

Fig. 13.1 Lund and Browder burns chart. Reproduced with permission from Hettiaratchy, S., et al. *British Medical Journal* 2004, **329**: 101–103.

- Full thickness burns:
  - Destroy the dermis and epidermis.
  - The surface has a dry leathery firm consistency with charring or pearly white discoloration.
  - Full thickness burns are not painful.
  - This tissue is avascular and there is a zone of ischaemia between the dead tissue above and the live tissue below.
  - Skin grafting is always required.
- Major burns are defined in different ways:
  - Partial thickness and full thickness with affected BSA >10% under 10 years old.
  - Partial thickness and full thickness with affected BSA >20% over 10 years old.
  - Full thickness with affected BSA >5%.
  - A partial thickness or full thickness burn involving face, hands, feet, perineum, or major joints.
  - A partial thickness or full thickness burn involving an electrical or chemical burn.
  - A partial thickness or full thickness burn involving an inhalational injury.
  - A partial thickness or full thickness burn associated with a pre-existing medical disorder.
- Morbidity and mortality ↑ with the size and the depth of the burn and with decreasing age.
- The most common cause of death within the first hour after a major burn is smoke inhalation.
- When assessing a child with a severe burn it is easy to become distracted and focus solely on the burn but other injuries could also be present. The structured ABC approach of APLS is followed and assessment of the burn takes place during the secondary survey.

Primary survey
- As the primary survey is starting, the patient should receive high flow oxygen from a face mask with a reservoir bag.
- A cervical collar should be applied if there is potential injury to the spine from a fall or escape attempt and if no history is available.
- Information should be sought from witnesses, firefighters, and paramedics as the primary survey is taking place. A history of exposure to smoke in a confined space for any length of time indicates a potential inhalational injury.
- There could be airway compromise related to a thermal injury to the upper airway from inhalation of hot gases or smoke, because of burns to the face or neck, from chemical injury to the lung, and from asphyxia. Look for singeing of facial hair and carbonaceous deposits in the oropharynx. Listen for wheeze and stridor.
- Oedema of the airway and face can occur very rapidly following significant smoke inhalation. If there is concern that the airway may deteriorate, the patient should be anaesthetized and the airway secured with an appropriately sized uncut ETT at an early stage in the assessment.

- A rapid sequence induction with thiopentone and suxamethonium is appropriate if respiratory function is inadequate and there are no concerns about the airway. If a difficult airway or endotracheal intubation is possible, an inhalational induction and endotracheal intubation without neuromuscular blockade should be performed.
- If the airway is adequate, breathing is assessed looking for abnormal chest movement, respiratory rate, wheeze, crepitations, and cyanosis. If there are signs of hypoventilation, and the patient is not already intubated and ventilated, this should be carried out.
- A full thickness circumferential chest burn can hinder respiratory movements of the chest. If this is present, escharotomies should be performed. Although the full thickness burn itself is insensate because the dermal nerve endings are destroyed by the burn, effective relieving incisions must extend in to innervated tissue and for this reason, anaesthesia is required.
- Large bore IV access on two limbs is secured as soon as possible. Burnt areas are avoided. The intraosseous route can be used for initial fluid resuscitation. Samples for FBC, U&E, and group and save are taken. An arterial blood gas is required to measure the percentage of carboxyhaemoglobin. This can cause a deceptively high S_pO_2 reading.
- Although major burns are associated with large volumes of fluid loss in the first 4–6 hours, any signs of hypovolaemia on initial presentation should not be assumed to be due to the burn only and other causes should be sought e.g. fractures of long bones or pelvis.

Secondary survey

- With a major burn, there is a rapid reduction in plasma volume due to loss of the skin's barrier function and oedema. Oedema is caused by an ↑ in microvascular permeability and tissue osmotic pressure that leads to interstitial fluid accumulation.
- In unburnt tissues there is oedema caused by a transient endothelial injury related to a rise in the concentration of systemic inflammatory mediators and the presence of hypoproteinaemia.
- The burnt areas should be covered to reduce heat and fluid loss and as a barrier against infection. Initially cling film can be used and later specialized dressings such as Paraffin gauze dressing are applied.
- There are a number of formulae for *estimating* fluid requirements relating to the size of the burn. One of the most straightforward is the Parkland formula:

% BSA burnt × weight in kg × 4 = volume of crystalloid fluid (mL) required in the first 24 hours *from the time of burn*.

- Usually given as Hartmann's solution.
- Half of the calculated volume is given in the first 8 hours, and the remainder given in the following 16 hours.
- Maintenance fluids are required in addition to resuscitation fluids.
- Fluid balance is assessed regularly. Urine output should be 1–1.5 mL/kg/hour and the fluid regimen adjusted as necessary to achieve this. Other signs of adequate resuscitation are rapid capillary refill, a decline in a high haematocrit and a normal or normalizing pH.

- Analgesia is required—morphine sulphate 200 mcg/kg IV followed by an IV infusion of 20–60 mcg/kg/hour (📖 Chapter 6).
- Urinary catheter.
- Once the child has been stabilized, a management plan for the treatment of the burn is made by a senior plastic surgeon. This is likely to involve skin grafting and multiple visits to theatre for assessment, staged grafting and dressing changes.

Anaesthesia for patients with burns and scalds

- Patients range from toddlers with small chest wall scalds caused by pulling a cup of hot liquid on to themselves who are well, feeding normally, and playing on the ward to children with extensive burns and smoke inhalation being ventilated on ITU.
- General anaesthesia is usually required for the initial cleaning and dressing of burns or scalds, subsequent skin grafts, and extensive changes of dressings.
- Minor changes of dressings are often performed on the ward with a combination of oral sedation and analgesia e.g. midazolam 500 mcg/kg oral and morphine sulphate 300 mcg/kg oral, ketamine given IV or IM or nitrous oxide (📖 Chapter 16).

Preoperative assessment

Patients may be on ITU intubated and ventilated with arterial and central venous access. Assess the history related to the burn, extent of burn, adequacy of resuscitation, as well as any co-morbidities. Correct electrolyte imbalances preoperatively. Anticipate significant blood loss during extensive grafting. Group and save or cross match of blood. Patients usually undergo a series of operations. Family members may have died in the fire. Minimize the psychological and physiological disruption as much as possible—quiet environment preoperatively and at induction, sedative premedication if necessary, minimize fasting time.

Nasogastric or nasojejunal feeds need not be stopped in intubated patients. Children often have chest symptoms from one or more of: infection, significant opioid consumption with cough suppression, and restriction of chest movement and coughing by circumferential dressings around the trunk. Patients are frequently infected and may be febrile and tachycardic.

Parents are usually devastated by the injury and require sensitive communication. In the aftermath of a house fire, it is not uncommon for the parents to be patients in an adult hospital and unavailable to give a history or to comfort the child.

Anaesthetic technique

- Intensive care patients are transferred to theatre with sedative and analgesic infusions continuing. Additional volatile anaesthetic is usually given.
- For other patients, if IV access is present, an IV induction is usually appropriate. Given that most patients are preschool, an inhalational induction is easier in most cases without IV access.
- Endotracheal intubation and IPPV are usually indicated although a LMA can be used with SV for minor scalds and burns.

- Although suxamethonium can be used safely during the initial treatment of a burn, it is later contraindicated for 3–6 months because of the hyperkalaemia it causes in patients with burns. There is often a relative resistance to non-depolarizing neuromuscular blockers for several weeks after a major burn.
- Dressing around the trunk may restrict ventilation and make airway management difficult.
- Application of monitoring equipment such as ECG leads, oximeter probes and NIBP cuffs may be difficult
- The application of circumferential dressings around the trunk requires a team of people to lift and hold the child off the operating table and for this reason, if no other, in many cases a secure ETT is the airway device of choice.
- Where endotracheal intubation is performed, the ETT may need to be tied with a bandage rather than taped to avoid tape on burns or grafted areas.
- Maintenance is with volatile in oxygen and air or nitrous oxide.
- Venous access is obtained once the child is anaesthetized. This is often very difficult if limbs are burnt. A femoral vein is often used (🕮 Chapter 5) as the groin skin creases are often spared. Cut-downs are avoided if possible because they ↑ infection risk. Consider the use of invasive monitoring for major cases.
- Skin grafts are usually taken from a thigh if this is unburnt and IV access is preferably not placed in the limb used to harvest the grafts. If the thighs are unavailable or the burn is very extensive, skin may be harvested from the back. This requires the child to be positioned lateral or prone.
- Patients are prone to hypothermia. Heat loss is minimized by increasing the ambient temperature in the theatre, using a warming mattress and warming IV fluids. A warming blanket over the patient is often not feasible given the extent of access to the patient required by the surgical team.
- Reduce infection risk to patient—minimal number of personnel in theatre, use aseptic techniques where possible.
- Major blood loss can occur during grafting of extensive burns. Adequate gauge venous access is required and equipment for a rapid transfusion prepared. Blood loss can be reduced by staging the necessary procedures and infiltrating the burn sites generously with a very dilute solution (1/500000) of adrenaline.
- For analgesia, harvest sites are covered with swabs soaked in a dilute solution of local anaesthetic. A bolus of opioid is also given (morphine sulphate 100–150 mcg/kg IV or fentanyl citrate 2–4 mcg/kg IV). Many children have been receiving regular opioids and other sedatives during the admission and may be resistant to normal doses of opioid. Further analgesia may be required in the recovery area after emergence from anaesthesia.
- The opportunity of a general anaesthetic is often used to perform procedures such as change of nasogastric tube, change of peripheral or central venous access or change of urinary catheter that would distress the child if performed when awake.

Postoperative care

The patient may be returned to ITU anaesthetized and ventilated. Otherwise, the child is extubated awake and observed closely to ensure circumferential dressings around the chest do not impede ventilation. Maintenance fluids are given until feeding resumes. FBC and U&E are checked after extensive grafting. Blood is transfused if necessary.

Analgesia requirements are very variable and depend on the extent of the burn and grafting and previous analgesia administration. For minor procedures a combination of morphine sulphate 200–300 mcg/kg oral 4-hourly and paracetamol 15 mg/kg oral 4-hourly is adequate.

In many cases, it is preferable to run an IV morphine infusion (📖 Chapter 6) for 24 hours to ensure as good analgesia as possible for these unfortunate children. NSAIDs are usually regarded as relatively contraindicated in patients at risk of gastric erosions and ulceration.

Analgesia for patients with burns and scalds

Burn pain can be very severe, and the pain threshold is ↓ because of the local inflammatory response. The patient will have background pain and procedural pain. Use a stepped approach using simple oral and opioid analgesics.

Initial presentation

- In the initial hypermetabolic state, ↑ doses of narcotic and sedative drugs are required.
- A bolus of morphine sulphate 200 mcg/kg IV is given followed by further boluses of 50 mcg/kg every 5–10 min if required until the child is pain free.
- An IV infusion of morphine sulphate 20–60 mcg/kg/hour is commenced.

Procedural pain

- Ketamine, nitrous oxide, benzodiazepines, and opioids (e.g. morphine oral solution, fentanyl lollipops) can be useful for attaining intense analgesia for short procedures such as dressing changes.

Postoperative care

Topical local anaesthetic is applied to graft donor sites intraoperatively.

Paracetamol 15 mg/kg oral four hourly, a NSAID e.g. ibuprofen 10 mg/kg oral 6-hourly (if no contraindications) and an opioid codeine phosphate 1 mg/kg oral 4-hourly or morphine 200–300 mcg/kg oral 4-hourly is an effective combination after smaller procedures.

IV infusion or PCA (in older children) with morphine sulphate (📖 Chapter 6) is used after large grafts.

Long term

- If symptoms of neuropathic pain occur, seek advice from a pain specialist. The patients may need low dose tricyclic antidepressants or gabapentin.
- Consider TENS machines and relaxation techniques in older children.
- Symptoms of anxiety and post-traumatic stress disorder require expert psychological input.

Neurosurgery

- The majority of non-elective paediatric neurosurgery concerns V-P shunts.
- There is a smaller workload from patients with head injuries who require resuscitation, CT scanning, surgical procedures and intensive care.

Blocked ventriculo-peritoneal shunt

- Ventriculo-peritoneal (V-P) shunts are placed to treat or prevent hydrocephaulus caused by ↑ CSF volume.
- This is caused by a variety of pathologies:
  - Excess CSF production (e.g. choroid plexus papilloma) is rare and the majority of cases are due to some type of obstruction to CSF flow or inability to absorb CSF.
  - Common causes include neonatal intraventricular haemorrhage, aqueductal stenosis trauma, previous infection, or previous tumour resection.
- The shunt drains excess CSF from a ventricle to the peritoneal cavity and keeps the ICP normal. Blockage or fracture of a V–P shunt is relatively common and requires either revision of one component or replacement of the whole thing.
- Shunts usually consist of three parts:
  - A proximal end placed into the ventricle.
  - A valve that allows unidirectional flow. This can have various opening pressures. It usually has a reservoir that allows for checking shunt pressure (indicative of ICP) and sampling of CSF.
  - A distal end placed into the peritoneum by tracking the tubing subcutaneously.
- A separate intraventricular CSF access device is often in place. This is a dome-shaped, self-sealing reservoir attached to a catheter. The reservoir is implanted underneath the skin and the catheter is inserted into the ventricle to provide access to cerebrospinal fluid. The reservoir volume is usually 1.5–2.5 mL. These devices provide access for the measurement of intracranial pressure, sampling of CSF, and occasionally the administration of antibiotics or chemotherapy.
- The median survival of a shunt (before need for revision) in a child less than two years of age is 2 years; over two years of age it is 8–10 years.
- Signs and symptoms of blockage or fracture include:
  - Headache
  - Drowsiness
  - Malaise
  - Vomiting
  - Bulging fontanelle
  - Cranial nerve palsies (especially sixth)
  - ↑ in seizures.
- Most commonly, the proximal ventricular end is obstructed with cells, choroid plexus, or debris. There also may be kinking of the tubing, disconnection or fracture of components or migration of the distal end.
- Diagnosis is based on signs and symptoms and is confirmed by CT scan of the head or shunt tap.
- Patients requiring surgery to deal with a blocked V–P shunt are generally well known to the paediatric neurosurgical unit and will often have had a number of procedures performed under general anaesthetic in the past.
- The parents of the patient are usually well informed and aware of the symptoms and signs of a rising ICP.

Preoperative assessment

In most cases, the raised ICP is reduced preoperatively by removing CSF via the access device. The child then comes to theatre with a normal or near normal ICP. In this case, the procedure is usually scheduled to take place once the child is fasted. IV access will usually have been secured on the ward before the patient reaches theatre. Rarely, a child with ↑ ICP must be anaesthetized as an emergency.

Anaesthetic technique

- On theoretical grounds, an IV induction is preferable to minimize ↑ in ICP.
- In reality, an IV or gaseous induction can be used depending on the circumstances. Many anaesthetists take the view that a gaseous induction is less detrimental to ICP than a difficult IV cannulation that causes crying and struggling.
- The airway is secured using an appropriately sized ETT and taped in position. A south facing RAE type ETT or an armoured ETT is used.
- The duration of the procedure can be difficult to gauge. It may be possible to replace the ventricular end without retunnelling a new peritoneal catheter. If the whole shunt is replaced this can take 1–2 hours
- The patient is positioned with the head remote from the anaesthetist and anesthetic machine to allow unrestricted surgical access. Connections between the ETT and circuit are checked and tightened before the head is draped.
- A warming mattress is used to maintain normothermia.
- Blood loss is minimal for this procedure. Fasting deficit and maintenance fluid requirements are given as isotonic crystalloid e.g. Hartmann's during the procedure.
- A solution of local anaesthetic plus adrenaline is usually infiltrated into the wound(s) for haemostasis and analgesia. This is supplemented by fentanyl 2–4 mcg/kg IV and paracetamol 15 mg/kg IV or 40 mg/kg rectal.
- The patient is extubated awake.

Postoperative care

Neurological observations are made for the first postoperative 24 hours and medical staff informed if there is any deterioration in the patient's clinical state or a drop in the appropriate coma scale of two points or more. Maintenance fluids are prescribed until oral intake resumes. Paracetamol 15 mg/kg oral 6-hourly and ibuprofen 10 mg/kg oral 6-hourly generally meet analgesic requirements, with codeine phosphate 1 mg/kg oral 4-hourly if required.

Head injury: initial resuscitation and management

- Anaesthetists are frequently involved in the early management of paediatric head injuries. This may involve:
    - Resuscitation and initial management in the hospital to which the child presents.
    - Escort during CT scan and transfer within the hospital.
    - Interhospital transfer.
    - Anaesthesia for a surgical procedure.
    - Ongoing intensive care.
- Head injury is the most common single cause of trauma death in children between the ages of 1–15 years.
    - It is the cause of death in 40% of injury related deaths.
    - In children, road traffic accidents are the commonest cause, followed by falls.
    - In infancy, the commonest cause is non-accidental injury.
- Damage to the brain is caused by primary or secondary effects of the injury.
- Primary damage includes:
    - Cerebral lacerations and contusions.
    - Intracerebral haematoma.
    - Dural tears.
    - Diffuse axonal injury.
- Secondary damage refers to consequences of the initial injury:
    - Ischaemia caused by inadequate cerebral perfusion as a result of raised intracranial pressure.
    - Ischaemia related to blood loss and hypovolaemia.
    - Hypoxia due to airway obstruction or chest injuries.
    - Hypoxia from hypoventilation caused by damage to the respiratory centre and loss of respiratory drive.
    - Hypoglycaemia and loss of metabolic homeostasis leading to cellular breakdown in cerebral tissues.
    - ↑ in the cerebral metabolic rate e.g. convulsions or fever.

Intracranial pressure homeostasis

- Once the cranial sutures have fused (at 12–18 months of age), the cranium is a fixed volume cavity.
- Cerebral oedema or haematoma after a primary injury will ↑ the volume of the contents of this fixed volume cavity and the pressure within it.
- Initially, this ↑ is compensated for by a reduction in the volume of blood and CSF in the skull.
- When these compensatory mechanisms fail, the ICP rises dramatically.

Cerebral perfusion pressure = Mean arterial pressure – Mean ICP

- A significant ↑ in ICP initially cause transtentorial herniation which if not halted or reversed continues to transforaminal herniation ('coning') and death.
- Cerebral oedema is the commonest cause of raised ICP in children.
- Haematoma formation can cause unilateral transtentorial herniation in which the third cranial nerve is pinched against the tentorium leading to a unilateral fixed dilated pupil.

Assessment

- The primary survey should follow the organized approach of APLS or ATLS guidelines.
    - **A**irway with cervical spine control
    - **B**reathing
    - **C**irculation assessment and intervention if necessary are the first priorities.
    - **D**isability—the pupils are examined for size and reaction to light and the level of consciousness assessed.
- The AVPU scale is a good rapid assessment tool in younger children
    - A—**A**lert to voice.
    - V—responds to **V**oice.
    - P—responds to **P**ain.
    - U—**U**nresponsive.
- During the secondary survey, the head is examined for bruises, lacerations and skull fractures. Signs of a basal skull fracture include a CSF leak from the ears or nose, haemotympanum, 'panda eyes', or Battle's sign (bruising behind the ear).
- A detailed assessment of conscious level is made using the Glasgow Coma Scale if older than 4 years or the Children's Coma Scale if younger. With these scales a 'snapshot' assessment is obtained and it should be repeated regularly to follow the trend in conscious level.
- The fundi are examined to look for papilloedema, which indicates a raised ICP and retinal haemorrhages, which raise the suspicion of non-accidental injury in a young child especially if there are other unexplained injuries.
- The limbs are examined looking for spontaneous movements, tone and reflexes that may reveal lateralizing signs indicating the presence of an intracranial bleed.
- Investigations: FBC, U&E, glucose, cross match, arterial blood gases to assess oxygenation and the adequacy of ventilation.

Initial management of severe head injury

- Aim to prevent secondary brain damage following the primary injury.
- Maintain adequate ventilation, oxygenation, and circulation.
- Maintain adequate CPP and minimize raised ICP.
- If spontaneous ventilation is inadequate, the patient should be anaesthetized and intubated with in-line stabilization of the cervical spine. Anaesthesia is induced with thiopental (2–5 mg/kg) and suxamethonium (1–2 mg/kg). IPPV is instituted. Ongoing sedation (midazolam 100 mcg/kg/hour or propofol 100–300 mcg/kg/hour) and neuromuscular blockade ± analgesia are required. Capnography is used and arterial blood gases checked to ensure the adequacy of IPPV. Normocapnia is the aim.

- Adequate mean arterial pressure should be maintained to ensure cerebral perfusion. This may require fluid resuscitation (20 mL/kg isotonic crystalloid or colloid repeated as required) or, if the patient is judged to be normovolaemic, a vasopressor e.g. noradrenaline 0.01–0.5 mcg/kg/min. Glucose containing solutions are avoided.
- The recommended MAP to maintain CPP varies with age
  - <3 months: 40–60 mmHg
  - 3–12 months: 45–75 mmHg
  - 1–5 years: 50–90 mmHg
  - 6–11 years: 60–90 mmHg
  - 12–14 years: 65–95 mmHg
- An arterial line is useful but this should not delay urgent investigation or treatment if it is difficult to insert.
- Focal seizures are regarded as a focal neurological sign in these circumstances. Generalized seizures are of less significance but are controlled as they ↑ the cerebral metabolic oxygen demand. Benzodiazepines such as diazepam (300–400 mcg/kg IV repeated if necessary) or lorazepam (100 mcg/kg IV repeated if necessary) are the first line therapy. A phenytoin infusion (18 mg/kg) over 30 min is given if there are persistent or prolonged seizures.
- The patient should be positioned 20–30° head-up position to improve venous drainage and lower ICP.

Imaging

- There is little point performing skull films if CT is also planned. Skull films are not always useful, as severe intracranial trauma can be present in the absence of a fracture.
- CT scanning is widely available and is routine in the type of child who requires anaesthetic input to their management.
- Neurosurgical referral is made if there is a deteriorating level of consciousness, focal neurological signs, a depressed skull fracture, a penetrating head injury, basal skull fracture, or a coma score of <12/15. Surgical options include evacuation of an intracerebral haematoma, insertion of a ventricular drain, or insertion of a bolt to measure ICP.
- If there are signs of ↑ ICP and definitive treatment will be delayed, then the patient should be hyperventilated to a pCO_2 of 3.5–4.0 kPa, given mannitol 0.5–1 mg/kg IV and Furosemide up to 1 mg/kg IV (urinary catheter required).
- Paediatric neurosurgery services are based in tertiary paediatric centres and an interhospital transfer is often required (📖 Chapter 14).

Table 13.1 Glasgow Coma Scale (4–15 years)

Eye opening	Score
Spontaneously	4
To verbal stimuli	3
To pain	2
No response to pain	1
Best motor response	
Obeys verbal command	6
Localizes to pain	5
Withdraws from pain	4
Abnormal flexion to pain (decorticate)	3
Abnormal extension to pain (decerebrate)	2
No response to pain	1
Best verbal response	
Orientated and converses	5
Disorientated and converses	4
Inappropriate words	3
Incomprehensible sounds	2
No response to pain	1

Table 13.2 The Childrens' Glasgow Coma Scale (<4 years)

Eye opening	Score
Spontaneously	4
To verbal stimuli	3
To pain	2
No response	1
Best motor response	
Spontaneous or obeys verbal command	6
Localizes to pain or withdraws to touch	5
Withdraws from pain	4
Abnormal flexion to pain (decorticate)	3
Abnormal extension to pain (decerebrate)	2
No response to pain	1
Best verbal response	
Alert, babbles, coos, words to usual ability	5
Less than usual words, spontaneous irritable cry	4
Cries only to pain	3
Moans to pain	2
No response to pain	1

Evacuation of intracranial haematoma

- This usually follows trauma and is an emergency procedure to reduce a raised ICP, maintain CPP and minimize the secondary damage that can occur after a head injury.
- The haematoma may be extradural, subdural or intracerebral.
- The patient will have been assessed and stabilized using the ABC approach of the APLS guidelines.
  - In the case of a head injury serious enough to cause an intracerebral haematoma, early management usually involves anaesthesia, endotracheal intubation, ventilation, sedation with infusions of morphine and midazolam, and IV fluid administration. These interventions are aimed at maintaining CPP and oxygenation of the tissues.
  - The patient may need interhospital transfer to a paediatric neurosurgical centre.

Preoperative assessment

This is usually brief and may be incomplete depending on the circumstances. If the child has already been anaesthetized and intubated then details of endotracheal tube size and length along with drugs given, known allergies, and vascular access are noted before taking responsibility for the child. Occasionally mannitol has been given to reduce ICP and this will produce a diuresis. It is important to determine the presence or absence of other injuries in addition to the head injury and to clarify the status of the cervical spine.

Anaesthetic technique

- The principles are to maintain CPP (minimize ICP and maintain blood pressure), provide adequate oxygenation and ventilation, and protect the lungs from aspiration.
- The recommended MAP to maintain CPP varies with age
  - <3 months: 40–60 mmHg.
  - 3–12 months: 45–75 mmHg.
  - 1–5 years: 50–90 mmHg.
  - 6–11 years: 60–90 mmHg.
  - 12–14 years: 65–95 mmHg.
  - If the MAP is low despite control of haemorrhage and resuscitation then an infusion of noradrenaline (0.1–0.5 mcg/kg/min) may be required to maintain this and hence CPP.
- Care must be taken on transferring the patient from the transfer trolley to the theatre table as there may be other associated injuries e.g. involving the cervical spine. The patient should be log-rolled if turning is necessary.
- If the child is not yet anaesthetized then a rapid sequence induction and endotracheal intubation with an armoured ETT is usually the preferred technique. Manual in-line stabilization of the cervical spine is required if a cervical spine injury has not been excluded.

- Moderate hyperventilation (arterial pCO_2 4.0–4.5 kPa) is normal. Anaesthesia is usually maintained with a volatile agent in oxygen and air or oxygen and nitrous oxide.
- Boluses of morphine (100 mcg/kg) or fentanyl (2–4 mcg/kg) can be given for intraoperative analgesia or an infusion of remifentanil (0.25–0.5 mcg/kg/minute) commenced. In this case, a bolus of morphine is given approximately 30 min before the end of the procedure if extubation is planned. The surgeon can infiltrate a long acting local anaesthetic around the skin suture line.
- Standard anaesthetic monitoring (capnography, S_pO_2, NIBP, ECG) may be supplemented with an arterial line for invasive blood pressure monitoring. An arterial line is often placed in the femoral artery but this should not delay emergency surgery unduly.
- Skin and/or rectal thermometers and a warming mattress are used.
- Blood loss is variable. IV crystalloid fluids are given initially to replace maintenance requirements and blood loss. A group and save sample should be taken preoperatively and blood can be cross-matched urgently if necessary. 'Haemacue' or blood gas samples can be used to monitor haemoglobin levels during the procedure and blood can be transfused if the haemoglobin falls below 7 g/dL. If blood loss is large, an urgent coagulation screen is required and blood products such as fresh frozen plasma or platelets transfused in the light of the results.
- Maintenance fluids are usually restricted to 50% of normal and given as an isotonic fluid e.g. Hartmann's solution. Blood glucose should be monitored and kept in the normal range. A loading dose of phenytoin (18 mg/kg) should be considered if there has been seizure activity at any stage.

Postoperative care

If the child was awake preoperatively and has undergone evacuation of an isolated extradural haematoma, then it is common to let them recover from anaesthesia and extubate. More commonly, transfer to an ITU with ongoing ventilation and sedation is appropriate particularly if the operation was prolonged, the ICP is raised, or there are associated injuries. Measurement of U&E and a FBC is required if not already done.

Ophthalmology

Considerations in non-elective ophthalmic surgery

- Ophthalmology comprises a relatively small part of the emergency workload in paediatric anaesthesia. Almost all of it is related to trauma.
- Children up to the age of 14 years comprise 20–30% of all patients with ocular trauma.
- Incidence is maximal between the ages of 8–14 and boys are affected more commonly than girls.
- Domestic accidents are commonest in pre-school children while sporting injuries and unintended contact comprise the main two causes in school children.
- During surgery, the anaesthetist is remote from the airway and has limited access to the airway, ETT, or LMA during the procedure.
- This type of surgery predisposes to severe postoperative nausea and vomiting and prophylactic antiemetics are given during anaesthesia.
- The oculo-cardiac reflex (☐ p.298) is particularly strong in children. Depending on preference atropine 20 mcg/kg IV or glycopyrronium bromide 10 mcg/kg IV can be given as prophylaxis or kept available for treatment if required.

Perforating eye injury

- Perforating eye injuries in the developed world are commonest in boys between the ages of 3–9 years.
- The commonest causes of perforating ocular injury are sharp tools (knives/scissors) poked by the child into their own eye, or objects thrown at the child. Injuries are most likely to occur at home.
- Wound closure with or without removal of a foreign body are required.

Preoperative assessment

Although repair of a perforated eye is an urgent operation, surgical repair is usually delayed until the child is technically fasted. Manoeuvres that cause crying and struggling and so ↑ IOP such as venous cannulation without topical analgesia should be avoided if possible. Analgesia should be administered as required for the same reasons.

There has been concern in the past that the use of suxamethonium, which is known to raise IOP, could cause extrusion of vitreous humour. This concern is likely to have been overemphasized and most anaesthetists will use suxamethonium under these circumstances if it is indicated. Thiopental and other IV induction agents ↓ IOP and the net effect is likely to be minimal.

Anaesthetic technique

- The ideal induction should avoid making the child cry or struggle. If the child is fasted then an 'elective' induction can be performed. A sedative premedication can be given if required and a smooth gaseous or IV (preceded by topical cutaneous analgesia) induction performed. A non-depolarizing relaxant is used to facilitate endotracheal intubation. A bolus of opioid e.g. fentanyl 1–2 mcg/kg IV or lidocaine 1.5 mg/kg IV may be given to attenuate the rise in IOP in response to laryngoscopy. If the patient can be treated in this elective manner then the issue of suxamethonium and IOP is irrelevant.
- If there is concern about regurgitation then a rapid sequence induction using preoxygenation, suxamethonium, and cricoid pressure should be performed.
- Maintenance of anaesthesia is with a volatile agent in oxygen and air. Nitrous oxide should be avoided because it may ↑ the size of any air bubbles present in the eye. It also potentiates the emetic effects of the surgery.
- This operation may be of long duration. Maintenance IV fluids are required. Temperature is monitored and a warming mattress used.
- LA drops are administered by the surgeon and provide good analgesia.
- A prophylactic antiemetic e.g. ondansetron 100 mcg/kg IV is given since the likelihood of PONV is high.
- Emergence from anaesthesia and extubation should be as smooth as possible to minimize coughing or straining that will ↑ IOP.

Postoperative care

IV maintenance fluids until oral fluids are tolerated and PONV is not a problem. Further antiemetic of a different class if required e.g. cyclizine 1 mg/kg IV. For analgesia a combination of paracetamol 15 mg/kg oral 4-hourly, ibuprofen 10 mg/kg oral 6-hourly and codeine phosphate 1 mg/kg oral 4-hourly is prescribed. Topical NSAID drops can also be used. Postoperative pain is not usually a major problem. If the duration of anaesthesia was prolonged or the surgery was performed 'out of hours', it is common to keep patients overnight for discharge the following day. This may also be necessary if further doses of topical ocular medication are required.

Retinal detachment

Retinal detachment is unusual in children (1–2% of all cases). It is classified as primary (or idiopathic) or secondary detachment, which is due to a condition that is not primarily retinal. They have different causes, treatments, and outcomes.

Primary detachment

- There is a defect in the retina, which allows fluid from the vitreous cavity to pass into the sub-retinal space.
- The defect is usually peripheral in the retina and risk factors include significant myopia (seen in Marfan's, Ehler's–Danlos, and Sticklers syndromes) and trauma.
- There may be a strong family history of idiopathic retinal detachment. There may be no obvious cause.
- Symptoms are visual and may not be reported by young children.
- Treatment is surgical.

Secondary detachment

- A collection of sub-retinal fluid may form as a transudate originating from the vitreous, retinal, or choroidal circulations.
- Causes include hypertension, chronic renal failure, uveitis, and various tumours including retinoblastoma. Alternatively, the retina may be displaced by fibrous bands that develop following trauma with vitreal haemorrhage or retinopathy of prematurity.
- The treatment of secondary retinal detachment is directed to the underlying cause.

Preoperative assessment

If there is a predisposing condition or syndrome then previous medical records may need to be obtained. Occasionally, further investigations e.g. cardiac ultrasound may be required although most complex children are known to local services and the relevant information is in the general paediatric notes. The surgical treatment of primary retinal detachment is delayed until the child is fasted.

Anaesthetic management

- If there is concern about the possibility of the patient having a full stomach especially after trauma, a rapid sequence induction should be performed.
- The airway is secured using an ETT. This is usually a south facing preformed RAE ETT.
- Particular care should be taken to tape the ETT securely in place. The anaesthetist is remote from the airway during surgery accidental manipulation, obstruction, or disconnection of the tube can occur under cover of the head drape.
- Surgery may be prolonged in the region of between 2–4 hours. The patient is usually ventilated, partly to maintain normocapnia and help provide optimal surgical conditions and partly because of the duration of surgery.

- Temperature should be monitored and a warming mattress used.
- Blood loss is minimal for this procedure. Crystalloid is given to replace the calculated fasting deficit and maintenance fluid needs.
- Most of the surgery is not stimulating to the patient. However, manipulation of the retina can be transiently very stimulating and a short acting opioid such as fentanyl or alfentanil can be used to cover these episodes. Alternatively, an infusion of remifentanil 0.25–0.5 mcg/kg/min provides intraoperative analgesia and allows low concentrations of volatile agent to be used so facilitating recovery.
- An antiemetic such as ondansetron 100 mcg/kg IV or cyclizine 1 mg/kg IV are given prophylactically.

Postoperative care

Maintenance IV fluids until drinking. Further antiemetic if required. Analgesic requirements in the postoperative period are generally low and oral analgesics such as ibuprofen 10 mg/kg oral 6-hourly and paracetamol 15 mg/kg oral 4-hourly generally give effective pain relief.

Dental abscess

- A dental abscess is an infection in the centre of a tooth that spreads through the tooth to infect supporting bone and other nearby tissues.
- Dental abscesses are common in children and are usually a complication of dental caries.
- The periapical abscess, which starts in the dental pulp, is the most common type in children.
- Symptoms include:
  - Pain (toothache). This can be severe and throbbing.
  - The affected tooth may become tender to touch, and may become loose.
  - Swelling of the gum.
  - Swelling of the face.
  - The skin over an abscess may become red and inflamed.
  - Pyrexia and malaise.
  - In severe cases there may be spasm of the jaw muscles with difficulty swallowing.
- Treatment requires extraction of one or more teeth, drainage of pus and IV antibiotics followed by oral antibiotics.
- In all but the most co-operative older child, a dental abscess is examined and treated under general anaesthetic.
- The airway of the patient is 'shared' with the dentist and the anaesthetist will not have immediate access to the airway if it becomes partially obstructed. Good communication between anaesthetist and dentist is essential.

Preoperative assessment

The patient is likely to be anxious and in pain and will need adequate analgesia in the preoperative period. If the child is febrile and toxic they may be dehydrated (especially if oral intake has been less than normal because of pain) and benefit from IV fluids while fasting.

The airway is inspected looking for signs of swelling around the jaw and neck, noting particularly if it crosses the midline. The degree of mouth opening is noted. The swelling is often impressive and children may be reluctant to open their mouths voluntarily because of pain. This can make the imprecise science of airway assessment more difficult than normal.

Anaesthetic technique
- If there is concern about the patient's airway, an inhalational induction is performed and spontaneous ventilation maintained until the trachea is intubated.
- Limitation of mouth opening because of pain or muscle spasm usually disappears when the child is anaesthetized and airway manoeuvres can usually be performed without difficulty.
- Rarely this may not happen in which case advanced airway management techniques may be required (📖 Chapter 5).

- Endotracheal intubation is usually the preferred method of airway management because of the potential for pus from the abscess to contaminate the trachea if an LMA is used. The airway is secured with a south facing preformed RAE ETT.
- A throat pack is inserted to prevent blood or pus soiling the airway.
- Once the tooth (or teeth) has been extracted and the abscess drained, the dentist may perform a nerve block. This is sometimes omitted in the presence of infection and systemic analgesia given instead e.g. fentanyl citrate 1–2 mcg/kg.
- An appropriate IV antibiotic is usually given during the case.
- The patient should be extubated awake after removal of the throat pack and suction of the oropharynx.

Postoperative care

Swelling and discomfort usually improve very quickly. Oral intake can usually resume. Paracetamol 15 mg/kg oral 4-hourly and ibuprofen 10 mg/kg oral 6-hourly usually provide adequate analgesia. A weak opioid such as codeine phosphate 1 mg/kg oral 4-hourly is prescribed if necessary. The patient may be kept in hospital for 24 hours to receive further doses of IV antibiotic before discharge of oral antibiotics.

Facial trauma

- Facial trauma covers a wide spectrum of injuries. About 70% of paediatric facial trauma comprises soft tissue injuries, 25% dental trauma, and 5% facial fractures.
- The nasal bones and mandible are the two most frequent sites of facial fracture, followed by the midface.
- Manipulation of nasal fractures is usually performed on an elective basis 2–5 days after the injury.
- Mandibular condylar fractures account for 60% of mandibular fractures in children. Trauma to the condylar growth centre beneath the articular disk may cause delayed growth of the affected side of the jaw. Most condylar fractures are treated conservatively.
- Midface fractures are classified as Le Fort I, II, or III. Le Fort I is a fracture separating the palate and alveolus from the rest of the maxilla. Le Fort II separates the midface from the skull, creating a free-floating pyramidal segment. This fracture includes a mobile palate. Le Fort III involves a complete separation of the face from the cranial base. The mobile segment includes the maxilla, palate, zygoma, and ethmoid bones. These fractures are indicators of considerable trauma and associated injuries are common.

Preoperative assessment

The treatment of facial fractures is delayed until after the primary survey, resuscitation, and treatment of more urgent injuries. Cervical spine injury should be excluded. If there is no urgency, the child is fasted and operated on during a daytime trauma list.

Fractures of the mandible are usually associated with tearing of the gingival tissue and haematomas on the buccal and lingual sides of the intra-oral aspect of the mandible. In patients with bilateral condylar fractures, the mandible is displaced posteriorly, which occasionally results in airway compromise. Mobile fracture segments, oedema, haemorrhage, vomit, bone fragments, and foreign bodies may cause obstruction of the airway. Loose teeth should be documented.

Anaesthetic technique

- If there is a possibility of the facial injuries compromising the patency of the airway an inhalational induction should be performed.
- Manipulation of a nasal fracture is a brief procedure but surgical reduction and fixation of other facial fractures is usually complex and prolonged.
- For manipulation under anaesthesia of a nasal fracture a LMA and spontaneous ventilation is usually used.
- For other cases, the airway is secured using an ETT. An armoured ETT is often used. Alternatively, a north or south-facing ETT is used depending on the site of injury and the proposed surgery.
- A throat pack is inserted if there is a possibility of airway soiling.

- Maintenance is with a volatile agent in oxygen and air or nitrous oxide. Morphine sulphate 100–150 mcg/kg IV or fentanyl 2–4 mcg/kg IV can be given. Alternatively, an infusion of remifentanil 0.25–0.5 mcg/kg/min provides cardiovascular stability and reduces the requirement for volatile anaesthetic agent. IPPV is the norm.
- Temperature is monitored and a warming mattress used.
- The fasting fluid deficit and maintenance fluid requirements are given as crystalloid such as Hartmann's solution.
- Blood loss is generally not significant unless arterial damage has occurred and is replaced with colloid or crystalloid.
- If remifentanil is used a bolus of morphine is required before the end of surgery. LA infiltration and/or specific nerve blocks performed by the surgeon may be helpful. A NSAID and paracetamol 15 mg/kg IV or 40 mg/kg rectal can also be given intraoperatively.

Postoperative care

Postoperatively the child should go to a ward used to looking after facial injuries. Admission to an HDU is appropriate if there is significant oral or facial swelling that could compromise the airway. If there is concern about airway patency in the postoperative period then admission to an ITU with continuing endotracheal intubation is required. Occasionally a tracheostomy will be required until the risk of postoperative airway obstruction has passed.

IV maintenance fluids are continued until oral intake is established. Analgesia depends on the extent of surgery. A combination of paracetamol 15 mg/kg oral 4-hourly, ibuprofen 10 mg/kg oral 6-hourly, and codeine phosphate 1 mg/kg oral 4-hourly will often be adequate. Occasionally an IV morphine infusion or PCA are necessary, especially if there are other injuries or the child cannot take oral drugs.

Section 6

Problems during anaesthesia, resuscitation, syndromes, and sedation

Problems during anaesthesia, resuscitation, and patient transfer

Carolyn Smith

Problems during anaesthesia

The anaesthetist is often best placed to notice the first signs of any developing problem regardless of its cause.

- The morbidity and mortality of critical incidents can be reduced by:
  - Getting help early.
  - Good communication.
  - Designating a team leader.
  - Delegating tasks to named individual(s).
  - Working together as a team.
- Following the ABC of resuscitation helps ensure the safety of the patient and will often help to identify the underlying problem.

Hypoxia

- Fundamentally this is a reduced availability of oxygen for tissue consumption.
- Classically, it is divided into:
  - Hypoxaemic hypoxia—inadequate arterial oxygen (P_aO_2).
  - Anaemic hypoxia—normal P_aO_2 but reduced availability of haemoglobin.
  - Stagnant (ischaemic) hypoxia—normal P_aO_2 and haemoglobin but reduced tissue blood flow.
  - Histiotoxic (cyotoxic) hypoxia—normal P_aO_2, Hb and oxygen delivery but inability of the tissues to utilize oxygen.
- All of these result in anaerobic metabolism, ↑ lactate formation, failure of cell membranes, impairment of the normal intracellular and extracellular ion balance, and eventually cell death.

Causes

- Hypoxic gas mixture:
  - Incorrect or inadequate flow.
  - Second gas effect.
  - Oxygen failure.
  - Equipment or anaesthetic machine malfunction.
- Hypoventilation (reduced alveolar ventilation) which may be due to a reduced respiratory rate and/or a reduced tidal volume:
  - Disconnection.
  - ETT or other equipment displacement.
  - Inadequate IPPV settings.
  - Incorrect mode of ventilation.
  - Drugs—opioids, anaesthetic agents.
  - Underlying medical conditions—metabolic disturbances, intracranial pathology, sleep apnoea syndromes, hypothermia.
  - Airway obstruction—↑ airway obstruction and/or ↓ FRC.
- Shunt:
  - Intrapulmonary—atelectasis, secretions, aspiration.
  - Extrapulmonary—congenital heart disease.
- Inadequate oxygen delivery:
  - Hypoperfusion e.g. sepsis.
  - Embolus.
  - Local problem e.g. limb ischaemia, hypothermia, patent ductus arteriosus.
- ↑ oxygen requirement:
  - Sepsis.
  - Malignant hyperthermia.

Management

- ↑ F_IO_2 to 100%.
- Measure F_IO_2 near patient end of the circuit.
- Observe patient, looking at respiratory rate and pattern and for signs of obstruction such as tracheal tug, use of accessory muscles, see-saw pattern, and noisy respiration.

- Hand ventilate with three or four big breaths to allow assessment of airway patency and the degree of airway resistance.
- If unsure whether it is a patient or a circuit problem give manual ventilation breaths with a simple bag and valve plus a reservoir attached to an external oxygen source.
- If resistance is high at the patient end suction down airway device to check its patency. Pull back ETT a short distance or adjust other airway devices while auscultating and observing chest movements. If in doubt take it out and revert to a face mask and manual ventilation.
- If patient continuing to deteriorate get help.
- Alert surgical colleague if not already aware.
- Determine and treat underlying cause.

Points to note
- Infants and neonates have a reduced FRC relative to closing volume and therefore less reserve in the event of apnoea or airway obstruction (📖 Chapter 1).
- Neonates and infants have a high oxygen consumption and fewer alveoli (~15% adult number) at birth.
- Neonates are unresponsive to the CO_2 stimulus to respiration at birth.
- Neonates and particularly ex-premature infants are more prone to apnoea, are more sensitive to opioids, and suffer more episodes of apnoea after opioids and general anaesthesia.
- Narrow airways have a high resistance to flow and any small reduction in circumference due to secretions produces a marked ↑ in resistance.
- Small ETTs are liable to kink, obstruct, and dislodge.
- The smaller LMAs are prone to twisting, displacement, and dislodgement.
- The work of breathing is high in a neonate and many anaesthetists feel that LMAs are inappropriate for all but the shortest of cases.
- If the hypoxia is showing no improvement with 100% oxygen and adequate ventilation the cause is likely to be a shunt.
- Although a patent ductus arteriosus usually closes within the first week of life, it can re-open in neonates during severe hypoxia.
- PEEP may exacerbate the hypoxia caused by a shunt.
- Atelectasis:
  - May occur with a high F_IO_2 due to absorption of nitrogen (required to splint the alveoli open).
  - Occurs in dependent parts of the lung during anaesthesia, it may occur with endobronchial intubation.
  - May persist into the postoperative period in those with poor lung function and difficulty clearing secretions.
- FRC is ↓ by anaesthesia, infection, atelectasis, respiratory distress syndrome, pulmonary infection, and oedema. It is ↑ by PEEP, CPAP, and in asthma.

Airway obstruction

- Airway obstruction may occur in the mouth, pharynx, larynx, trachea, and large bronchi.
- Airway obstruction leads to hypoventilation and ↑ work of breathing.
- During spontaneous ventilation it may present as:
  - Noisy respiration.
  - Stridor.
  - Use of accessory muscles.
  - Tracheal tug, indrawing, and paradoxical see-saw movement of the chest and abdomen.
- Tachypnoea, tachycardia, hypoxia, hypercapnia, and poor movement of the reservoir bag may all be indicative of the problem.
- Pulmonary oedema may occur if intrathoracic pressures are excessive or prolonged.
- During IPPV, warning signs include:
  - ↑ airway pressures with ↓ chest movement.
  - Noisy respiration or wheeze.
  - Hypoxia.
  - Hypercapnia.

Causes

- Tongue.
- Hypotonia of pharyngeal muscles involved in upper airway maintenance.
- Laryngospasm.
- Secretions.
- Strictures, tumours, soft tissue swelling, oedema, infection, and foreign bodies including teeth and anaesthetic equipment.
- Laryngomalacia and tracheomalacia.
- Mechanical obstruction at any point along the breathing circuit.

Management

- In spontaneous ventilation:
  - ↑ F_iO_2.
  - ↑ fresh gas flow.
  - Airway opening manoeuvres—mouth opening, head tilt and chin lift, check patency and position of airway device.
  - Remove secretions.
  - CPAP.
  - Endotracheal intubation.
- In IPPV:
  - ↑ F_iO_2.
  - Ventilate by hand.
  - Check ventilator tubing for obstruction.
  - Pass suction catheter down ETT.
  - Auscultate chest to exclude bronchospasm or pneumothorax.
  - Withdraw ETT slightly and if no improvement remove and use face mask.
  - Consider inadequate neuromuscular blockade.
- Treat any underlying cause.

Laryngospasm

- Laryngospasm is a common (up to 3% of infants) and potentially serious problem in paediatric anaesthesia.
- It is the result of reflex closure of the glottis by adduction of the true and/or false cords.
- It may persist after cessation of the causative stimulus.
- Laryngospasm can cause complete or partial airway obstruction. Partial obstruction causes inspiratory stridor.
- Severe episodes with profound hypoxia and bradycardia are more likely in infants <12 months of age.
- It may present with inspiratory stridor, hypoxaemia, hypoventilation, and rarely pulmonary oedema.

Causes

- Local stimulation of the larynx: blood, saliva, vomit, foreign body, including laryngoscope, airway, LMA, or ETT.
- Inadequate depth of anaesthesia and response to stimulation: surgery, movement.
- Tracheal extubation at a light plane of anaesthesia.
- More common in children with active or recent (2–4 weeks) respiratory tract infection.

Management

- Stop or remove stimulus.
- 100% oxygen.
- CPAP/PEEP by partially closing expiratory valve. Risk of gastric distension if the vocal cords are closed.
- Deepen anaesthesia or awake depending on circumstance.
- Drugs: bolus of propofol and/or suxamethonium.
- Endotracheal intubation if not recovering or deteriorating.
- If the child is intubated or reintubated then extubate when fully awake.

Point to note

- The use of suxamethonium in severe hypoxia may lead to profound bradycardia and/or cardiac arrest.

Bronchospasm

- Bronchospasm during anaesthesia presents as:
  - Hypoxia.
  - ↑ airway pressures.
  - ↑ expiratory time.
  - ↓ movement of the reservoir bag.
  - Audible wheeze.
- It occurs more frequently in those with a history of asthma, allergy, active or recent respiratory infection, or when anaesthesia is inadequate.

Causes

- Surgical stimulation.
- Airway stimulation: oropharyngeal airway, LMA, ETT, or suction.
- Pharyngeal, laryngeal, bronchial secretions or blood.
- Foreign body inhalation.
- Aspiration of gastric contents.
- Anaphylactic or anaphylactoid reactions.
- Pulmonary oedema.
- Histamine releasing drugs.
- Consider and exclude the following as they form part of the differential diagnosis:
  - Pneumothorax.
  - Mechanical obstruction within the circuit or ETT.
  - Laryngospasm.
  - Oesophageal intubation or displacement of ETT.
  - Pulmonary oedema.

Management

- ↑ F_iO_2.
- ↑ inspired concentration of volatile agent.
- Treat primary cause.
- Nebulized salbutamol 2.5 mg.
- Salbutamol 5–15 mcg/kg IV over 10 min, then infusion of 1–5 mcg/kg/min.
- Aminophylline 5 mg/kg over 30 min, then infusion 0.8–1 mg/kg/hour (if no recent doses).
- Hydrocortisone 4 mg/kg IV. 1 month–1 year: 25 mg; 1–6 years: 50 mg; 6–12 years: 100 mg; 12–18 years: 100–500 mg.

Points to note

- If patient remains unresponsive to treatment adrenaline 10 mcg/kg IM or an adrenaline infusion of 0.02–0.1 mcg/kg/min may be helpful.
- Ketamine 2 mg/kg IV may be useful, as may magnesium sulphate 40 mg/kg IV (maximum 2 g).

Hypotension

When working out the causes of hypotension it is useful to remember the physiological equations:
- Mean arterial pressure (MAP) = cardiac output (CO) × systemic vascular resistance (SVR).
- CO = HR × stroke volume (SV).

Causes

Reduction in cardiac output
- Reduction in heart rate:
  - Vagal reflexes.
  - Drugs e.g. halothane, remifentanil, neostigmine.
  - Dysrhythmias.
- Reduction in stroke volume:
  - Reduction in venous return: hypovolaemia, head up position, aorto-caval compression, tension pneumothorax, cardiac tamponade, PEEP.
  - Dysrhythmias.
  - ↑ after load: aortic stenosis, pulmonary embolus, tension pneumothorax, cardiac tamponade.
  - reduced myocardial contractility: drugs, hypoxia, hypercapnia, acidosis, hypothermia, cardiomyopathy, myocarditis, cardiac failure

Reduction in systemic vascular resistance
- Drugs: volatile and IV anaesthetic agents.
- Adverse drug reactions.
- Sepsis.

Management
- ↑ F_1O_2.
- Treat underlying cause.

Points to note
- Hypovolaemia is a reduction in circulating blood volume. This may be a result of:
  - Blood loss.
  - Plasma loss as in burns.
  - Extracellular and/or intracellular fluid loss as in dehydration, 'third space' loss during surgery, or in sepsis.
  - Evaporative loss during surgery or in pyrexia.
- Relative hypovolaemia occurs when there is vasodilatation and pooling of blood as in sepsis or drug allergy.
- Treatment consists of replacement of appropriate fluid.
- Neonates have a relatively fixed stroke volume and are dependent on heart rate to maintain cardiac output (📖 Chapter 1).
- Neonates have little or no ability to constrict capacitance vessels.
- The baroreceptor reflexes of infants, especially those born prematurely, are immature and limit the response to hypovolaemia.
- Systolic blood pressure in an infant is closely related to the circulating volume.

Dysrhythmias

- Bradycardia, junctional rhythm, and ventricular ectopics are common during anaesthesia but usually benign.
- Certain condition are associated with an ↑ incidence of dysrhythmias during general anaesthesia:
  - Pre-existing cardiac disease.
  - Hypoxia.
  - Hypercarbia.
  - Acid–base disturbance.
  - Electrolyte abnormalities especially potassium, calcium and magnesium.
  - Some drugs e.g. high concentrations of halothane combined with hypercarbia or catecholamines, suxamethonium.
  - Insertion of CVP lines into the cardiac chambers.
  - Activation of reflex pathways e.g. dental surgery, neurosurgery, oculo-cardiac reflex, visceral manipulation, tracheobronchial suction.

Management

- ↑ F$_I$O$_2$.
- Correction of any underlying cause.
- Drug therapy and cardioversion will be discussed under resuscitation (📖 p.502).

Anaphylaxis

- Anaphylaxis is an IgE mediated type B hypersensitivity reaction of rapid onset with circulatory collapse.
- Risk factors include:
  - Known allergy or previous allergic reaction.
  - History of atopy or asthma.
  - Cross sensitivity e.g. latex and kiwi fruit, melon and bananas, aspirin and NSAIDs.
  - Some drugs e.g. radiographic contrast media, penicillin, arachis oil (purified peanut oil) and neuromuscular blockers.
- Diagnosis: signs usually consist of a mixture of stridor, wheeze, cough, hypoxia, respiratory distress, cardiovascular collapse, rash, urticaria, and oedema.

Management

- Every department has an anaphylaxis protocol to guide treatment and prevent omissions during the episode.
- Initially follow the ABC of resuscitation. 100% oxygen and endotracheal intubation if indicated.
- Remove trigger agent if possible.
- Adrenaline 10 mcg/kg IM (10 mcg/kg is 0.1 mL/kg of a 1/10,000 solution) or a dose from the patient's EpiPen[®]. Repeat every 5 min as necessary.
- Fluid resuscitation: 20 mL/kg of crystalloid/colloid. Repeat as required.
- Further IV access should be established and, if the reaction is severe, invasive monitoring should be established.
- Infusions of inotropes may be required to maintain blood pressure in a severe reaction:
  - Adrenaline 0.3 mg/kg in 50 mL 0.9% saline.
    - —1 mL/hour = 0.1 mcg/kg/min.
    - —Infusion rate 0.1–5 mL/hour (0.01–0.5 mcg/kg/min).
  - Noradrenaline if blood pressure not maintained by adrenaline. Same dilution and infusion rate as adrenaline.
- Bronchodilator therapy may be necessary:
  - Salbutamol 2.5 mg nebulized.
  - Aminophylline 5 mg/kg IV over 20 min followed by infusion of 0.8–1.0 mg/kg/hour.
- Review airway periodically to identify any oedema formation, intubate early or if in doubt.
- Antihistamines (chlorphenamine 250 mcg/kg) and hydrocortisone 4 mg/kg have little or no effect in the acute phase but should be given as they are thought to reduce the incidence of late relapse.
- Blood samples:
  - Arterial blood gases.
  - Clotting screen.
  - Plasma tryptase (sample needs to be stored on ice).

- Exclude the following differential diagnoses:
  - Tension pneumothorax.
  - Latex allergy.
  - Sepsis.
  - Acute severe asthma.
- ITU admission after a severe reaction.

Hyperthermia

- A temperature of >38°C is a pyrexia and implies an intact temperature regulatory mechanism.
- A body temperature >41.6°C implies impaired thermoregulation regulation.

Causes

- Hypothalamic lesions.
- ↑ heat production: drug induced (malignant hyperthermia, neuroleptic malignant syndrome, salicylate poisoning, cocaine poisoning), hyperthyroidism, phaeochromocytoma, tetanus, status epilepticus, fever, or sepsis
- Impaired heat loss: autonomic neuropathy, drug induced (anticholinergics, phenothiazines, neuroleptic malignant syndrome), dehydration.
- Excessive warming: warming mattress, warming blanket, fluid warmer.

Management

- Remove or switch off warming devices.
- Cooling with tepid water.
- Irrigation of body cavity with cold fluid e.g. peritoneal lavage.
- Paracetamol 15 mg/kg IV over 15 min.
- Specific treatment e.g. dantrolene for malignant hyperthermia.

Malignant hyperthermia (MH)

Malignant hyperthermia (MH)

- MH is a pharmacogenetic disease of skeletal muscle, induced by exposure to certain anaesthetic agents such as suxamethonium and all the volatile agents.
- It is an autosomal dominant condition where exposure to triggering agents leads to loss of normal calcium homeostasis at some point along the excitation–contraction coupling process. Any defect along this complex pathway can result in the clinical features of MH and may explain the heterogeneity seen. The t-tubule, dihydropyridine receptor, and sarcoplasmic reticulum are all thought to be involved culminating in abnormal calcium efflux from the ryanodine receptor channel.
- Incidence is 1:10,000–1:15,000.
- Mortality is 2–3% compared with 70–80% when first described due to ↑ awareness and changing anaesthetic practice.
- A previous uneventful anaesthetic with triggering agents does not preclude MH (75% have had a previous anaesthetic).
- Affects mainly young adults ♂>♀.
- Presentation varies from a life-threatening classic fulminant episode with severe hyperthermia and metabolic derangement through severe masseter muscle rigidity to elevation of end-tidal carbon dioxide, tachycardia, or hyperthermia of unknown cause. It may rarely develop 2–3 days postoperatively with myoglobinuria and/or renal failure due to rhabdomyolysis.

Risk factors

- Family history.
- Exposure to triggers.
- Central core disease.
- Scoliosis.
- Squint surgery.

Pathophysiology

- ↑ metabolism: tachycardia, ↑ CO_2 production, tachypnoea, metabolic acidosis, pyrexia.
- Dysrhythmias.
- Disseminated intravascular coagulation.
- Muscle signs: masseter spasm after suxamethonium, generalized muscle rigidity.
- Hypercalcaemia.
- High creatine kinase.
- Myoglobinuria.
- Renal failure.

Diagnosis

- Masseter spasm after suxamethonium.
- Unexplained tachycardia.
- Unexplained rise in end-tidal carbon dioxide or minute volume.
- Falling S_pO_2 despite ↑ F_iO_2.
- Cardiovascular instability including peaked p waves.
- Generalized muscle rigidity.
- A rise in core temperature of more than 2°C/hour.

Management

- Every department has a malignant hyperthermia protocol to guide treatment and prevent omissions during the episode.
- ABC.
- Discontinue volatile agent.
- Get help.
- Endotracheal intubation if not already intubated.
- Hyperventilate with 100% oxygen using high fresh gas flow (2–3 times estimated minute volume).
- Dantrolene 1 mg/kg IV repeated every 10 min up to a total of 10 mg/kg. Falling heart rate and central temperature are evidence of a response.
- Depending on circumstances stop surgery, convert to TIVA for duration of surgery, and use a volatile free machine if available.
- ↓ body temperature: warming mattress or blanket set to cool, ice in groins and axillae, peritoneal lavage, cold IV fluids (do not induce shivering). Fluids must be potassium free.
- Check arterial blood gases and potassium. Sample for creatine kinase.
- Institute invasive monitoring.
- Urinary catheter.
- Urine for myoblobin measurement.
- May need to treat hyperkalaemia (📖 Table 15.3)
- May need postoperative IPPV.
- Postoperative care in ITU.

Hypothermia

- Core temperature <36°C.
- Usually due to heat loss during anaesthesia.
- Prevention is important because of the adverse effects of hypothermia and because of the ↑ postoperative oxygen consumption caused by shivering (up to 10 times). Duration of action of neuromuscular blockers is prolonged and drug excretion is delayed.
- It is particularly important to avoid in neonates due to their reduced reserves.

Causes

- Prolonged surgery.
- ↑ heat loss through radiation (patient uncovered, vasodilated, surrounded by cold objects), convection (uncovered), evaporation (open body cavity, low environmental humidity, unhumidified inspired gases), and conduction (cold irrigating fluids).
- Reduced heat production.
- Impaired temperature regulation through peripheral mechanisms (vasodilation, shivering, impaired piloerection) or central mechanisms (drug effects).

Prevention

- Identification of patients at high risk—ill, prolonged surgery, major blood loss, neonates, and open body cavity.
- Temperature monitoring for all but very brief procedures.
- Cover during transfer from anaesthetic room to operating theatre.
- Maintenance of ambient temperature of 22–24°C and humidity about 50%.
- Cover patient with drapes, blanket, and hats in neonates.
- Warming of solutions for skin cleaning.
- Humidification of inspired gases.
- Warming of IV fluids.
- Warming mattress and/or blanket.
- Warming of bed for recovery period.

Management

- If hypothermia does occur during anaesthesia, treatment is along the same lines as prevention.

Failed intubation

- The key to management of failed intubation is to anticipate problems if possible and plan accordingly.
- Despite careful assessment, approximately 50% of airway difficulties arise unexpectedly.
- Problems may arise from:
  - Difficult or failed intubation.
  - Difficult or failed mask ventilation.
  - Both.
- Unexpected difficulty is more likely during emergency cases and during anaesthesia by inexperienced anaesthetists.
- The Difficult Airway Society (DAS) algorithms and clinical simulation have been developed to reduce the incidence of serious morbidity and mortality in these situations.
- When difficulties do occur, patients do not die from failure to intubate but from failure to oxygenate.
- Failed intubation is defined as inability to intubate the trachea. The commonest cause is difficulty in viewing the larynx. Many paediatric syndromes are associated with difficult intubation and/or ventilation. Some of these improve with age e.g. Pierre Robin syndrome and some deteriorate with age e.g. Goldenhar syndrome and the mucopolysaccharidoses.
- Failed intubation can be thought of as a four-step process:
  1. Primary intubation attempt (optimal anaesthesia, optimal position, optimal blade, optimal laryngeal manipulation, use of a gum elastic bougie or stylette).
  2. Secondary intubation attempt (includes intubation via a LMA or intubating LMA, use of a flexible or rigid fibreoptic system, light wand or retrograde intubation depending on the experience of the anaesthetist).
  3. Oxygenation and ventilation with face mask ventilation or supraglottic adjuncts.
  4. Invasive techniques (needle or cannula cricothyroidotomy, surgical airway).
- Decisions to proceed from A–B–C–D depend on failure of each technique. In most cases senior help should be called when plan A fails. Plan D should be reserved for '*Can't Intubate, Can't Ventilate (CICV)*' (📖 p.500) situations with progressive desaturation despite optimal attempts at oxygenation.

Points to note

- Consider if it is in the patient's best interest to continue anaesthesia and surgery.
- If not then abandon procedure and reschedule for another occasion ensuring appropriate help and equipment is available.
- Retain a high degree of suspicion of misplacement of ETT after difficult intubation. Confirm position by capnography, auscultation, observation of chest, and/or fibreoptic visualisation.

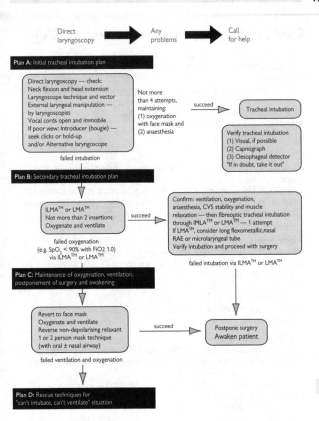

Fig. 14.1 Unanticipated difficult airway intubation. Reproduced with permission from the Difficult Airway Society.

Can't intubate, can't ventilate (CICV)

- Inability to intubate the trachea and ventilate the lungs is a life-threatening situation. Managed badly it will lead to morbidity or death.
- It is more common during emergency anaesthesia, intubation in the emergency department, after multiple attempts at intubation, and with inexperienced anaesthetists. Fortunately it is rare in children.
- This is 'Plan D' of the DAS guidelines.

Rescue techniques for CICV

LMA

- Insertion of an appropriate LMA will rescue the airway in >90% of cases.
- Once the LMA is inserted it should be left in place during tracheal access, as it may allow oxygenation and provides a route for exhalation that will be needed if a needle cricothyroidotomy is performed or jet ventilation used.

Cricothyroidotomy

- Options are needle or surgical cricothyroidotomy.
- In children <12 years, needle cricothyroidotomy is preferred to surgical cricothyroidotomy.
- In the adolescent either technique can be used. The surgical technique allows better protection of the airway.
- In a very small baby, or if a foreign body is below the cricoid ring, direct tracheal puncture using the same technique can be used.

Needle cricothyroidotomy

- This technique is simple in concept but far from easy in practice as the child may be struggling and attempts to breathe or swallow may result in the larynx moving up and down.
- It is, however, quicker than a formal tracheostomy.
- It is performed at the level of the cricothyroid membrane.
- Appropriate techniques include a cannula over needle technique (e.g. <2 mm ID, non-kinking cannula, such as the Ravussin cannula, VBM GmBH®, Sulz, Germany) or larger catheters placed using a Seldinger technique (e.g. Cook Melker® cricothyroidotomy catheter, 5.0 mm cuffed or 4.0/6.0 mm uncuffed, Cook, Letchworth, UK)
- Cannulae of <4.0 mm ID require jet ventilation for adequate ventilation and rely on exhalation through the upper airway. It is essential to ensure that there is no obstruction to expiration otherwise barotrauma will result.
- Aspiration of air from the cannula must be confirmed prior to connection to an oxygen delivery system.
- If a jet ventilator is not available then a Y-connector attached to the wall oxygen with a flow rate (in litres) equal to the child's age in years is used. Occlude the open end of the Y-connector for 1 sec, to allow oxygen to insufflate the chest, and allow passive exhalation by taking the thumb off the connector for 4 sec.

- In the event of complete upper airway obstruction, reduce the flow rate to 1–2 L/min. This will provide some oxygenation by insufflation but no ventilation.
- Catheters >4.0 mm internal diameter permit conventional ventilation but may only provide adequate ventilation if they are cuffed or the upper airway is obstructed.

Surgical airway

- This should only be considered in older children (>12 years).
- The technique allows introduction of an appropriately sized endotracheal or tracheostomy tube into the trachea through the cricothyroid membrane.
- A scalpel is used to make a horizontal skin incision and an incision through the cricothyroid membrane. The hole in the latter may be enlarged with the handle of the scalpel.
- Insert an appropriate sized ETT or tracheostomy tube (usually a slightly smaller size than would have been used for an oral or nasal tube).
- Having completed emergency airway management, arrange to proceed to a more definitive airway procedure such as a tracheostomy.

Complications

- Aspiration of blood or secretions (empty the stomach).
- Haemorrhage or haematoma.
- Creation of a false passage(s) into the tissues.
- Surgical emphysema (subcutaneous or mediastinal).
- Pulmonary barotrauma.
- Subglottic oedema or stenosis.
- Oesophageal perforation.
- Infection.

Points to note

- Multiple intubation attempts may lead to airway trauma and ↑ the likelihood of a CICV situation.
- If an airway technique has failed twice it is unlikely to work at all.
- CICV is associated with an ↑ incidence of aspiration. Empty the stomach with a nasogastric tube when there is an opportunity.
- After prolonged upper airway obstruction anticipate post-obstructive pulmonary oedema.

See also 📖 Chapter 5.

Resuscitation

Resuscitation Council (UK) guidelines and protocols updated in 2005 are used in the UK.

Basic life support

- This provides the foundation for advanced life support.
- The most common arrest situation in children is bradycardia proceeding to asystole as a response to profound hypoxia and acidosis.
- Basic life support aimed at restoring oxygenation is therefore a priority of management.
- Adopt a **SAFE** approach:
  - **S**hout for help.
  - **A**pproach with caution.
  - **F**ree from danger.
  - **E**valuate the patient's ABCs.
- Gentle stimulation should be used to obtain a response.
- Airway opening manoeuvres consist of mouth opening, head tilt, and chin lift unless head or neck injury is suspected in which case a jaw thrust should be used with in-line stabilization of the neck. Optimal position of the head is 'neutral' under 1 year and 'sniffing the morning air' in older children.
- Breathing should be assessed for up to 10 sec. Five rescue breaths should be given (ensure that the chest is seen to rise and fall) and each breath should take about 1–1.5 sec.
- Circulation should be assessed for 10 sec by feeling for a carotid pulse in children >1year and a brachial or femoral pulse in those <1 year. If no pulse is present or it is <60/min then CPR should be commenced.
- CPR should be performed at a ratio of 15 compressions to 2 ventilations in all age groups. Landmarks for compression are the lower third of the sternum, using two fingers or thumbs for those <1 year and the heel of one or two hands in older children. The depth of compressions should be half to one-third the depth of the chest and the rate should be 100/min.
- CPR should be continued for 1 min before reassessing the patient and checking that help is on the way. CPR should then continue until help arrives, the patient recovers or the provider is exhausted.

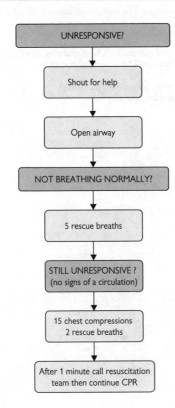

Fig. 14.2 Paediatric basic life support. Reproduced with permission from the Resuscitation Council (UK) 2005.

Choking

- Usually affects younger children, boys more frequently than girls.
- It often presents with sudden onset of coughing in a previously well child.
- CPR 15:2 as in basic life support (📖 p.503).
- Repeatedly assess for deterioration.

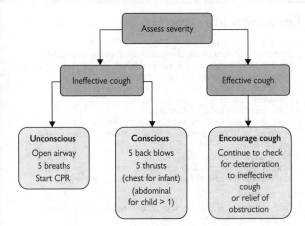

Fig. 14.3 Paediatric foreign body airway obstruction (choking). Reproduced with permission from the Resuscitation Council (UK) 2005.

Advanced life support

- The priority is to restore oxygenation.
- Establish basic life support. Oxygenate, ventilate, and start chest compressions. Ventilate—5 breaths with high concentration of oxygen.
- Endotracheal intubation as soon as feasible.
- Establish IV or intraosseous (IO) access. When no IV is present immediate IO access is recommended.
- Consider IV fluid bolus of 20 mL/kg.
- Once the airway has been secured, chest compressions should be continued at 100/min uninterrupted with breaths administered at a rate of 10/min.
- Attach a defibrillator or monitor.
- Assess rhythm and check for signs of a circulation (signs of life). Assess pulse in a child at carotid, in infant at brachial artery.

Points to note

- Place monitoring electrodes in the conventional chest positions.
- If using a defibrillator:
  - Place one defibrillator pad or paddle on the chest wall just below the right clavicle, and one in the left anterior axillary line.
  - Pads or paddles for children should be 8–12 cm in size, and 4.5 cm for infants. In infants and small children it may be best to apply the pads or paddles to the front and back of the chest.
  - A standard automated external defibrillator (AED) may be used in children >8 years of age.
  - Purpose-made paediatric pads, or programs which attenuate the energy output of an AED, are recommended for children between 1–8 years.
  - There is insufficient evidence to support a recommendation for or against the use of AEDs in children aged <1 year.
- All drugs should be flushed with 2–5 mL of 0.9% saline due to the small volumes of drugs often required.
- Useful to take blood for FBC, U&E, and blood glucose when establishing IV access.

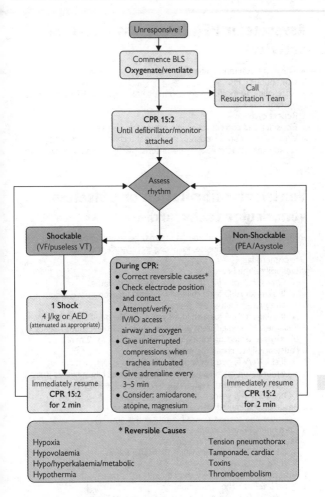

Fig. 14.4 Paediatric advanced life support. Reproduced with permission from the Resuscitation Council (UK) 2005.

Asystole or PEA (pulseless electrical activity)

- The more common scenario in children.
- Continuous CPR.
- Adrenaline 10 mcg/kg every 3–5 min (100 mcg/kg via ETT if no other option).
- Repeat cycle.
- Consider and correct reversible causes (Hs and Ts).
- When circulation is restored, ventilate the child at a rate of 12–20 breaths/min to achieve a normal arterial pCO_2 and monitor end tidal CO_2.

Ventricular fibrillation or pulseless ventricular tachycardia

- These rhythms are uncommon but may be seen in children with underlying cardiac disease, following ingestion of tricyclics or in hypothermia.
- Defibrillate the heart:
  - One shock of 4 J/kg if using a manual defibrillator.
  - If using an AED for a child of 1–8 years, deliver a paediatric attenuated adult shock energy.
  - If using an AED for a child >8 years, use the adult shock energy.
- Resume CPR immediately with chest compression without reassessing the rhythm or feeling for a pulse. Continue CPR for 2 min.
- Pause briefly to check the monitor.
  - If still VF/VT, give a second shock at 4 J/kg if using a manual defibrillator, or the adult shock energy for a child >8 years using an AED, or a paediatric-attenuated adult shock energy for a child between 1–8 years.
- Resume CPR immediately after the second shock.
- Consider and correct reversible causes (Hs and Ts).
- Continue CPR for 2 min.
- Pause briefly to check the monitor.
  - If still VF/VT, give adrenaline 10 mcg/kg followed immediately by a third shock.
- Resume CPR immediately and continue for 2 min.
- Pause briefly to check the monitor.
  - If still VF/VT, give an IV bolus of amiodarone 5 mg/kg over at least 3 mins and an immediate fourth shock.
  - Continue giving shocks every 2 min, minimizing the breaks in chest compression as much as possible.
  - Give adrenaline immediately before every other shock (i.e. every 3–5 min) until return of spontaneous circulation.

- After each 2 min of uninterrupted CPR, pause briefly to assess the rhythm.
  - If still VF/VT continue CPR and the shockable (VF/VT) sequence.
  - If asystole continue CPR and switch to the non-shockable (asystole or pulseless electrical activity) sequence as above.
- If organized electrical activity is seen, check for a pulse.
  - If there is return of spontaneous circulation, continue post-resuscitation care.
  - If there is no pulse, and there are no other signs of a circulation, give adrenaline 10 mcg/kg and continue CPR as for the non-shockable sequence as above.
- Repeat cycles of shock, CPR and adrenaline while other alternatives are considered and administered.
  - Amiodarone loading dose 5 mg/kg; infusion 5–15 mcg/kg/min.
  - Atropine 20 mcg/kg; minimum 100 mcg, maximum 600 mcg.
  - Magnesium 25–50 mg/kg (maximum 2 g).

Dysrhythmias

Dysrhythmias are divided into fast tachyarrhythmias and slow bradyar-rhythmias.

Bradyarrhythmias

The rate is slow and the rhythm usually irregular.

Causes

- Preterminal event in hypoxia or shock.
- Raised ICP.
- After conduction pathway damage during cardiac surgery.
- Congenital heart block (rare).
- Long QT syndrome.
- Poisoning with β blockers or digoxin.

Treatment

- ABC.
- High flow oxygen.
- Bag valve mask ventilation or endotracheal intubation.
- Volume expansion 20 mL/kg.
- If the above measures are ineffective give adrenaline 10 mcg/kg IV.
- May require an infusion of adrenaline 0.05–2 mcg/kg/min IV.
- If there is bradycardia treat with adequate ventilation, atropine 20 mcg/kg IV or IO (minimum dose 100 mcg; maximum dose 600 mcg), repeat after 5 min (maximum dose 1.0 mg in a child, 2.0 mg in an adolescent).
- If poisoning obtain expert advice.

Tachyarrhythmias

The rate is fast but the rhythm is usually regular.

Causes

- Re-entrant congenital conducting pathway abnormality (common).
- Poisoning.
- Metabolic disturbance.
- After cardiac surgery.
- Cardiomyopathy.
- Long QT syndrome.

Presentations include:

- History of palpitations.
- Poor feeding.
- Heart failure.
- Shock.

Features suggesting a cardiac cause of respiratory inadequacy include:

- Cyanosis that does not correct with oxygen.
- Tachycardia out of proportion to respiratory difficulty.
- Raised jugular venous pulse.
- Gallop rhythm or murmur.
- Enlarged liver.
- Absent femoral pulses.

Ventricular tachycardia

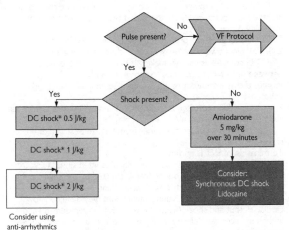

Fig. 14.5 Ventricular tachycardia

Supraventricular tachycardia (SVT)

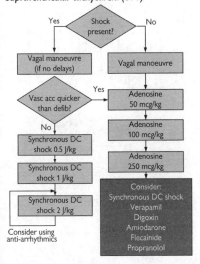

Fig. 14.6 Supraventricular tachycardia (SVT)

Points to note

- SVT is the most common non-arrest dysrhythmia during childhood and the most common dysrhythmia that produces cardiovascular instability during infancy.
- SVT in infants generally produces a heart rate >220/min and often 250–300/min. Lower rates may occur in children during SVT.
- The QRS complex is narrow making it difficult to differentiate between sinus tachycardia due to shock and SVT.
- In sinus tachycardia heart rate is usually <200/min in infants and children.
- P waves are difficult to see but upright in I and aVf in sinus tachycardia and negative in II, III and aVf in SVT.
- In sinus tachycardia heart rate varies from beat to beat and often responds to stimuli.
- Termination of SVT is abrupt.
- A history consistent with shock is usually present in sinus tachycardia.
- Cardiopulmonary stability during SVT is affected by the child's age, duration of SVT, prior ventricular function, and ventricular rate.
- SVT may be undetected in young infants until they develop a low cardiac output and shock (from ↑ myocardial oxygen demand and limitation in oxygen delivery during the short diastole of very rapid heart rates).
- If baseline myocardial function is impaired, SVT can produce signs of shock in a relatively short time.

Hypothermia

- A core temperature (rectal or oesophageal) reading should be obtained as soon as possible and further cooling should be prevented.
- Hypothermia is common following drowning, and adversely affects resuscitation attempts unless treated.
- Not only are dysrhythmias more common but some, such as ventricular fibrillation, may be refractory at temperatures <30°C. According to CPR guidelines, defibrillation may be attempted at temperatures <30°C. If unsuccessful, further shocks should be delayed until the temperature is >30°C.
- Resuscitation should be continued until the core temperature is at least 32°C.
- Rewarming strategies depend upon the core temperature and signs of circulation. External rewarming is usually sufficient if the core temperature is above 30°C.
- Active core rewarming should be added in patients with a core temperature of <30°C, but beware of *rewarming shock*.
- Most hypothermic patients are hypovolaemic. During rewarming the peripheral vascular resistance falls more rapidly as core rewarming is accomplished. As a result of vasodilatation and impaired myocardial function, hypotension ensues.
- External rewarming:
  - Remove cold, wet clothing.
  - Warm blankets.
  - Infrared radiant lamp.
  - Heating blanket.
  - Warm air system.
- Core rewarming:
  - Warm IV fluids to 39°C.
  - Warm ventilator gases to 42°C.
  - Gastric or bladder lavage with normal saline at 42°C.
  - Peritoneal lavage with potassium—free dialysate at 42°C (20 mL/kg cycled every 15 min).
  - Pleural or pericardial lavage.
  - Endovascular warming.
  - Extracorporeal blood warming.
- The temperature is generally allowed to rise by 1°C per hour to reduce haemodynamic instability.
- Recent evidence suggests that in post-cardiac arrest patients after restoration of adequate spontaneous circulation mild hypothermia (32–34°C) for 12–24 hours has a beneficial effect on neurological outcome when the initial rhythm was ventricular fibrillation.

Newborn life support

At birth the baby must change, within a matter of moments, from an organism with fluid-filled lungs whose respiratory function is carried out by the placenta to a separate being whose air-filled lungs can successfully takeover this function. Preparation for this begins during labour, when fluid-producing cells within the lung cease secretion and begin re-absorption of that fluid.

The Apgar score comprises five components: heart rate, respiratory effort, muscle tone, reflex irritability, and colour, each of which is given a score of 0, 1, or 2. The score (from 0–10) is recorded at 1 and 5 min after birth and provides a convenient shorthand for recording the status of the newborn infant and the response to resuscitation if required.

Points to note
- Food grade plastic wrapping may be used to maintain body temperature in very premature babies.
- Attempts to aspirate meconium while the head is on the perineum are no longer recommended.
- Ventilation may start with air but oxygen is added quickly if there is a poor response.
- Adrenaline should be given IV (not via the ETT).

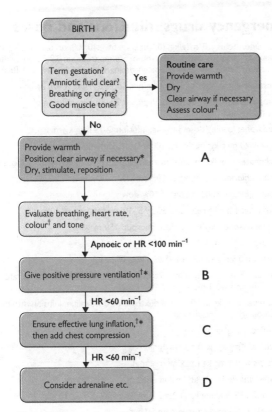

* Tracheal intubation may be considered at several steps
† Consider supplemental oxygen at any stage if cyanosis persists

Fig. 14.7 Newborn life support. Reproduced with permission from the Resuscitation Council (UK) 2005.

Emergency drugs: dilutions and doses

Adrenaline: bolus 10 mcg/kg (0.1 mL/kg of 1:10,000 or 0.01 mL/kg of 1:1,000); infusion 0.3 mg/kg in 50 mL of 5% dextrose or 0.9% saline. Infusion rate of 1 mL/hour gives 0.1 mcg/kg/min; nebulized 1–5 mL of 1:1000.

Alprostadil: initial dose of 3–5 ng/kg/min, increasing to 10–20 ng/kg/min.

Aminophylline: loading dose 5 mg/kg over 20–30 min; infusion of 0.8–1 mg/kg/hour.

Amiodarone: loading dose 5 mg/kg; infusion 5–15 mcg/kg/min.

Atropine: 20 mcg/kg; minimum 100 mcg, maximum 600 mcg.

Bicarbonate: 1 mL/kg of 8.4% for resuscitation (1–2 mmol/kg for acidosis).

Calcium chloride: 0.2 mL/kg of 10% slowly.

Calcium gluconate: 0.5 mL/kg of 10% slowly.

Dantrolene: 1 mg/kg repeated every 5–10 min; maximum 10 mg/kg.

Dexamethasone: single oral dose in croup 150 mcg/kg.

Dextrose: 10% 5 mL/kg.

Diazepam: 0.5 mg/kg PR; 0.1–0.25 mg/kg IV or IO.

Dobutamine: 3 mg/kg in 50 mL 5% dextrose or 0.9% saline. Infusion rate of 1 mL/hour gives 1 mcg/kg/min.

Dopamine: 3 mg/kg in 50 mL 5% dextrose or 0.9% saline. Infusion rate of 1 mL/hour gives 1 mcg/kg/min.

Ketamine: 2 mg/kg.

Lidocaine: 1 mg/kg as antiarrhythmic.

Lorazepam: 0.1 mg/kg (maximum 4 mg).

Magnesium: 25–50 mg/kg (maximum 2 g).

Mannitol: 250–500 mg/kg (1.25–2.5 mL/kg of 20%) over 30 min.

Midazolam: 0.5 mg/kg (maximum 20 mg).

Naloxone: 10 mcg/kg.

Neostigmine: 50 mcg/kg.

Paraldehyde: 0.4 mL/kg PR; 0.1–0.15 mL/kg IM.

Phenytoin: loading dose 18 mg/kg IV over 30–45 min.

Prednisolone: 1–2 mg/kg (maximum 40 mg).

Salbutamol: nebulized 2.5–5 mg; IV bolus 5 mcg/kg; infusion 1–5 mcg/kg/min.

Principles of stabilizing a critically ill child in a general hospital

- The patient should be assessed and resuscitated along ABC principles.
- Immediate management includes:
  - ABC.
  - 100% oxygen via a non-rebreathing mask ± ventilatory support/endotracheal intubation.
  - IV or IO access (preferably two cannulae).
  - Fluid boluses of 20 mL/kg crystalloid or colloid repeated twice if required to restore normovolaemia.
  - Correct any underlying hypoglycaemia with 5 mL/kg of 10% dextrose.
  - Commence appropriate therapy for underlying condition.
  - Bloods taken for FBC, U&E, LFT, glucose, arterial blood gases, clotting screen, and group and save or cross match.
- If fluid boluses are ineffective at maintaining blood pressure consider inotrope infusion e.g. dobutamine (up to 20 mcg/kg/min).
- Consider antibiotic therapy.
- Obtain senior help early.
- Patient discussed by referring clinician with ITU and receiving specialist in regional centre.
- Invasive monitoring should be established, if possible, once patient is stable.
- Take careful notes of timings, drugs given and any intervention(s) required.
- Obtain chest X-ray, any other X-rays required and a 12-lead ECG.
- Obtain detailed history from parents/guardian including drug history and allergies.
- Avoid hypothermia.
- The patient should be reassessed following the ABCD rapid clinical assessment and kept in a high dependency area.
- Use of a checklist helps ensure a safe transfer and avoid omissions.

Pre-transfer checks

- Airway/respiratory: ETT, humidification, ventilation parameters, chest X-ray, blood gas results.
- Cardiovascular: Circulatory status, hepatic size, use of inotropes, ECG, chest X-ray.
- Neurological: GCS, pupils, use of sedation, analgesia and paralysis, imaging, neuroprotection for raised ICP.
- Gastroenterological: Nasogastric tube, nutrition, antacid prophylaxis, ileus.
- Renal and fluids: Urine output, fluid balance, U&E, need for renal support.
- Hepatic: Liver function tests.
- Biochemistry: U&E, blood sugar, calcium, magnesium.
- Haematology: Hb, clotting studies.
- Infection: Temperature, WCC, review of cultures/swabs, CRP, specific PCR, antibiotics.
- Skin/joints: Skin, mouth, and eye care, rashes, passive movements.
- Drugs: Complete list of enteral and IV drugs, drug levels.
- Lines and tubes: Access for monitoring, blood sampling and IV drugs security of catheters and drains.
- Parents and family: Communications, concerns, support

- Transport of any patient either within the same hospital or between hospitals requires experienced personnel and attention to detail.
- Important considerations for any transfer are:
  - How urgent is the transfer?
  - Is the child in the optimal condition for transfer?
  - Does the benefit of transfer out weigh the risks involved?
  - Who are the most appropriate people to transfer this child?
  - What type and mode of transport is required for this child?

Interhospital transfer to a paediatric intensive care unit

- In the UK, the Paediatric Intensive Care Society has set a standard of practice for the transport of critically ill children.
- Specialized transport teams improve outcome but are not always available or appropriate.
- Referring and receiving units should make notes on their conversations, as well as the names and contact details of the clinicians responsible for current and ongoing care.
- Joint management by the referring hospital and the transport team should commence immediately, since successful initial resuscitation and stabilization is crucial to ultimate outcome. It is the responsibility of the referring hospital to resuscitate and stabilize with the help and guidance of the receiving hospital.
- The transport team has the responsibility to ensure that they have the appropriate equipment and drugs. Drugs and infusions, where appropriate, should be made up prior to transfer and labelled.
- The ability to monitor and record the following vital functions is essential during transport:
  - End-tidal CO_2.
  - Arterial oxygen saturation.
  - ECG and heart rate.
  - Non-invasive blood pressure.
  - Temperature (core and peripheral).
  - Respiratory rate.
- All the equipment must be kept in a constant state of readiness and checked at frequent intervals. Batteries must be capable of supporting full function for a period of at least twice the maximum anticipated length of the transfer.
- Dangers of transfer include:
  - Deranged physiology made worse by movement (acceleration/ deceleration leads to cardiovascular instability) and 15% of patients develop avoidable hypoxia and hypotension.
  - Vibration leads to failure and inaccuracy of non-invasive blood pressure monitoring. Use invasive monitoring if possible.
  - Cramped conditions with poor access to the patient, isolation, changes in temperature and pressure.
  - Hypothermia especially in the infant. Use of warming mats, 'bubble wrap' and hats help to minimize this.
  - Vehicle crashes.
- The transport vehicle:
  - Should have adequate space, light, gases, electricity, and communications.
  - Mode of transport: consider urgency, mobilization time, geography, weather, traffic, and costs.
  - Consider air transfer if the distance is >150 miles.

- Air transfers:
  - Helicopters fly at relatively low altitude and therefore avoid some of the problems of airplanes.
  - High altitude ↓ the partial pressure of oxygen—at 1500 m above sea level the P_aO_2 is ~10 kPa (75 mmHg).
  - Most aircraft are pressurized to a cabin altitude of 1500–2000 m.
  - ↓ barometric pressure leads to expansion of gas filled spaces—pneumothoraces, distended bowel.
  - Pressurizing the cabin to sea level can ↓ these problems but ↑ fuel consumption and costs.
  - Air in the ETT cuff should be replaced by saline.

Syndromes and conditions with implications for anaesthesia

Anthony Moores

Arthrogryposis multiplex congenita

- Arthrogryposis is a descriptive term for the occurrence of multiple congenital joint contractures.
- It is not a single diagnosis but is a syndrome with multiple aetiologies. The true aetiology is unknown but is thought to relate to the effect of early fetal akinesia on joint and muscle development.
- Causes of this can be classified into external mechanical factors (oligohydramnios, twin pregnancy, amniotic bands, fibroids), neuropathic, myopathic (central core disease, myotonic dystrophy, congenital myasthenia), and abnormal connective tissue.
- The most common diagnostic subgroup is associated with hypoplastic muscle (amyoplasia congenita) probably arising from a developmental defect in fetal muscle. Amyoplasia has no recognizable pattern of inheritance and tends to occur sporadically. Those affected have fatty and fibrous tissue replacement of their limb muscles. The neuropathic forms show denervation atrophy of muscles and reduced number and size of anterior horn cells in the spinal cord. Demyelination may also be seen in the pyramidal tracts and motor roots.
- In addition to these causes there are many other conditions and syndromes associated with congenital contractures that are accompanied by anomalies of other systems e.g. Pierre Robin syndrome, Potter syndrome, cerebral palsy, Turner's syndrome and spina bifida.
- There may be other congenital anomalies—cardiac, gastrointestinal, and genitourinary.
- The incidence of AMC varies from 1:3000 to 1:10000 live births.

Clinical features

- There is often involvement of all four limbs.
  - The upper limbs have internally rotated shoulders, extended elbows, flexed fingers and wrists.
  - The lower limb abnormalities are more variable, but usually severe equinovarus deformities of the feet are present.
  - The hips are usually flexed and dislocated, the knees hyper-extended and dislocated.
  - Contractures are non-progressive.
  - Distal muscles are usually small and wasted with absent reflexes. There may be webbing of soft tissues.
- The skin is often thickened and tense with dimples over the affected joints and a lack of normal skin creases.
- Children with AMC are usually of normal intelligence.
- Other abnormalities may be present—micrognathia, congenital heart defects, scoliosis, cleft palate, and hypoplastic lungs.

This group of patients commonly present for orthopaedic procedures to release contractures or correct deformities, ENT, oral surgical procedures, and diagnostic muscle biopsies.

Anaesthetic problems and management

- Potential airway difficulties may be encountered because of micrognathia, temporomandibular joint involvement, trismus, cleft palate, and cervical spine involvement (scoliosis, Klippel–Feil syndrome).
- Children may have chronic lung disease from recurrent aspiration (secondary to dysphagia) and the restrictive effect of scoliosis on ventilation. Postoperative atelectasis and pneumonia may result.
- Limb contractures and deficiencies of subcutaneous tissue can make IV access very difficult.
- AMC has been associated with hypermetabolic responses to anaesthesia although this is more likely to be due to an underlying primary neuromuscular disorder. Patients with an associated myopathy may be at risk of malignant hyperpyrexia. A link between AMC and malignant hyperthermia remains unproven. Volatile anaesthetics are administered routinely to these patients without any malignant hyperthermia type reactions.
- Positioning requires careful padding of pressure point areas.
- Regional anaesthesia may be difficult due to difficulty in positioning and abnormal bony landmarks.
- Suxamethonium should be avoided in patients with a recognized underlying myopathic cause of their AMC due to the risk of an exaggerated hyperkalaemic response. There is a slight increased sensitivity to non-depolarizing muscle relaxants.

Branchial (pharyngeal) arch syndromes

Goldenhar syndrome

- Also known as hemifacial microsomia or oculoauriculovertebral dysplasia. This is a congenital defect of the first and second branchial arch derivatives resulting in asymmetric craniofacial anomalies.
- Cardiac, vertebral, and central nervous system defects may also exist.
- Cases tend to occur sporadically but rarely are inherited in an autosomal dominant manner.

Clinical features

- Patients present with unilateral hypoplasia of malar, mandibular, and maxillary development accompanied by epibulbar dermoids, congenital heart defects (VSD, TGA, or tetralogy of Fallot) and vertebral anomalies (40%).
- The ear on the affected side may be absent or abnormal in shape or size. There may be atresia of the external auditory canal, preauricular skin tags, pretragal fistulae, and a high incidence of unilateral deafness.
- Coloboma of the upper eyelid is common. There may be defects of the extraocular muscles, cataracts, or atrophy of the iris.
- Patients may have cleft lip and/or palate.
- Often, but not always a low IQ.
- Facial asymmetry may worsen with age.

Patients tend to present for reconstructive surgery of their ear, ophthalmic surgery, or for mandibular advancement surgery.

Anaesthetic problems and management

- The main issues are with airway management which may become more difficult with age as the child grows and the facial asymmetry becomes more pronounced.
- Facial asymmetry may result in difficulty in achieving a seal with a facemask. Laryngoscopy and intubation can be difficult especially if the right side is affected. Fibreoptic endotracheal intubation, retrograde intubation, and tracheostomy have all been used to overcome difficult endotracheal intubation.
- Congenital heart disease and craniovertebral anomalies require assessment.

Treacher Collins syndrome (mandibulofacial dysostosis)

- This is an autosomal dominant disorder of craniofacial development resulting from developmental anomalies of the first arch. It results in symmetrical malformations.
- Nager syndrome presents similar anaesthetic problems.

Clinical features

- Hypoplasia of the facial bones (mandible and zygomatic complex), down-slanting palpebral fissures, colobomata of the lower eyelids, and absent eyelashes medial to the defect.
- Abnormalities of the external pinnae, auditory canals, and middle ear ossicles resulting in a high incidence of conductive deafness.

- There may be a high-arched or cleft palate, macroglossia, and malocclusion of the teeth.
- Associated defects include CHD, mental retardation, and skeletal abnormalities.
- Chronic upper airway obstruction and apnoea (awake, asleep, or during anaesthesia) are also problems.

Anaesthetic problems and management

- The risks of apnoea and upper airway obstruction mean that sedative premedication is relatively contraindicated. An antisialogogue reduces secretions during induction.
- Inhalational induction can be difficult. It may be necessary to get an assistant to pull the mandible and tongue forward.
- Unless the child has been laryngoscoped previously and the laryngoscopic view is known, a difficult endotracheal intubation is anticipated. A fibreoptic endotracheal intubation is often necessary (📖 Chapter 5).
- Awake extubation.
- Monitor postoperatively on HDU or ITU due to a high incidence of respiratory complications.

Cerebral palsy

- Cerebral palsy (CP) is a term used to represent a spectrum of non-progressive disorders of motor function and posture that present early in life. They are the result of lesions or anomalies that occur in the motor pathways during the early stages of brain development.
- There is a wide range in clinical severity from a mild monoplegia to severe spastic quadriplegia. The motor defects are often accompanied by intellectual impairment, developmental delay, speech difficulties and epilepsy.
- The incidence of cerebral palsy is 2.5:1000.
- The causes of CP may be prenatal (congenital infection e.g. rubella, toxoplasmosis, cytomegalovirus, herpes or cerebral malformation), perinatal (asphyxia) or postnatal (IVH, cerebral ischaemia, trauma, non-accidental injury, or meningitis).
- It is often associated with low birth weight and premature infants.

Clinical features

- Cerebral palsy is classified according to the predominant type of motor defect i.e. spasticity, ataxia, or dyskinesia.
- Spasticity can present as a hemiplegia, diplegia, or quadriplegia.
- Ataxic patients have poor balance, tremor, hypotonia, and may have uncoordinated movements.
- Dyskinesia may present with involuntary movements (athetosis, dystonia), poor postural tone, or fluctuating muscle tone.
- Patients may develop a progressive scoliosis that impinges on respiratory function or makes sitting difficult.
- Gastro-oesophageal reflux (GOR) and poor swallowing result in recurrent chest infections.
- A multidisciplinary approach to the care of these patients aims to preserve motor function and mobility in those who can walk, but also improve ease of care in those more severely affected. This is achieved with regular physiotherapy, splinting of limbs, and medical therapy to control spasms and so slow the onset of contractures.
- Drugs used to control spasms include centrally acting drugs—baclofen (oral or intrathecal), diazepam, vigabatrin, and tizanidine. The main side effects of these drugs are sedative. Peripherally acting drugs include botulinum toxin type A and dantrolene. Botulinum toxin is injected into muscles causing a functional denervation by inhibiting the release of acetylcholine at the motor end-plate. The effect lasts for about 3 months and aims to improve range of movement or pain from contractures.
- Patients often present for orthopaedic surgery for muscle releases, muscle transfers, and osteotomies of the feet or femurs to maintain mobility and range of movement. Patients in wheelchairs are at risk of recurrent hip dislocations causing problems with sitting and often chronic hip pain. Femoral and pelvic osteotomies and correction of their scoliosis may be necessary to improve position in the wheelchair. Patients may also require surgery for feeding gastrostomies, fundoplication for GOR, and dental procedures.

Anaesthetic problems and management

- These children have often had multiple admissions for surgery or medical problems related to chest infections or seizures. Information about their previous anaesthetic management is important to help plan perioperative management. Despite marked deformity, some patients may have normal intelligence but difficulties with communication.
- The main problems are associated with recurrent chest infections, poor nutritional status, control of seizures, and an increased incidence of latex allergy. Patients are often on anticonvulsant or antispasmodic medication.
- IV access can be difficult due to previous scarring and limb contractures.
- Increased secretions and drooling may require an antisialogogue to help with a gas induction.
- GOR disease is common and often requires a rapid sequence induction. Patients often undergo surgery to manage severe reflux (Nissen fundoplication). Laparoscopic surgery reduces the morbidity associated with postoperative chest complications in this group.
- Patients are positioned carefully on the operating table with padding on pressure areas to prevent pressure sores.
- Hypothermia in poorly nourished patients can be minimized by active warming measures—warming mattress, warm air blanket, warming IV fluids.
- Patients may be more sensitive to suxamethonium. Resistance to non-depolarizing muscle relaxants may be related to anticonvulsant therapy.
- Postoperatively pain and muscle spasms can be difficult to manage. Epidurals can be difficult to site in patients with scoliosis but are particularly effective in controlling pain and spasm. Regional blocks, morphine infusions, and oral benzodiazepines can also be effective. IV midazolam may be required for distressing spasms.
- Feeding and medication are restarted as soon as possible postoperatively.

Diabetes mellitus

- Diabetes mellitus is the most common metabolic disease of childhood. 90% of cases are due to type 1 insulin-dependent diabetes mellitus (IDDM) resulting from pancreatic beta-cell destruction and insulin deficiency.
- Aetiology is uncertain but is partly autoimmune in origin. 80% of patients have islet cell antibodies at presentation and there is an association with other autoimmune diseases (thyroid disease). There are also genetic and environmental components. An increased incidence occurs in children whose parents or siblings have diabetes.

Clinical features

- Clinical presentation may be a short history of a few weeks of polydipsia, polyuria, fatigue, anorexia, and weight loss. There is hyperglycaemia, glycosuria, and possibly ketosis. Some patients present acutely with ketoacidosis and coma.
- Diagnosis is confirmed in symptomatic patients with:
  - A random venous plasma glucose of >11.1 mmol/L *or*
  - A fasting plasma glucose >7.1 mmol/L *or*
  - Plasma glucose >11.1 mmol/L 2 hours after a 75 g glucose load.
  - In asymptomatic patients, a plasma glucose > 11.1 mmol/L repeated on another day (fasting, random or 2 hours post 75 g glucose load).
- Impaired glucose tolerance refers to a condition where the fasting plasma glucose is <7.0 mmol/L and plasma glucose 2 hours after a 75 g glucose load is >7.8 but < 11.1mmol/L.
- Treatment of IDDM is with insulin. Most insulin preparations are derived from animals (porcine), humans, or produced biosynthetically by recombinant DNA technology using bacteria or yeast. The three types of insulin preparation are short, intermediate, and long acting. Each treatment regimen is personalized to the individual patient and usually combines an intermediate or long-acting insulin with a short-acting one.
- Monitoring of blood glucose aims to achieve a level of 4–9 mmol/L, while avoiding hypoglycaemia. Glycosylated haemoglobin gives a better measure of glycaemic control over the preceding 6–8 weeks. In children, a level of 6.5–7.5% or less is ideal, although achieving this target can run the risk of hypoglycaemia.
- Diet, adequate exercise, and avoidance of obesity are important in long-term management.
- Optimal glycaemic control helps to avoid complications. Retinopathy, neuropathy, and nephropathy are rare in children but are usually screened for 5 years after first being diagnosis or annually from the age of 12 years.

Type II (maturity-onset diabetes)

This is due to reduced levels of insulin or peripheral resistance to insulin and tends to occur in the adult population (age >40 years). It is rare in children but the incidence is increasing as obesity becomes more common. Maturity onset diabetes in the young (MODY) is characterized by

impaired glucose tolerance and treatment aims at weight reduction.
Oral hypoglycaemic agents are not used and only occasionally is insulin
required in symptomatic or hyperglycaemic patients.

Anaesthetic problems and management

- Management should involve a team approach and requires communication between the surgeon, anaesthetist, and diabetic team. Surgery
  results in a stress response characterized by increased catabolism,
  increased metabolic rate, protein and fat breakdown, periods of
  starvation, and glucose intolerance. The type and duration of surgery
  and presence of infection can influence the response. In diabetes,
  the stress response is exaggerated and can result in ketogenesis,
  hyperglycaemia, ketosis, or ketoacidosis.
- The aim of perioperative management is to maintain normoglycaemia
  (target range 4–10 mmol/L), avoid electrolyte abnormalities (↓K, ↓Mg,
  ↓phosphate), and get the patient back to normal oral intake as soon as
  possible postoperatively.
- Patients are admitted the day before surgery for elective procedures.
  If possible, they should be placed first on the list and preferably, this
  should be a morning list.
- Management depends on the type and duration of the surgical procedure. Minor procedures are regarded as lasting up to 30 min where
  patients are expected to eat within 4 hours postoperatively. Patients
  who are poorly controlled, undergoing emergency procedures, or
  having major surgery are managed with infusions of glucose, insulin,
  and potassium.
- A common approach to perioperative glycaemic control is outlined
  below. Most hospitals have a protocol agreed between diabetologists,
  surgeons, and anaesthetists. Expert diabetic advice should be obtained
  to fine tune management as required.

Minor procedures

- Patient should, if possible, be first on the list.
- Check blood glucose. Ideal range is 4–10 mmol/L.
- If >15 mmol/ L check urine for ketones. If negative or small trace,
  continue but monitor. If positive for ketones, surgery may need to
  be postponed and advice sought from the diabetic team.

Morning list

- Normal insulin on day before surgery.
- Fast from midnight.
- Omit normal morning dose of insulin. Give instead 20% of total dose
  as long acting analogue (*insulin detemir*) subcutaneously when starting
  IV fluids.
- Start IV fluids at 08.00 0.45% NaCl/5% dextrose at maintenance rate.

Afternoon list

- Normal insulin on day before surgery.
- 20% of total daily insulin dose as long acting analogue (*insulin detemir*)
  and 10% of total daily dose as soluble insulin (Actrapid®) before
  breakfast.
- Give breakfast on morning of surgery then fast.

- Start IV fluids 0.45% NaCl/5% dextrose at maintenance rate.
- Monitor blood glucose hourly after giving insulin.

Postoperative
- If patient can eat or drink within first 2 hours postoperatively:
  - After eating give 20% total daily dose as soluble insulin (Actrapid®)
  - Return to normal insulin regimen after second meal is eaten.
  - Once tolerating fluids and food stop IV fluids.
  - Monitor blood glucose until stable.
- If patient is not going to eat within 2 hours:
  - Either a combined infusion of glucose, insulin, and potassium or separate infusions of glucose and insulin (as for major surgery) is required.
  - The combined infusion is along the lines: 500 mL 0.45% NaCl/5% dextrose + 10 mmol KCl + 10 units soluble insulin. Infuse at the maintenance rate. Blood glucose should be monitored hourly until awake and stable then 2-hourly. Change insulin as follows: if blood glucose >21 mmol/L increase to 16 units in 500 mL; if blood glucose <7 mmol/L decrease to 8 units in 500 mL.

Major or emergency surgery
- This is best managed with a continuous infusion of insulin and separate IV fluids.
  - Insulin: 50 units of soluble insulin dissolved 50 ml 0.9% NaCl. Infusion rate = 0.05 units (mL)/kg/hour if blood glucose < 15 mmol/L; 0.1 units (mL)/kg hour if blood glucose is 15 mmol/L or more. This should maintain the blood glucose between 5 and 12 mmol/L.
  - IV fluids: 0.45% NaCl/5% dextrose + 10 mmol KCl per 500 mL bag. Infusion rate = 2.5mL/kg/hour.
  - If the insulin and IV fluids are going into the same cannula, an anti-syphon/anti-reflux valve must be used to separate the infusions.
- Blood glucose should be measured hourly before, during, and after surgery. Urea and electrolytes should be measured preoperatively and at least daily while on IV fluids.
- IV insulin has a half-life of 3–4 min and should not be stopped unless hypoglycaemia occurs (blood glucose < 3 mmol/L). It is stopped for 15 min. If hypoglcaemia continues to be a problem, change to 10% glucose solutions.
- The IV regimen should be used until the child starts eating and drinking again. The usual subcutaneous dose of insulin should be given after the first meal and the infusion stopped 1 hour later. Insulin requirements may initially be higher than normal in the postoperative period. The diabetic team will review and advise on management of patients during this period.

Hypoglycaemia

- This is the most common acute complication of IDDM.
- It may result from missed meals, unexpected exercise, or errors in insulin administration.
- Awake patients tend to get symptoms of feelings of hunger, sweating, tremor, tachycardia, anxiety, weakness, change in affect, slurred speech and confusion. This can progress to convulsions and coma if not treated.
- If the patient is conscious and able to eat then give oral carbohydrate. If unconscious, give 2 ml/kg of 10% dextrose solution initially followed by IV fluids containing 5% or 10% glucose.

Down's syndrome

- Down's syndrome (DS) is the most common chromosomal abnormality and occurs in approximately 1:700 live births. This figure is similar for most populations and changes mainly in relation to maternal age. The incidence for mothers aged 25 years is 1:1400, increasing to 1:46 for mothers aged 45 years.
- 95% of children with DS have trisomy 21 caused by meiotic non-disjunction. The remainder arise from chromosomal translocations (2–3%) or mosaic trisomy 21 (2–3%).
- Life expectancy for patients with DS has improved due to a more pro-active attitude towards managing life-threatening congenital abnormalities. About 20% die in the first year and 45% are expected to survive to 60 years of age (86% of the general population survive to 60 years) compared to a generation ago when approximately two-thirds would die in early childhood.

Clinical features

DS gives rise to characteristic craniofacial features often leading to diagnosis at birth. Patients are intellectually impaired and there are often anomalies of other organ systems.

General appearance

- Small head circumference, brachycephaly (the head is disproportionately wide), often a third fontanelle, short thick neck, upwardly sloping palpebral fissures, epicanthic folds, Brushfield's spots (small white spots on the periphery of the iris), flat nasal bridge, large protruding tongue, small mouth and ears.
- A single transverse palmar (Simian) crease in both hands (50% DS).
- Patients usually have low birth weights but tend towards obesity in childhood.
- Often small in stature.

Congenital heart disease

- Occurs in 40–60%.
- Most common abnormalities are atrioventricular canal and ventricular septal defects. Others include atrial septal defects, patent ductus arteriosus and tetralogy of Fallot.
- Pulmonary hypertension is more severe and earlier in onset in DS patients with defects resulting in left to right shunts. Without early corrective surgery, this may progress to Eisenmenger's syndrome where the shunt becomes right to left.

Respiratory tract

- Obstructive sleep apnoea is relatively common (50%).
- Subglottic stenosis (2–6%).
- Chronic lower respiratory tract infections are relatively common often secondary to reduced immunity and gastro-oesophageal reflux.

Gastrointestinal tract
- Gastrointestinal anomalies occur in 7% of DS patients.
- One-third of patients with duodenal atresia have DS.
- Gastro-oesophageal reflux, oesophageal atresia, Hirschsprung's disease and coeliac disease are all more common in this group.

Neurological
- Neonates with DS may be hypotonic.
- Intellectual function is limited with an ultimate population mean IQ of about 50. A steady decline in IQ with age in adults has been attributed to a presenile (Alzheimer's) dementia.
- Up to 10% have epilepsy.

Haematological
- Leukaemias have 10–18-fold higher incidence than normal in DS.
- Neonates may show a transient leukaemoid reaction.
- In the first year of life, acute non-lymphoblastic leukaemia predominates.
- In older children, acute lymphoblastic leukaemia predominates.

Immune system
- There are defects in cell mediated immunity, granulocyte abnormalities, and a decreased adrenal response.
- Infections are more common than in non-Down's children secondary to these deficiencies.
- This population have a higher incidence of hepatitis B than normal.

Endocrine
- Hypothyroidism without antibodies occurs commonly in childhood.
- Hypothyroidism is common in adults with DS.

Skeletal
- High incidence of atlanto-axial instability (30%) due to a lax transverse ligament and/or malformation of the odontoid peg.
- Subluxation or dislocation may result in cord compression.

Anaesthetic problems and management
- This group of patients tend to have a higher incidence of perioperative morbidity and so thresholds for referral to HDU or ITU for postoperative care should be lower than normal.
- It may be useful to prescribe sedative premedication (midazolam 0.5 mg/kg oral; maximum 20 mg) and have a supportive parent or carer present at induction. Low IQ and a failure to understand the induction process may result in a scared, sizable uncooperative patient who may injure themselves or theatre staff.

- Several airway issues exist with DS:
  - Although they may have several craniofacial abnormalities that suggest they may be difficult to intubate (macroglossia, micrognathia, short neck), this is rarely the case.
  - Potential subglottic stenosis should prompt the anaesthetist to choose an ETT 0.5–1.0 mm smaller than predicted for the age of the patient. It is essential that an audible leak is heard with positive pressure ventilation to avoid any post extubation airway oedema with stridor and respiratory distress.
  - Atlanto-axial instability is common (15% incidence with screening) but not always symptomatic. Lateral cervical spine X-rays are no longer carried out routinely unless there is a history of neurological symptoms of spinal cord compression e.g. ataxia, abnormal gait, exaggerated reflexes, clonus, quadriplegia. New symptoms require investigation before elective surgery. Excessive neck movement should be avoided in patients with DS by both the anaesthetist during laryngoscopy and the surgeon for positioning on the table.
- Cardiac anomalies should be assessed. Patients are usually under the care of a paediatric cardiologist and, if appropriate, cardiac lesions have been corrected. Patients may be on medications to treat cardiac failure or reduce the incidence of cyanotic spells in tetralogy of Fallot. It is useful to have information from recent cardiology follow-ups and echocardiograms. Antibiotic prophylaxis is often required.
- Chronic chest infections are common as is postoperative atelectasis and respiratory tract infection. Infections are treated preoperatively and postoperative chest physiotherapy may be prescribed to minimize chest complications.
- Obstructive sleep apnoea is common and may result in airway obstruction during anaesthesia or in the recovery area.
- Antacid prophylaxis should be given for a history of gastro-oesophageal reflux.
- Pain assessment and management is not always straightforward. Regional techniques may avoid the respiratory depressant effects of opioids and improve compliance with chest physiotherapy. Some patients are able to use PCA.
- Post-operative agitation may be a problem often warranting the use of sedation or early presence of their carer.
- Information from a parent or carer and their presence can be invaluable in the perioperative management of these patients.

Epidermolysis bullosa

- Epidermolysis bullosa is the name given to a group of genetic diseases where blistering and shearing of the skin occurs from minimal trauma.
- Patients present to theatre for plastics procedures (syndactaly release and dressing changes), excision of squamous cell carcinoma with split skin grafts, dental surgery and oesophageal dilatation.

Clinical features

Three main types exist, each with several subtypes.

Epidermolysis bullosa simplex

- Most common form.
- Autosomal dominant inheritance.
- Non-scarring intra-epidermal blisters form on arms, legs, hands, feet, scalp, palms, and soles.
- Tends to improve with age.

Epidermolysis bullosa letalis

- Severe form.
- Autosomal recessive inheritance.
- Blisters in lamina lucida.
- All parts of skin affected with blistering of the respiratory and gastrointestinal tracts.
- Patients rarely survive through infancy often dying of septicaemia.

Dystrophic epidermolysis bullosa

- Two types exist both caused by mutations in the COL7A1 gene responsible for synthesis of type VII collagen. This collagen anchors the lamina densa within the superficial dermis.
- The **autosomal dominant** variant is less severe than the recessive form.
- The more **severe autosomal recessive** form can present at birth or in infancy and includes widespread atrophic scarring blisters resulting in limb contractures, fusion of digits and mouth contractures. Blistering of the mucosal membrane of the oesophagus results in strictures, problems with oral feeding, malnutrition, and iron deficiency anaemia. Oesophageal strictures increase the risk for reflux, regurgitation, and pulmonary aspiration. Nails are dystrophic, teeth are malformed, hair sparse, and corneal ulceration occurs. There is an increased incidence of squamous cell carcinoma, porphyria, and amyloidosis.

Anaesthetic problems and management

Should aim to minimize any unnecessary pressure or shearing trauma.

- Airway management:
  - Vaseline gauze should be used to pad facemasks and areas of skin where anaesthetic fingers support the chin to avoid facial bullae.
  - Intubation with a lubricated laryngoscope blade and a smaller than normal size ETT minimize laryngeal problems.
  - Cricoid pressure is not contraindicated but should be applied evenly.

- Oropharyngeal suctioning can result in life-threatening bullae formation. More commonly, poorly placed oropharyngeal airways may result in bullae in the mouth.
  - Laryngeal masks airways have been used successfully with a case report of a lingual bulla. A smaller size should be used and the shaft wrapped with gauze to protect the lips. Remove under deep anaesthesia.
  - Atropine or glycopyrronium bromide can be useful to dry secretions.
- Venous access:
  - Can be difficult due to scarring.
  - Cannulae can be secured by covering with vaseline gauze and wrapping with a crepe bandage.
  - A central line may be necessary. This is sutured in place.
- Positioning:
  - Allow patient to position themselves on the table if appropriate.
  - Avoid friction from movement on sheets.
- Monitoring:
  - Pulse oximeter probe on digit or ear lobe.
  - Avoid adhesive electrode pads and instead use petroleum jelly gauze over the ECG leads in contact with the patient
  - Place more gauze between the BP cuff and skin.
- Avoid adhesive tapes:
  - ETT and LMA tied in rather than taped.
  - Lubricating eye ointments can be used instead of tape to avoid corneal damage.
- Antacid prophylaxis if history of reflux or oesophageal stricture.
- Adrenal suppression from long-term steroids may require peri-operative supplementation with hydrocortisone.
- Regional anaesthesia can avoid many of the potential problems in these patients:
  - Brachial plexus block for hand surgery.
  - Central blocks if indicated.
  - Topical on split skin graft donor sites.
- Postoperative analgesia:
  - IV, rectal, regional all acceptable.
  - Oral is the preferred method when appropriate using liquid or effervescent preparations because of swallowing difficulties.

Epilepsy

- Abnormal paroxysmal bursts of neuronal activity give rise to seizure activity which can be seen clinically as altered consciousness, motor, sensory, or autonomic events.
- The recurrence of unprovoked seizure activity is diagnosed as epilepsy.
- The incidence of epilepsy in childhood is about 4–9:1000 and about 60% of all patients with epilepsy are diagnosed in childhood.
- Epilepsy is classified according to the clinically observed features of the seizure. The two main groups are generalized seizures and partial seizures.

Clinical features

- Generalized seizures usually involve loss of consciousness and show no evidence of localized onset. Generalized seizures are further subdivided into:
  - Absence seizures where there is loss of consciousness without evidence of abnormal motor activity. They are sometimes accompanied by reduced tone and automatic behaviour.
  - Seizures with abnormal motor activity. This may be atonic, myoclonic, tonic, clonic, or a combination of tonic–clonic.

Patients may have a prodromal period with behavioural change or aura before the seizure. Following the seizure they may remain unconscious and sleepy (postictal phase).

- Partial seizures have a localized onset in the brain sometimes spreading to become generalized.
  - Simple partial seizures may present with jerking of a limb, altered sensation involving a strange taste or smell, a hallucination, or paraesthesia. Activity may spread to involve other limbs or areas of the body.
  - Complex partial seizures are localized seizures with an impaired conscious level.
- There is an extensive range of '*epilepsy syndromes*' including:
  - Infantile spasms
  - Juvenile myoclonic epilepsy
  - Temporal lobe epilepsy
  - Childhood absence epilepsy
  - Benign rolandic epilepsy.
- Febrile convulsions occur in 2–5% of children under 5 years. They are seizures related to a febrile illness that may recur in up to a third of sufferers. There is an associated increased risk of developing epilepsy later (1% in general and up to 10% with family history of epilepsy).
- Diagnosis is made from the history and by observation of a seizure. EEGs can help confirm the diagnosis and often localize epileptic foci in the brain. MRI, single photon emission computed tomography (SPECT), and positron-emission tomography (PET) scans can all be used to locate abnormal brain lesions and look at local cerebral blood flow during seizures. These may provide useful information for surgical resection of foci in patients with intractable seizures.

- Medical therapy for epilepsy is started only once two or more seizures have occurred. The main drugs are sodium valproate, carbamazepine, ethosuximide, phenytoin, and phenobarbital. Clobazam, clonazepam, and nitrazepam may be added to any of these for resistant seizures. Newer agents are now available and include gabapentin, lamotrigine, topiramate, and vigabatrin.
- Some patients with intractable epilepsy improve with the introduction of a ketogenic diet. This is a high fat low carbohydrate diet. IV fluids without glucose should be given to these patients intraoperatively with monitoring of there plasma glucose levels to avoid hypoglycaemia.
- Surgical management for intractable seizures is becoming more common. The four main types are lesionectomy, anterior temporal lobectomy, hemispherectomy, and division of the corpus callosum. Cervical vagus nerve stimulation also appears to be effective in some patient groups.
- The anaesthetic implications of epilepsy are concerned with the effects of anaesthetic drugs on seizure activity and drug interactions affecting anaesthetic drug metabolism.

Anaesthetic problems and management
- A history of seizure type, frequency, last seizure, and medication is useful to establish how well controlled the patient is.
- It is important to ensure that the patient continues to get their anticonvulsant medication preoperatively and that it is started again as soon as possible postoperatively. If oral intake is delayed, some medications may be given rectally (carbamazepine), intramuscularly (phenobarbital) or intravenously (phenytoin or sodium valproate).
- It is common for this group of children to have learning difficulties and behavioural problems. Sedative premedication with midazolam may help produce a smooth induction in uncooperative patients.
- Anaesthetic drugs may raise or lower the threshold for seizures.
  - Thiopental has powerful anticonvulsant properties.
  - Propofol is associated with abnormal movements during induction that may be confused for seizure like activity. It is known to suppress EEG seizure activity.
  - Methohexitone and enflurane (especially with hyperventilation) are both associated with causing seizures.
- Anticonvulsant drugs may induce liver enzymes so that drugs normally metabolized in the liver (vecuronium) may have a shorter than expected duration of action. Atracurium may be a better choice of muscle relaxant in these cases.
- Regional analgesia techniques may allow a more rapid return to oral intake and medication.
- Status epilepticus is a seizure lasting >30 min or when intermittent seizure activity occurs over a 30 min period without regaining consciousness. It is a medical emergency with a mortality rate of up to 4% in children. Complications of prolonged convulsions include cardiac dysrhythmias, hypertension, pulmonary oedema, disseminated intravascular coagulation, and myoglobinuria.

Haemophilia and von Willebrand's disease

Haemophilia refers to the three most common hereditary bleeding disorders—haemophilia A (factor VIII deficiency), haemophilia B (factor IX deficiency), and von Willebrand's disease (vWD)—von Willebrand factor (vWF) deficiency.

Haemophilia A

- Haemophilia A is an X-linked recessive bleeding disorder affecting 1:5000 males arising from a mutation on chromosome Xq28. There is a positive family history in two-thirds of cases.
- There is a range in severity, which correlates with the level of factor VIII coagulation activity (VIIIc) measured by clotting assay. Levels are commonly expressed as a percentage of the normal expected level and severity is inversely related to the amount of factor present (<1%—severe; 2–5%—moderate; 5–30%—mild; 50–200%—normal). The proportions of patients who are severe, moderate, or mild are 50%, 10%, and 40% respectively.
- Age at presentation depends on the level of severity and the type of trauma.
  - Patients commonly present with spontaneous bleeding into joints (ankles, knees, hips, and elbows) and muscles. This results in painful swelling that reduces function and leads to degenerative arthritis and deformity in the joints and possibly necrosis and contractures in the muscles.
  - The more severely affected may suffer intracranial haemorrhage with mild head trauma.
  - Haematuria occurs quite commonly.
  - Even in mildly affected patients, haemorrhage from operative trauma can be life threatening e.g. dental extraction, circumcision, tonsillectomy, and childbirth.
- Preoperative blood tests elicit abnormalities of the intrinsic coagulation pathway with a prolonged partial thromboplastin time (PTT), normal thrombin time (TT), prothrombin time (PT), and fibrinogen. Bleeding time is normal except in the most severe cases. It is important to have a baseline factor VIIIc assay.

Anaesthetic problems and management

- Patients are usually under the care of a consultant haematologist and haemophilia nurse specialist who advise on the haematological aspects of care. Good communication is essential in coordinating management in the perioperative period.
- IV access can be difficult. Patients usually have a portacath in situ for their regular treatment. Strict asepsis when accessing this is essential.
- Manufactured recombinant factor VIII concentrate is the mainstay of treatment for this condition. It is useful to establish preoperatively how much, how often and what affect a dose has on factor VIIIc assay levels. It is essential to know if there are factor VIIIc antibodies. Factor VIII has a half-life of 8–12 hours and may have to be given 2 or 3 times daily. Generally, maintenance therapy is given 3 times each week from walking age to minimize long-term joint damage.

- Sustained levels of over 50% are required for surgery. Approximately 15 IU/kg will raise the level by 30%. Usually about 50 IU/kg are given just before surgery followed by 25 IU/kg that evening and twice daily thereafter for the first week. The peak level should be measured approximately 20 minutes post dose with the aim of having a level above 100% post-infusion. Factor VIII assays are repeated daily for the first week post surgery to ensure that levels do not fall below 50%.
- Dental surgery usually requires a single dose of factor VIII (25 IU/kg). Tranexamic acid can also be given. This inhibitor of fibrinolysis is usually continued for about 1 week post procedure.
- Desmopressin (DDAVP) causes the release of stored factor VIII and vWF from endothelial cells. In mild or moderate haemophiliacs undergoing minor surgery (e.g. dental extractions) there may be an adequate rise in factor VIII levels from DDAVP for haemostasis during the procedure. The dose is 0.3 mcg/kg IV.
- 10–15% of patients develop antibodies to factor VIII that decrease its effectiveness. Surgery in this group of patients should only be performed for important procedures. Recent data suggests that using recombinant factor VIIa may be an alternative method for managing perioperative haemostasis in this difficult group. It acts by activation of the extrinsic coagulation pathway forming a complex with tissue factor at the site of bleeding.
- IM injections, NSAIDs and regional techniques are avoided. Oral analgesia, PCA or IV infusions are preferable.
- The incidence of hepatitis B and C in haemophiliacs should be falling with the use of recombinant factor VIII concentrate.

Haemophilia B (Christmas disease)

- This X-linked disorder is due to a deficiency of factor IX.
- It is 4 times less common than haemophilia A.
- Clinically it resembles the features of haemophilia A and can only be distinguished from it by assay of factors VIIIc and IX. Other results include a long PTT, normal PT, TT, fibrinogen, and bleeding time.
- Treatment is with heat-treated factor IX concentrate. This has a long half-life (>18 hours) and so can be given once daily for bleeds.
- Desmopressin is not effective in treating haemophilia B.

Von Willebrand's disease

- vWD is the most common inherited bleeding disorder affecting approximately 1% of the population.
- It is caused by deficiency or dysfunction of von Willebrand factor (vWF) due to a defect on chromosome 12 and occurs in both sexes.
- This large glycoprotein has two main roles in haemostasis.
  - Firstly, it promotes platelet aggregation and adherence at the sites of vascular injury forming a platelet plug.
  - Secondly, it acts as a carrier protein for factor VIII in the plasma, protecting it from premature activation and degradation. A problem with transporting and stabilizing factor VIII results in a secondary deficiency of factor VIII. The effect of vWF deficiency is to produce a defect in both platelet plug formation and in fibrin formation.

- vWD is classified into three main phenotypes varying in severity from mild to severe:
  - Type I. This is the mildest and most common variant (60–80%). It is characterized by moderate deficiencies of vWF and factor VIII (reduced to 5–30% of normal levels). Inheritance is autosomal dominant. Patients may present with bruising after trauma or surgery. They usually do not bleed spontaneously but may suffer epistaxis or menorrhagia. Symptoms are often so mild that a person is never diagnosed.
  - Type II (10–30%). Inheritance can be autosomal dominant or recessive and results in a qualitative abnormality of vWF. It has several subtypes IIA, IIB, IIM, and IIN. Type IIB has a reduced vWF associated with decreased platelet survival and a thrombocytopenia. Patients may present with spontaneous skin and mucosal bleeding e.g. gastrointestinal tract, epistaxis or dental.
  - Type III is the most severe form of the disease. Inheritance is autosomal recessive. Bleeding is more frequent and severe due to an absence of vWF and factor VIII. This group also suffers bleeding into joints and muscles.
- Test results may vary in an individual and may need to be repeated to exclude or confirm a diagnosis. Tests that are used to diagnose vWD include:
  - The bleeding time which tends to be grossly prolonged (normal in haemophilia A).
  - The PTT that is elevated while PT, TT, and fibrinogen are normal.
  - Platelet aggregation and adhesion are reduced.
  - Factor VIII and vWF antigen levels are reduced. The disease is considered mild if vWF antigen level is between 20–40% normal and severe if it is below 10%.
  - vWF activity can be measured by the ristocetin co-factor activity test.
  - Analysis of the vWF multimers helps classify the type of vWD and has implications for treatment.
- The mainstays of treatment are desmopressin (intravenously, subcutaneously, or intranasal) which induces autologous secretion of factor VIII and vWF into plasma, plasma concentrates (cryoprecipitate), recombinant factor VIII, or purified vWF concentrate. Fibrinolysis inhibitors, platelet concentrates, and the oral contraceptive pill may be useful as adjuvant therapy.
  - Desmopressin is not effective in some type II and all type III patients. In type IIB, it can lead to platelet aggregation and thrombocytopenia.
  - In those patients who respond to desmopressin, tachyphylaxis limits use to 3 doses in a 48-hour period.
- Patients with type III vWD may require prophylaxis if they have recurrent bleeding into mucosa or joints.
- In types I and II prophylactic treatment is only given before invasive procedures or if spontaneous bleeding occurs.

Anaesthetic problems and management
- Good communication between the haematologist, anaesthetist and surgeon is essential to ensure these patients receive appropriate and safe management tailored to their individual needs.
- For a surgical procedure involving mucosal membranes, it is important to normalize the bleeding time.
  - The pharmacological agents most commonly used are desmopressin and tranexamic acid.
  - Desmopressin is given intravenously (0.3 mcg/kg IV) diluted in 10 mL of normal saline and given over 10 min. Patients should be monitored for side effects (tachycardia, hypotension, facial flushing). desmopressin can also be administered by intranasal spray.
  - For elective surgery, patients are often admitted for a trial of treatment to assess the efficacy of desmopressin. Blood is taken 45–60 min post-dose and it is hoped that factor VIII and vWF levels exceed 50% of normal values following treatment.
  - If treatment is to be administered for >2 days, these levels should be monitored as tachyphylaxis can occur.
  - Desmopressin is not given to known 'non-responders', patients with type IIB or III disease, and children <2 years.
  - It has an antidiuretic effect and if several doses are given fluid balance and electrolytes should be monitored. Children under 2 years are at ↑ risk from hyponatraemia.
  - A combination of desmopressin with a fibrinolytic inhibitor (tranexamic acid—15–25 mg/kg orally) can be used for dental extractions.
  - Tranexamic acid can be given orally and as a mouth wash for up to 7 days afterwards.
  - For patients who do not respond to desmopressin, a single dose of recombinant factor VIII or vWF is given.
- For major surgery, haematological advice is taken on the appropriate use of cryoprecipitate, vWF concentrate, pasteurised factor VIII preparation (Humate-P) and platelet transfusion.
- Aspirin and other NSAIDs that reduce platelet function are avoided.
- Universal precautions are used, as there is a higher incidence of hepatitis C and HIV from multiple blood product transfusions.
- IM injections are avoided.

HIV/AIDS

- Paediatric acquired immune-deficiency syndrome (AIDS) was first reported in 1982 and today represents 5% of the total number of cases worldwide. It refers to those under 13 years old who are infected with HIV. Approximately 90% of cases are found in developing countries in south and central Africa and southern Asia.
- The causative agent, human immunodeficiency virus (HIV) was identified in 1983. HIV is a retrovirus belonging to the lentivirus group. Retroviruses contain the enzyme reverse transcriptase that allows genetic material encoded on RNA to be converted into DNA and then incorporated into the host cell genome. HIV preferentially infects T-helper cells (CD4$^+$ T cells) and destroys them. This has a direct effect on cell-mediated immunity and results in increased susceptibility to opportunistic infections and malignancies. Two distinct types of HIV exist—HIV-1 and HIV-2. HIV-2 is found almost exclusively in West Africa. Disease progression is slower and vertical transmission from mother to child is less common.
- 80% of paediatric HIV results from vertical transmission from an infected mother to the fetus during the intra-partum period, labour, and delivery or from breast feeding. Transmission rates vary from 30% in Europe to 50% in developing countries. Perinatal antiretroviral therapy may reduce transmission rates to 8%. The combination of elective Caesarean section and antiretroviral therapy can further reduce the risk to about 2%. Less commonly nowadays, AIDS may result from receiving infected blood or blood products and rarely sexual abuse by an infected individual.
- Children born to HIV antibody-positive mothers acquire HIV antibodies by passive transfer across the placenta. These may remain for the first 12–18 months of life. This makes diagnosis in the first 15 months of life difficult. Enzyme-linked immunoassays and Western blot analysis are used to test for antibody activity but are limited in their ability as a reliable predictor of future infection. A more sensitive method for detecting HIV in early infancy is the polymerase chain reaction (PCR) technique.
- Only 30–40% of those infants with maternal antibodies actually go on to make their own antibodies and develop AIDS. However, if antibodies persist beyond 15 months, the child should be assumed to be infected.

Clinical features

- Incubation period is 6 months to several years. Patients may present with non-specific signs and symptoms—failure to thrive, oral thrush, recurrent diarrhoea and respiratory infections, unexplained fever, anaemia, lymphadenopathy, dermatitis, hepatosplenomegaly, and thrombocytopenia.
- Vertically acquired infection behaves in a more aggressive manner than other forms. 20–30% develop profound immune deficiency and an AIDS defining illness before 1 year of age. More commonly the disease is slowly progressive with 75% of infected infants surviving at 5 years of age.

Infection

- Respiratory sepsis, meningitis, osteomyelitis, cellulitis, gastrointestinal and urinary tract infections all occur. Causative organisms include *Streptococcus pneumoniae*, *Haemophilus influenzae*, *Salmonella* species, *Escherichia coli*, *Staphylococcus aureus*, and *Pseudomonas* species.
- The commonest opportunistic infection is *Pneumocystis carinii* pneumonia. Candidal, tubercular and viral pneumonias can occur. Opportunistic infections may also occur with cytomegalovirus, varicella-zoster virus, herpes simplex, *Candida albicans*, *Toxoplasma gondii*, and atypical mycobacteria.
- *Pneumocystis carinii* pneumonia is treated with high dose co-trimoxazole. Systemic prednisolone therapy (1 mg/kg/day) is advised for patients with a $P_aO_2 < 9.3$ kPa. Respiratory support and oxygen therapy may be required. Prophylaxis with co-trimoxazole or inhaled pentamidine is recommended for children who have had an episode of *Pneuomocystis* pneumonia, those born to infected mothers but not yet diagnosed HIV antibody-positive and for infected children with low CD4 lymphocyte counts.

Respiratory system

- Respiratory disease is the main cause of morbidity and presents the biggest challenge for anaesthetic management. Opportunistic infections (*Pneumocystis* pneumonia, *Aspergillosis*, herpes simplex, cytomegolovirus), mycobacterial infections (mycobacterium tuberculosis) and bacterial infections (*Streptococcus pneumoniae*, *Haemophilus influenzae*, *Staphylococcus aureus*, and *Pseudomonas aeruginosa*) may progress to acute respiratory failure. *Pneumocystis carinii* is a particularly virulent organism in children and is associated with a poorer prognosis than in adults.
- Lymphoid interstitial pneumonitis presents with dyspnoea on exertion, a non-productive cough, diffuse reticulonodular shadowing on CXR, and finger clubbing. Onset is insidious with an uncertain pathophysiology. Treatment is with steroids and bronchodilators. Opportunistic infection is less common in these children and the overall prognosis is improved. These children may also get episodes of parotid gland enlargement and lymphadenopathy.

Cardiovascular system

- Cardiovascular involvement is common. Myocarditis may result from infection with coxsackie B virus, cytomegolovirus, cryptococcus, aspergillosis or HIV. This may progress to a dilated cardiomyopathy with myocardial dysfunction and rhythm disturbances.
- Infective endocarditis, pericardial effusions and autonomic neuropathy may also be present.

Central nervous system

- Most infected children have an encephalopathy that may be progressive with developmental delay, symmetrical motor deficits (abnormal gait, tone, and reflexes), behavioural changes, and seizures.
- Abnormal brain growth results in microcephaly and cerebral atrophy with early demyelination of cerebral white matter.

- *Cryptococcus neoformans*, HIV and tuberculosis can cause meningitis.
- Patients have an increased susceptibility for primary CNS lymphomas and cerebrovascular accidents.

Gastrointestinal system
- With disease progression patients may fail to thrive or lose weight. Adequate nutritional intake is made difficult by pain from oral and oesophageal candidiasis and recurrent diarrhoea due to infection or HIV-enteropathy.

Haematological
- Microcytic anaemia, thrombocytopenia and a leucopenia may be seen secondary to the disease or drug therapy.

Other features
- Recurrent skin infections: bacterial (staphylococcal), fungal and viral (molluscum contagiosum).
- Kaposi's sarcoma is only seen in about 10% of children.
- Between 5 and 10% may develop nephrotic syndrome secondary to a focal glomerulosclerosis.

Drug therapy and side effects
Antiretrovirals are used to slow the progression of HIV disease but are toxic and complicated regimens make compliance difficult. They suppress viral replication and are given as a combination therapy to reduce drug resistance. Three categories of drug are used:
- Nucleoside analogue reverse transcriptase inhibitors e.g. zidovudine (bone marrow suppression, gastrointestinal upset), lamivudine (anaemia), didanosine (peripheral neuropathy, pancreatitis). They act as a false nucleotide and prevent reverse transcriptase from synthesizing DNA.
- Non-nucleoside reverse transcriptase inhibitors e.g. nevirapine (rash, hepatitis), efavirenz (rash). These bind to reverse transcriptase and inhibit enzyme activity.
- Protease inhibitors e.g. saquinavir (diarrhoea, ↑transaminases), ritonavir, and lopinavir (gastrointestinal upset, hyperlipidaemia, circumoral paraesthesia). They prevent the processing of viral proteins into their functional forms.

Infected children may be taking other drugs that may be nephrotoxic (amphotericin B, aciclovir, pentamidine) or cause thrombocytopenia (zidovudine, co-trimoxazole, ketoconazole).

Anaesthetic problems and management
Children with HIV commonly present for central line insertion, gastrostomy feeding tubes, drainage of infected lesions and diagnostic procedures (lung, liver biopsies). As survival in paediatric AIDS improves, more children are presenting for other types of surgery e.g. dental, ENT, and day case general surgery. HIV can damage almost every organ and evidence of this should be sought in the history and examination.

- Risk of transmission of infection.
  - Patient to anaesthetist. Universal precautions (gloves, gown, mask, eye protection) during anaesthesia for high risk patients. Spillage of infected body fluids is avoided and the disposal of needles without resheathing into sharps containers is essential. The risk of HIV transmission from a significant needle-stick injury from an infected patient is approximately 0.31%.
  - Patient to patient. HIV is destroyed by heat and chemicals (glutaraldehyde or sodium hypochlorite). Disposable airway devices, HME filters and circuits are used. Other anaesthetic equipment should be routinely cleaned and decontaminated.
  - Post exposure prophylaxis. A significant needle-stick injury from a high risk patient should be immediately discussed with occupational health. Post exposure prophylaxis should be started within 1–2 hours of exposure. Toxicity and compliance with treatment are sometimes a problem.
- Respiratory function is assessed looking for the presence of infection. CXR useful.
- Cardiovascular involvement (myocarditis, cardiomyopathy, dysrhythmias, autonomic neuropathy) are assessed with the help of an ECG and echocardiograph if indicated. Abnormal ECGs are common (>90%).
- Blood tests include FBC, U&E, and LFTs for evidence of abnormalities related to HIV or side effects from drug therapy. Laboratory personnel should be notified of the high risk specimen.
- Central neuraxial blockade is usually avoided in the presence of neurological signs or symptoms. Regional anaesthesia in this immunocompromised group of patients may carry a higher risk of CNS infection.
- Children with HIV/AIDS often come from complex social backgrounds and may not present with their biological parents. It is important to ascertain (sensitively) who has legal guardianship for these children in order to obtain informed consent.
- Postoperative mortality is not higher in this group. The incidence of postoperative fever, anaemia, and tachycardia is higher in HIV patients.

Juvenile chronic arthritis

- Juvenile chronic arthritis (JCA) is a descriptive term used to encompass a heterogeneous group of disorders characterized by arthritis of childhood onset (age <16 years), unknown aetiology, and persisting for a minimum of 3 months.
- It represents one of the most common connective tissue disorders in children with a bimodal peak age onset of 1–3 years and 8–12 years.
- Unlike adult rheumatoid arthritis, JCA is usually seronegative for rheumatoid factor (RhF) and is likely to have a different pathophysiology.
- Classification is based upon the distribution of joints involved and the presence or absence of systemic symptoms at presentation.

Clinical features

Pauciarticular onset JCA

- Up to 50% of children present with 1–4 joints involved in the first 6 months. In some cases, monoarthritis may persist and this most commonly affects the knee.
- Unlike polyarticular onset disease, the small joints of the hand and feet, cervical spine, or temporomandibular joints (TMJ) are rarely involved.
- Two subgroups exist. The first predominantly affects females under 4 years of age. It is uncommon for it to progress to severe disease and polyarthritis (20%) but 30% will develop iridocyclitis as a serious problem.
- The second subgroup mainly affects boys over 9 years, predominantly involves large joints of the lower limb, with a significant number going on to develop ankylosing spondylitis. 10% may develop an acute iridocyclitis.

Polyarticular onset JCA

- 40% have 5 or more joints affected at presentation. The knees, wrists, ankles, and the small joints of the hands and feet are most commonly (symmetrically) involved.
- Cervical spine involvement occurs in up to 70% of cases presenting with pain, limitation of movement, or torticollis.
- Bilateral TMJ involvement may limit mouth opening and mandibular development resulting in micrognathia.
- Systemic manifestations are usually mild (fever, anaemia, lymphadenopathy, rash).
- Two subgroups exist—those who are seronegative for RhF and a smaller group who are seropositive. Those children who are seropositive tend to be girls aged over 8 years with a more severe destructive joint disease of hands, feet, and hips. They may have rheumatoid nodules and are less likely to respond to treatment.
- The seronegative group have asymmetrical joint involvement of small and large joints, especially the TMJ and cervical spine. Progression to the destructive disease is unlikely.

Systemic onset JCA

- This group of children present with fever, rash, and arthritis at any age in childhood with an equal gender incidence.
- The fever is intermittent, in the range of 39.5–40.5°C, often occurs daily and the child generally appears very unwell during these episodes.
- The rash is maculopapular and salmon-pink in colour. It is non-puritic, variable in appearance, and most obvious when the child is febrile.
- Arthritis may not present for several weeks or months after the initial symptoms.
- Diagnosis is based on clinical features and exclusion of other causes of the presenting symptoms (infection, malignancy, and another connective tissue disease).
- Hepatosplenomegaly, generalized lymphadenopathy, and less commonly pericarditis, pleuritis, and pericardial effusion may occur. Children often have anaemia of chronic disease, thrombocytosis, a raised ESR and WCC, and are RhF negative.

Management for these patients combines physiotherapy with pharmacological agents to control symptoms and preserve joint function. NSAIDs are first line agents. Disease modifying drugs include methotrexate, ciclosporin, gold, and penicillamine. These are used as second line for systemic and polyarticular onset disease. Morbidity associated with chronic use now limits the use of steroids. They are indicated for use in acute febrile episodes, carditis and Coombs' positive haemolytic anaemia as oral or IV pulsed methylprednisolone.

Anaesthetic problems and management

- Patients should be positioned carefully with appropriate padding to protect pressure points.
- Arthritis of the temporomandibular joint may result in reduced mouth opening and mandibular hypoplasia. Laryngoscopy may be difficult. Fibreoptic endotracheal intubation may be necessary (📖 Chapter 5). There may also be cricoarytenoid joint involvement presenting with hoarseness, stridor, and the complaint of difficulty in swallowing.
- Manipulation of the cervical spine during intubation requires a careful preoperative neurological and radiological examination of the patient looking for evidence of instability, atlanto-axial subluxation, or cervical ankylosis.
- Side effects of drug therapy include anaemia and platelet dysfunction (NSAIDs), leucopenia, nephritis and hepatitis (gold therapy), cirrhosis and pulmonary fibrosis (methotrexate), and Cushingoid side-effects (steroids).
- Rarely there may be pulmonary (pleuritis) or cardiovascular (pericarditis) involvement requiring preoperative investigations— ECG, CXR, echocardiography.

Liver failure

Acute liver failure

- Acute liver failure or fulminant hepatitis is a rare complex disease with mortality greater than 70% without supportive treatment and/or liver transplantation.
- The adult disease is a well-defined clinical syndrome consisting of the acute onset of encephalopathy, coagulopathy, and evidence of acute liver necrosis with hepatic dysfunction starting within 8 weeks of the first signs of liver disease. This assumes the absence of any pre-existing liver disease.
- However, in infants and children encephalopathy may be absent, late, or undiagnosed even in severe disease. Acute liver failure may also be the first presentation of an underlying metabolic (Wilson's disease) or autoimmune disease.
- Paediatric definitions place more emphasis on the presence of a significant coagulopathy due to acute hepatic dysfunction unresponsive to parenteral vitamin K. It may be defined as hyperacute (up to 10 days), acute (11–30 days) or subacute (over 30 days) in onset depending on the duration of liver dysfunction. Jaundice is more commonly seen in subacute onset acute liver failure and encephalopathy, if seen, tends to be a pre-terminal event.

Clinical features

Aetiology

Aetiology varies with age of the child. Neonatal haemochromatosis is a rare disorder of iron handling and is the most common cause of acute liver failure in infants. Viral hepatitis accounts for 80% of cases of fulminant hepatic failure in children of all age groups.

Neonates and infants

- Infection: septicaemia, hepatitis B, adenovirus, parvovirus B19, echovirus, coxsackie, non-A-G hepatitis, EBV, HIV.
- Metabolic: neonatal haemochromatosis, tyrosinaemia type I, mitochondrial disorders, fatty acid oxidation defects, α1-antitrypsin deficiency.
- Drugs: paracetamol, iron, vitamin A, salicylates, anticonvulsants, isoniazid.
- Vascular: CHD, asphyxia, Budd–Chiari syndrome.
- Others: neuroblastoma, hepatoblastoma, leukaemia, familial erythrophagocytic syndrome.

Older children

- Infection: viral hepatitis A-G, EBV, CMV, HSV, leptospirosis, bacterial sepsis.
- Metabolic: Wilson's disease.
- Drugs: paracetamol, isoniazid, salicylates, valproic acid, drugs of abuse in adolescents (glue sniffing, ecstasy), halothane hepatitis.
- Toxins: carbon tetrachloride, Amanita phalloides (death cap mushroom), iron poisoning.
  - Neoplastic: lymphoma, leukaemia, hepatocellular carcinoma.
  - Vascular: sequelae of cardiac surgery, shock, sickle cell anaemia.

Presentation

- Jaundice is the most common presenting symptom. It is often preceded by a prodromal flu-like illness. Anorexia, nausea, vomiting, and ascites are common.
- Encephalopathy is not always obvious especially in neonates and infants where jaundice and coagulopathy may be the presenting features. Encephalopathy in infants may present with irritability and altered sleep time patterns while older children may present with aggressive behaviour.
- Hepatic encephalopathy is graded according to severity and this correlates with disease severity and worsening outcome:
  - Grade 1: lethargy, slightly reduced conscious level.
  - Grade 2: stupor, disorientated, combative.
  - Grade 3: unresponsive to command but responds to pain.
  - Grade 4: unresponsive to command or pain; extensor posturing and rigidity.
- Acute liver failure is a multisystem disorder associated with numerous complications—sepsis, acute renal failure, severe coagulopathy, gastro-intestinal bleeding, ascites, cerebral oedema, high cardiac output failure (with a low systemic vascular resistance), hypoglycaemia, hypokalaemia, and a metabolic acidosis. These patients are only anaesthetized for emergency procedures as perioperative morbidity and mortality is high.

Chronic liver failure

Incidence is 6:100,000 live births and it is suspected in any infant with jaundice continuing beyond 14 days.

Clinical features

Aetiology

- The most common cause of chronic liver disease in infants and children is extrahepatic biliary atresia. Infants undergo hepatic portoenterostomy (Kasai procedure) within their first eight weeks of life. If successful, the procedure may achieve a 90% 10 year survival. Failure of this procedure represents the commonest indication for liver transplant worldwide.
- Other causes of chronic liver disease in children include:
  - Biliary obstruction: choledochal cyst, cystic fibrosis, sclerosing cholangitis.
  - Infective: acute viral hepatitis B, chronic active hepatitis, CMV.
  - Metabolic: Wilson's disease, alpha-1-antitrypsin deficiency, tyrosinaemia, haemochromatosis.
  - Autoimmune: chronic active hepatitis.

Presentation

- Patients may be asymptomatic, present with symptoms of acute liver failure, or there may be a more insidious onset of symptoms.
- Features suggesting chronicity are a small hard liver, splenomegaly, jaundice, cutaneous manifestations (palmar erythema, spider naevi, caput medusae), ascites, fluid retention, impaired renal function, growth failure, or muscle wasting.

- Encephalopathy can be precipitated by sedative medication, infection, gastrintestinal bleeds, high protein diets, hypokalaemia, and surgery. A deteriorating conscious level may mark the onset of cerebral oedema necessitating intubation and intensive care management.

Anaesthetic problems and management

Patients with liver dysfunction represent a significant risk when presenting for surgery. Child's classification, later modified by Pugh is a scoring system that assesses the severity of chronic liver disease and can be used to predict prognosis and the risk of major surgery.

Table 15.1 Child–Pugh risk assessment in liver disease

Mortality	Minimal (<5%)	Modest (5–50%)	Marked (>50%)
Bilirubin (micromoles/L)	<25	25–40	>40
Albumin (g/L)	>35	30–35	<30
PT (sec prolonged)	1–4	4–6	>6
Ascites	None	Moderate	Marked
Encephalopathy	None	Grades 1 & 2	Grades 3 & 4

- In chronic liver disease serum bilirubin, serum albumin, and prothrombin time are accurate markers of disease progression. Rising bilirubin and prothrombin time with a falling albumin are poor prognostic signs.
- Assessment of encephalopathy, nutrition, and ascites, although subjective, are still useful.
- Standard liver function tests are poor markers of function and have no prognostic value. Alanine aminotransferase and aspartate aminotransferase serve as markers for liver damage but may fall in the late stages of disease. Alkaline phosphatase is elevated in cholestasis and biliary obstruction.
- Mortality in this patient group may result from sepsis, massive haemorrhage, renal failure or deterioration in hepatic function with encephalopathy.

Haemorrhage

- The liver is responsible for the synthesis of all coagulation factors except vWF (VIII). PTT and INR are usually prolonged and are good indicators of liver function.
- There is often a quantitative and qualitative drop in platelets primarily from splenic sequestration.
- Children are therefore at risk of massive haemorrhage especially from oesophageal, gastric, or rectal varices secondary to portal hypertension. Children are screened on a regular basis for varices. They may be treated medically with prophylactic β-blockers, undergo sclerotherapy or banding of varices or a porto-systemic shunt may be performed.

- Patients tend to have an anaemia related to chronic disease, chronic bleeding and malnutrition.
- Preoperatively a FBC, coagulation screen, appropriate cross-match and adequate platelets and clotting factors are required.

Ascites

- Oedema and ascites indicates advanced liver dysfunction.
- Raised intra-abdominal pressure may cause diaphragmatic splinting and respiratory distress. FRC is reduced.
- Patients may be on diuretics (spironolactone) or may have a peritoneovenous shunt.
- Intra-operative drainage of the ascites may result in marked hypovolaemia and hypotension postoperatively as the ascites recollects. Extra fluid should be given to account for this loss.

Respiratory

- P_aO_2 may be low because of intrapulmonary shunts, ventilation-perfusion mismatch, pleural effusions, and ascites (↓ FRC and diaphragmatic splinting).
- Atelectasis and chest infections are more common perioperatively.

Cardiovascular

- Patients have a hyperdynamic circulation with a high cardiac output and low systemic vascular resistance.
- A variety of shunts occur (cutaneous, porto-pulmonary) and portal hypertension results in ascites and varices.

Renal function

- Common with liver failure and carries a poor prognosis.
- A reduced SVR with low perfusion pressures activates the renin–angiotensin–aldosterone axis causing a further reduction in GFR. Antidiuretic hormone secretion is also increased in response to hypoperfusion and urine output falls further.
- There is the risk of hepatorenal syndrome with renal failure in the presence of liver failure and this is characterized by a hyperosmolar urine and low urinary sodium (<10 mmol/L). Sodium and water retention may occur.
- Renal failure in liver disease may also occur secondary to sepsis or acute tubular necrosis.

Metabolic

- Reduced glycogen stores and impaired gluconeogenesis mean there is a risk of hypoglycaemia. Blood glucose should be closely monitored.
- Acid–base balance may be influenced by renal dysfunction or diuretic therapy.

Infection

- Patients have reduced immunological function and are at increased risk of sepsis.
- Procedures should be carried out aseptically.
- A high index of suspicion should exist for the presence of infection as a cause for cardiovascular instability or worsening encephalopathy.

Altered drug pharmacokinetics

- The liver plays a major role in drug metabolism. Drugs are converted into their active or inactive metabolites and converted from lipid soluble compounds to water soluble compounds which are excreted in the urine or bile.
- Phase I reactions are carried out by the mixed function oxidase system (cytochrome P-450). The drugs undergo hydrolysis, oxidation or reduction.
- Phase II reactions involve conjugation of the products of the phase I reactions with glucuronide, sulphate, acetate, glycine, or methyl groups.
- Liver disease reduces the hepatic clearance of drugs reliant on these reactions e.g. opioids and benzodiazepines.
- Obstructive disorders may result in reduced biliary excretion and clearance of drugs or their metabolites in bile e.g. pancuronium, resulting in prolonged neuromuscular blockade.
- Reduced plasma albumin will increase the free active portion of drugs in the plasma resulting in a greater drug effect for a given dose e.g. thiopental.
- The volume of distribution for protein bound drugs in hypoalbuminaemia is increased as the free portion is more able to redistribute in the body compartments. Ascites, sodium, and water retention also increases the volume of distribution of drugs.
- Drugs which reduce cardiac output and hepatic blood flow during anaesthesia have a deleterious effect on hepatic metabolism. Halothane is avoided. Desflurane, sevoflurane, and isoflurane are safe to use.

Preoperative investigations

- FBC, coagulation, U+E, LFTs, blood glucose, CXR, ABGs, hepatitis B serology.

Anaesthesia

- Midazolam and diazepam premedication should be used with caution as they may precipitate encephalopathy.
- Increased intra-abdominal pressure from ascites will increase the potential for reflux, regurgitation, and aspiration. H_2 receptor antagonists or proton pump inhibitors should be given.
- A rapid sequence induction may be necessary.
- There should be a low threshold for invasive monitoring (CVP, intra-arterial blood pressure, urine output) and booking a HDU or ITU bed for postoperative care.
- The clearance of thiopentone is unchanged (high fat solubility and rapid redistribution). However, patients may be sensitive to it and the induction dose should be reduced.
- Propofol similarly has an unchanged clearance. With prolonged infusions, the half-life is prolonged in liver failure. Induction doses should be reduced to avoid hypotension.

- Cisatracurium or atracurium are the muscle relaxants of choice. Rocuronium, vecuronium, and pancuronium all have extended durations of action. Decreased synthesis of plasma cholinesterase prolongs the effect of suxamethonium and mivacurium. Monitoring of neuromuscular blockade should be used.
- Maintenance with isoflurane, sevoflurane (theoretical risk of compound A), or desflurane can be used. Halothane reduces hepatic blood flow and so should be avoided.
- Patients have an increased sensitivity to morphine, fentanyl, and alfentanil. The half-life of morphine is prolonged and so the frequency of administration will need to be reduced. PCA lockout times should be increased. Metabolism of remifentanil is unaffected by liver failure as it is broken down by blood and tissue esterases. NSAIDs should be avoided perioperatively.
- Regional anaesthesia is a good option for providing postoperative analgesia in some patients. Coagulation studies should be checked and LA doses reduced due to their reliance on hepatic clearance.
- Attention to detail with fluid balance, replacing blood loss, insensible losses and ascites is important to avoid the risk of developing renal failure. Lactate solutions should be avoided and dextrose solutions should be used to avoid hypoglycaemia. Losses are often best replaced with albumin solutions to maintain an adequate intravascular volume. Patients who have a coagulopathy may need fresh frozen plasma as their primary replacement fluid. Urine output should be maintained at 1 mL/kg/hour. Mannitol may be necessary to achieve this if fluid balance is correct.

Klippel–Feil syndrome

- Klippel–Feil syndrome is a congenital anomaly characterized by a failure of formation or segmentation of the cervical vertebrae.
- The clinical triad consists of short neck, low posterior hairline, and limited neck movement.
- Numerous other associated abnormalities of other organ systems may also be present. Less than 50% of patients demonstrate all three clinical features.
- Most cases occur sporadically although inheritance has been reported to be both autosomal dominant and recessive.

Clinical features

Early classification systems recognized three morphological types of cervical fusion in Klippel–Feil syndrome.

Type I
- Extensive fusions of cervical and upper thoracic vertebrae into bony blocks.
- Most often associated with other severe syndromic abnormalities.

Type II
- Fusions occur at only one or two cervical interspaces.
- C2/3 is the most common site of fusion.
- Often associated with other skeletal deformities e.g. Sprengel's deformity (congenital upward displacement of the scapula), cervical rib, hemivertebrae, occipitoatlantal fusion.

Type III
- Fusions both at cervical and lower thoracic or lumbar spine.
- Types I and III have a higher risk of development and progression of scoliotic curves (60% patients).
- Studies looking at affected families have shown that types I and III commonly have an autosomal dominant inheritance pattern, whereas type II is commonly autosomal recessive.

Klippel–Feil syndrome may also be associated with: spina bifida (45%), profound deafness (30%), rib abnormalities e.g. fused ribs (30%), cleft lip or palate (15%), renal aplasia or other genitourinary abnormalities, CHD (10%—usually VSDs). Less commonly: cervical rib, micrognathia, syringomyelia, Moebius syndrome (congenital facial palsy with impairment of ocular abduction), webbing of soft tissues (neck and syndactyly), and flattening of the base of skull (platybasia). Anomalies are present at birth but often not diagnosed until a later stage.

Patients may present for surgery to resect fused or cervical ribs, lower elevated scapula, genitourinary procedures, and neurosurgical procedures for neck instability or cord compression.

Anaesthetic problems and management

- Children with undiagnosed Klippel–Feil syndrome can present as an unexpected difficult intubation due to their short stiff neck. If a diagnosis has already been made before presenting for anaesthesia, the areas of spinal fusion should be identified and cervical stability assessed. If there are signs or symptoms of spinal cord compression, an MRI should be performed. Cervical spine instability may result in spinal cord injury if the neck is manipulated for tracheal intubation.
- Airway management may require fibreoptic intubation. LMAs have been used successfully in these patients with minimal neck movement for insertion.
- If CHD is present prophylactic antibiotics may be required.

Marfan's syndrome

- This is an inherited disease of fibrous connective tissue caused by a mutation in the fibrillin-1 gene on chromosome 15. This mutation reduces the tensile strength of collagen.
- The incidence is about 1:10000 live births.
- Inheritance is autosomal dominant although about 25% of affected individuals arise as new mutations.
- The cardinal features affect three systems: skeletal, ocular, and cardiovascular. The syndrome shows wide clinical variability of expression.
- Diagnosis is based on typical clinical features and a positive family history.
  - In the absence of a positive family history, involvement of the skeletal and at least two other systems with a minimum of one major manifestation (ectopia lentis, aortic dilatation/dissection, or dural ectasia) are required.
  - If there is a positive family history, only two organs need be involved for the diagnosis.

Clinical features

- Skeletal: tall, thin, arachnodactyly, ligamentous laxity, pectus excavatum, scoliosis ± kyphosis (10%), narrow high arched palate with crowding of teeth.
- Ocular: subluxation of the lens (ectopia lentis), myopia, increased axial globe length, retinal detachment.
- Cardiovascular: mitral valve prolapse, mitral regurgitation (most common reason for cardiac surgery), aortic root dilatation, and aortic regurgitation.
  - Aortic aneurysm and dissection are the commonest cause of death.
  - Affected pregnant patients are at particular risk during the third stage of labour.
  - Echocardiograms show that about one-third of affected people have mitral valve prolapse, aortic root enlargement or both despite a normal clinical examination.
- Other features include pulmonary blebs (predisposing to spontaneous pneumothorax), dural ectasia (widening of the spinal canal with erosion of the sacral bone), spinal arachnoid cysts or diverticula and obstructive sleep apnoea (lax pharyngeal wall).

Anaesthetic problems and management

- Cardiovascular assessment of these patients should include an echocardiogram to detect any aortic root dilatation, aortic regurgitation, or mitral valve prolapse before any surgery. Patients are now being treated with prophylactic beta-blockers to slow the rate of aortic dilatation and improve long-term survival. Labile intraoperative blood pressure can be controlled with sodium nitroprusside or glyceryl trinitrate infusion.
- Risk of bacterial endocarditis requires antibiotic prophylaxis.

- Careful positioning, handling, and padding to protect lax joints and avoid dislocation.
- Surgical repair of the ascending aorta is common. Complete replacement with a composite aortic valve-ascending aorta conduit is undertaken for moderate aortic regurgitation or dilatation of the aortic root greater than 5.0–5.5 cm.
- Pulmonary blebs increase the incidence of spontaneous pneumothoraces and perioperative lung complications. It is advisable to minimize peak airway pressures during anaesthesia.

Muscular dystrophies

- The term muscular dystrophy refers to a group of inherited disorders of muscle resulting from an abnormality or absence of the protein dystrophin.
- Affected muscle fibres undergo a degenerative process and are replaced with fat or connective tissue.
- Patients present with progressive weakness of the muscle groups involved. In the severe Duchenne form this is ultimately fatal.

Clinical features

The X-linked dystrophinopathies:

Duchenne muscular dystrophy
- This sex-linked recessive muscular dystrophy is the most common and most severe type affecting 1:3000 live male births.
- Patients normally present between the ages of 1–4 years with falls and an abnormal waddling (Trendelenberg) gait. Characteristically, children pick themselves up after falls by using the hands to climb up the legs (Gower's sign) due to a weakness of the proximal limb muscles and pelvic girdle. With disease progression, the calf muscles become pseudohypertrophied due to deposition of fat and connective tissue. Weakness worsens, flexion contractures of the limbs develop and 95% of affected children are wheelchair bound by the age of 12 years. Once wheelchair bound, the onset of scoliosis is rapid, forced vital capacity is reduced, distortion of the diaphragm may result in oesophageal reflux and combined with a poor cough the risk of aspiration pneumonitis is increased.
- 30% of patients are mentally retarded. This is not progressive.
- Cardiac muscle is affected. ECG changes are common with tall R waves, deep Q waves in V3–6, a prolonged P–R interval, and sinus tachycardia. Patients present with persistent tachycardias, mitral valve prolapse (25%), hypertrophic cardiomyopathy (over age 10 years), ventricular wall motion abnormalities, and sudden death.
- Death usually occurs as a result of cardiorespiratory failure in the third decade of life.
- Diagnosis of this condition is based on clinical findings, creatinine phosphokinase (CPK) levels (10 times normal) in children not walking by 18 months or showing a deterioration of gait, genetic testing (abnormality chromosome Xp21.3) and muscle biopsy.

Becker's muscular dystrophy
- This disorder is also sex-linked recessive but less common (1:60000) and milder than Duchene muscular dystrophy; the abnormality occurs on the same gene, dystrophin, located at Xp21.
- The onset of disease is later and progresses more slowly than Duchenne's. Up to 50% of patients survive beyond 40 years.
- Mental retardation is not as common as in Duchenne's.
- Cardiac muscle may be affected.
- Creatinine phosphokinase levels, EMG patterns, and muscle biopsy results may all be similar to those seen in Duchenne's.

Emery-Dreifuss muscular dystrophy
- Sex-linked recessive affecting humeral, peroneal, and cardiac muscle.
- Cardiac involvement may result in heart block and sudden death. Contractures of the Achilles tendon and elbows occur.
- CPK can be normal.
- The gene abnormality is at Xp28.

Congenital muscular dystrophy
- Presents as a floppy baby or a myopathic form of arthrogryposis.
- Autosomal recessive.
- The severe form may be fatal whereas the more benign form usually presents with orthopaedic complications (contractures, scoliosis).

Facioscapulohumeral muscular dystrophy
- This autosomal dominant disorder shows marked variations in severity in families.
- It is relatively benign and slowly progressive. Onset is later and affects abductors of the upper limb, causes facial muscle weakness, winging of the scapula, sensorineural deafness and a retinopathy.

Autosomal recessive limb girdle dystrophy
- A wasting weakness with a variable rate of progression. Patients are often wheelchair bound by 30 years.
- Both sexes affected.
- Calf hypertrophy may occur and CPK is high.

Anaesthetic problems and management
- The pattern and severity of muscle weakness should be established to help ensure that the benefits of surgery justify the risks associated with surgery and anaesthesia.
- Cardiac function should be assessed (ECG and echocardiography). Left ventricular ejection fraction should be above 0.5 for elective surgery. Invasive monitoring should be considered.
- Respiratory function tests may help to predict the need for postoperative ventilation. Patients who have a poor cough, kyphoscoliosis and respiratory muscle weakness are more prone to recurrent chest infections. Physiotherapy should optimise these patients for surgery and continue during the postoperative period. Desired targets before elective surgery are a FVC > 25% predicted and PEFR > 30% predicted.
- Suxamethonium is contraindicated in this group of patients. There is a risk of rhabdomyolysis, rigidity, hyperkalaemia, and cardiac arrest.
- The response to non-depolarizing muscle relaxants is variable but their use is safe. Reduced doses with neuromuscular monitoring recommended.
- Volatile agents may cause significant myocardial depression. Halothane has been responsible for serious dysrhythmias and myoglobinuria in several case reports.

- There is no proven link between malignant hyperthermia and muscular dystrophy. Occasionally, patients with muscular dystrophy may develop dysrhythmias and muscle damage on exposure to volatile anaesthetic agents. The effects are related to release of potassium from the cells or to release of cellular constituents such as myoglobin. The clinical picture may resemble malignant hyperthermia. For this reason volatile agents are often avoided and a TIVA technique used, although this may not be possible or appropriate in some cases.
- Antacid premedication (omeprazole 20 mg oral once daily if over 20 kg or ranitidine 2–4 mg/kg maximum 150 mg oral twice daily) and avoidance of gastric dilatation during IPPV with a face mask at induction will reduce the risk of aspiration.
- Regional anaesthesia and analgesia should be considered in an attempt to reduce the need for respiratory depressant analgesic drugs postoperatively and improve compliance with chest physiotherapy.
- Postoperative monitoring of ECG even after minor surgery.
- There should be a low threshold for postoperative care in a HDU or ITU.

Myasthenia gravis

- Myasthenia gravis is an autoimmune disease with IgG antibodies directed against postsynaptic acetylcholine receptors at the nicotinic neuromuscular junction.
- There is a reduction in the number of functional receptors due to antibodies blocking attachment of acetylcholine molecules, increasing the rate of degradation of the receptors and complement induced damage of the receptors.
- Myasthenia gravis is characterized clinically by muscular weakness and fatigue after exertion. It affects 1:10000 of the general population. Childhood (age <16 years) onset myasthenia gravis accounts for about 11% of these patients. Three forms are recognized in childhood:
  - Juvenile myasthenia gravis
  - Transient neonatal myasthenia gravis
  - Congenital myasthenia gravis.

Clinical features

Juvenile myasthenia gravis
- Girls are affected four times more often than boys.
- The most common presentation in this age group is ophthalmic with strabismus, ptosis, diplopia, and ophthalmoplegia due to involvement of the extra ocular muscles. If symptoms are confined to these muscles then spontaneous remission occurs in about 30% of patients.
- Onset may also be with bulbar, facial, generalized limb, or rarely respiratory muscle weakness. The disease tends to be slowly progressive often fluctuating in severity.
- Symptoms may worsen with infection, pyrexia, surgical, or emotional stress and in response to certain drugs (aminoglycosides and anticonvulsants).
- Thymic hyperplasia is implicated in the pathogenesis of myasthenia. Thymomas are found only in adults. Juvenile myasthenia gravis is often associated with other autoimmune diseases such as thyroiditis, systemic lupus erythematosus and rheumatoid arthritis.
- Diagnosis of juvenile myasthenia gravis
  - Anticholinesterase test: a dose of edrophonium results in a rapid improvement of muscle strength lasting for about 5 min. Atropine is given first.
  - Radioimmunoassay for acetylcholine receptor antibodies. Highly specific. A negative result does not rule out diagnosis.
  - Electrophysiological studies show a decremental response to repetitive nerve stimulation.

Treatment
- Anticholinesterases are the first line choice. They inhibit enzymatic hydrolysis of acetylcholine at the synapse, increasing the concentration present and prolonging activity at the neuromuscular junction. Pyridostigmine bromide (1 mg/kg 4-hourly initially) is the agent of choice due to its longer half-life and better side-effect profile than neostigmine.

- Immunosuppression with steroids can be used short term for acute exacerbations not responding to increased doses of anticholinesterase. Occasionally azathioprine, ciclosporin, or cyclophosphamide are used.
- Plasmapheresis can be used to optimize a patient preoperatively by removing acetylcholine receptor antibodies from the circulation. Occasionally it may be required during acute myasthenic crises with respiratory failure.
- IV immunoglobulin preoperatively or for myasthenic crises.
- Thymectomy in children may lead to a marked improvement of symptoms and remission in 60–90% of patients.

Neonatal transient myasthenia gravis

- Affects 15% infants born to myasthenic mothers. It is caused by antibodies to the acetylcholine receptor crossing the placenta.
- Symptoms usually occur in the first few hours of life, but can take several days. The neonate may be hypotonic, generally weak, have feeding difficulties, apnoeic episodes, or respiratory distress. They may have weakness of the facial muscles with ptosis. Edrophonium may confirm the diagnosis.
- Treatment is supportive. Ventilation may be necessary initially. Neostigmine is used in this group. Symptoms improve over 4–6 weeks.
- There is no increased incidence of myasthenia gravis later in life.

Congenital myasthenia gravis

- This is an autosomal recessive disorder of the neuromuscular junction. There is no autoimmune component to disease.
- Presentation is often at birth but may not present until adolescence. Newborns present with severe weakness, hypotonia, recurrent apnoeas, feeding difficulties, and ocular muscle weakness.
- The response to anticholinesterases is variable. Patients do not improve with immunosuppressive therapy or thymectomy. The course is often non-progressive with lifelong mild disease.

Anaesthetic problems and management

- A multidisciplinary approach involving neurologists, surgeons, intensivists, and anaesthetist is important in the perioperative management of these patients.
- Preoperative management:
  - Establish the muscle groups affected. In particular, assess respiratory and bulbar involvement. Lung function tests are performed.
  - The neurologist and patient should ensure that their muscle function is optimal on anticholinesterase therapy. It may be necessary in some patients to arrange IV immunoglobulin or plasmapheresis prior to surgery if weakness is severe.
  - Anticholinesterases are omitted the night before surgery and the child put first on the morning list. If weakness is severe then therapy is continued up to the time of surgery and glycopyrronium bromide given to reduce excessive salivation and vagal actions.

- Patients receiving steroids may need an additional dose intraoperatively.
- ITU or HDU admission for ventilation or observation postoperatively should be available and discussed with the patient and/or parents. This is especially likely after surgery in a major body cavity.
- Patients are usually intubated and ventilated during anaesthesia because of the respiratory depressant effects of most anaesthetic agents.
- Suxamethonium is avoided. There is an increased resistance to the drug and 3–4 times the normal dose is often required. The incidence of non-depolarizing phase II block is high. Anticholinesterases and plasmapheresis may prolong the action of suxamethonium.
- Non-depolarizing muscle relaxants can be used safely but should be titrated with neuromuscular monitoring. As ocular muscles are commonly affected and so sensitive to muscle relaxants, facial nerve monitoring is recommended. Atracurium and mivacurium are the agents of choice—dose 10–20% of normal. Reversal should be given and the patient extubated once their airway and respiratory muscle function have returned to normal. Head lift for 5 sec, vital capacity, and measured inspiratory force can help with assessment. Patients with known bulbar muscle weakness may need airway protection until muscle tone has returned.
- Muscle relaxation for endotracheal intubation and surgery can be achieved without the use of muscle relaxants. Volatile agents increase muscle weakness. Opioids such as remifentanil also produce a degree of muscle relaxation.
- Muscle weakness is exacerbated by hypothermia, hypokalaemia, aminoglycoside antibiotics, and anticonvulsants.
- Parenteral opioids (infusion or PCA), regional techniques, NSAIDs and paracetamol are all appropriate analgesic options.
- Oral anticholinesterase therapy is restarted as soon as possible postoperatively. If this is not possible, a nasogastric tube may be passed for enteral administration. If the patient has an ileus, IV neostigmine may be needed. This should be titrated slowly to effect up to a maximum equivalent to the patient's normal dose of oral pyridostigmine. 1 mg of IV neostigmine is equivalent to 30 mg of oral pyridostigmine.
- Postoperative muscle weakness may result from a myasthenic or cholinergic crisis. A dose of edrophonium will help differentiate between these and determine the appropriate therapy. Some patients may require postoperative immunoglobulins, plasmapheresis or an IV infusion of neostigmine.

Myopathies

This is a group of inherited diseases affecting muscle function. Classification is based on identifying specific molecular and enzyme defects often associated with particular histological changes seen in the muscle. There can be marked phenotypic variation in families affecting age of onset and severity.

Myopathies are divided into three groups:
- Morphologically defined congenital myopathies:
  - Central core disease
  - Nemaline myopathy.
- Mitochondrial myopathies:
  - MELAS
  - MERRF syndrome
  - Kearnes–Sayre
  - Leigh syndrome.
- Metabolic myopathies:
  - Muscle glycogenoses.

Morphologically defined congenital myopathies

Central core disease
- This inherited autosomal dominant condition is characterized morphologically by the presence of well-defined round cores of myofibrils exclusively in type 1 fibres.
- Patients may be hypotonic at birth with proximal muscle weakness. They may have associated skeletal deformities such as congenital dislocation of the hips, pes cavus, kyphoscoliosis, joint hypermobility, short neck, and mandibular hypoplasia. Symptoms may be mild and muscle biopsy may be required to confirm the diagnosis.
- The condition is non-progressive and intelligence is normal.
- The gene mutation is located on chromosome 19 in close proximity to the gene that encodes for the ryanidine receptor responsible for controlling calcium release in skeletal muscle during contraction.

Anaesthetic problems and management
- Central core disease is closely associated with malignant hyperpyrexia and patients are treated a susceptible. Trigger agents are avoided.
- Muscle weakness is assessed preoperatively.

Nemaline myopathy
- Nemaline myopathy is characterized by abnormal thread-like or rod-shaped structures called nemaline bodies (mostly alpha-actinin protein) in muscle fibres. All skeletal muscle can be affected.
- Weakness usually involves proximal muscle, facial, bulbar, and respiratory muscle groups.
- Inheritance may be both autosomal recessive and dominant. Several mutations have been found in association with nemaline myopathy on chromosomes 1, 2, and 19. There is a wide phenotypic spectrum of disease affecting onset age and severity.

- Two distinct clinical groups have been identified—typical and severe. The '*typical*' group is the most common and presents as infantile hypotonia and muscle weakness which is usually non-progressive. The '*severe*' form presents at birth with severe hypotonia, respiratory failure, arthrogryposis, and death in the first few months of life. Less commonly the disease may present later in childhood or in adults.
- Dysmorphic features are common. Micrognathia, hypertelorism, high arched palates, and cardiac abnormalities (septal defects, patent ductus arteriosus, aortic regurgitation) may be present.

Anaesthetic problems and management

- Patients are prone to recurrent aspirations and chest infections. Preoperatively, lung function should be optimized with chest physiotherapy and treatment of infection. Respiratory function and cough are assessed.
- Tracheal intubation may be difficult.
- There is no association with malignant hyperthermia.
- Abnormal responses may be seen with muscle relaxants—resistance to suxamethonium and increased sensitivity to non-depolarizers.
- Patients may require a period of postoperative ventilation following major procedures. Respiratory complications are the most common cause of death.

Mitochondrial myopathies

These are disorders of energy production resulting from defects of the mitochondrial respiratory chain enzymes and the five complexes of oxidative phosphorylation. ATP production is impaired and lactic acidosis is common at presentation. They are multisystem disorders.

MELAS (Mitochondrial myopathy, Encephalopathy with lactic Acidosis and Stroke)
- Present with stroke.
- Focal or simple partial seizures, dementia and deafness occur. The neurological symptoms may be episodic and stroke-like symptoms transient, possibly made worse by the lactic acidosis. Spongy brain degeneration.

MERRF syndrome (Myoclonus Epilepsy Associated with Ragged-Red Fibres)
- Myoclonus, mixed seizures, ataxia, and myopathy.
- Cerebral and cerebellar atrophy. Deafness. Elevated lactate

Kearnes–Sayre syndrome
- Ophthalmic symptoms (progressive ophthalmoplegia, retinitis pigmentosa).
- Deafness.
- Cardiac conduction defects including complete heart block, cardiomyopathy.
- Mental retardation, short stature, and limb weakness. Spongy degeneration of brain.

Leigh syndrome

- Autosomal recessive subacute necrotising encephalomyelopathy. Progressive degeneration of grey matter and focal brainstem necrosis.
- Presents in infancy and early childhood with developmental delay, hypotonia, seizures, brainstem dysfunction (apnoea, abnormal breathing pattern, and sudden infant death syndrome), lactic acidosis, short stature, and hypertrophic cardiomyopathy.
- Patients are very sensitive to the respiratory depressant effects of volatile and IV anaesthetic agents.

Anaesthetic problems and management

- Patients may be sensitive to induction agents and muscle relaxants. Use short acting muscle relaxants in reduced doses with neuromuscular monitoring.
- Suxamethonium may result in hyperkalaemia.
- Monitor blood glucose and avoid prolonged periods of fasting. Ensure administration of glucose throughout perioperative period.
- Monitor acid–base status and treat severe lactic acidosis if necessary with bicarbonate.
- Postoperative monitoring for apnoea is important in Leigh syndrome.

Metabolic myopathies

Muscle glycogenoses

The glycogen storage diseases are disorders resulting in the abnormal accumulation of glycogen in tissues. Specific enzyme defects give rise to over twelve identifiable types. Only four of these result in myopathy. Patients often present for liver and muscle biopsy to aid diagnosis.

Type II (Pompe's disease)

- Affects mainly cardiac and skeletal muscle.
- Infants may present with hypotonia, failure to thrive, macroglossia, and cardiomyopathy.
- Death is usually in the first year of life from cardiac or respiratory failure.
- A later onset form presents as a progressive myopathy with death in puberty.
- Diagnosis is from muscle biopsy or identification of the enzyme defect in leucocytes.

Type V (McArdle's disease)

- Presents in adolescence with muscle cramps and pain after exercise. Myoglobinuria may occur after severe exercise.
- Myophosphorylase deficiency and consequent inability to breakdown glycogen.
- Muscle biopsy and enzyme assay for diagnosis.

Anaesthetic problems and management

- Fasting may result in hypoglycaemia in types I (Von Gierke's disease), III (Forbe's disease), and IV (Andersen's disease). Glucose containing IV fluids are required when fasting.
- Assess for cardiac involvement with ECG and echocardiogram.
- Macroglossia may make laryngoscopy difficult.

- It is probably sensible to avoid suxamethonium due to theoretical risk of hyperkalaemic response.
- Patients are often sensitive to non-depolarizing muscle relaxants. Monitor neuromuscular function.
- Tourniquets on limbs should be avoided in McArdle's disease as may result in myoglobinuria.
- Patients with Pompe's disease often have poor respiratory reserve and may need a period of postoperative ventilatory support.

Myotonic syndromes

- The myotonias are a group of autosomal dominant inherited disorders characterized by the inability of muscles to relax following voluntary contraction or stimulation.
- Patients may have difficulty releasing their grip when shaking hands or present with myotonia in response to cold, suxamethonium, or surgical stimulation.
- Three distinct diseases exist—myotonic dystrophy, myotonia congenita, and paramyotonia.

Myotonic dystrophy

- This is the most common of the myotonias with a prevalence of 3–5:100000 and usually presents in the second or third decade. Inheritance is autosomal dominant with variable penetrance resulting from a defect on chromosome 19.
- It is characterized by myotonia and a characteristic distribution of muscle wasting and weakness. The muscles of the face (sunken temples, ptosis, hanging jaw), muscles of mastication, sternomastoid, bulbar muscles (dysarthria and dysphagia), and the distal limb muscles are affected. Muscle weakness is progressive.
- The disease is a multisystem disorder with extra muscular features including premature male-pattern frontal baldness, cataracts, low IQ, cardiomyopathy and conduction abnormalities (atrio-ventricular block, atrial fibrillation), mitral valve prolapse, restrictive lung disease, central and obstructive sleep apnoea, delayed gastric emptying, infertility, adrenal insufficiency, hypothyroidism, and diabetes mellitus.
- Neonates may present as a floppy baby with respiratory distress requiring ventilation for up to several months. They may have a weak cry, difficulty swallowing (often requiring tube feeding for the first few weeks of life), and a characteristic facial appearance with a facial diplegia (droopy face) and a tent shaped mouth. Arthrogryposis affecting feet or hands may be severe. The disease progresses with myotonia and muscle wasting and becomes similar to the adult form in later childhood. Mothers suffering from dystrophia myotonica may only be diagnosed after delivering an affected infant.
- Diagnosis relies on family history and electromyography of the small muscles of the hand. Electromyography demonstrates repetitive electrical activity causing muscle contraction and delayed relaxation following a stimulus. The discharge gradually decreases in amplitude and frequency. Muscle biopsy in neonates or examination for lens opacities in adults may also have prognostic value.
- Treatment is supportive with drugs used to increase the depolarization threshold and reduce the incidence of myotonia e.g. phenytoin, carbamazepine, quinine, procainamide.
- Death usually occurs in the fifth or sixth decade of life.

Myotonia congenita (Thomsen's disease)
- Autosomal dominant. 2:50000.
- This is myotonia without the dystrophy and presents in children as stiffness especially after rest. Persistent muscle contraction gives the child a muscular appearance.
- Life expectancy is normal.
- Symptoms may improve with age or require treatment with antimyotonic drugs (quinine, procainamide).

Schwartz–Jampel syndrome
- Autosomal recessive disorder.
- Patients have short stature, skeletal abnormalities, persistent muscular contraction, and hypertrophy.
- These patients have a higher risk of malignant hyperthermia and so trigger agents should be avoided.

Paramyotonia
A rare autosomal dominant disorder where myotonia is induced by cold. It is important to ensure these patients remain warm.

Anaesthetic problems and management
- Preoperative evaluation of affected patients should establish the distribution and extent of muscle weakness with emphasis on respiratory and cardiovascular involvement.
- Respiratory muscle weakness, poor cough, bulbar palsy, and recurrent aspirations result in an impaired respiratory reserve. Lung function tests show a restrictive lung defect with reduced vital capacity, expiratory reserve volume, maximum breathing capacity, and maximal inspiratory pressure. Consider measuring blood gases in advanced disease or for major surgery.
- Patients are usually intubated during anaesthesia and have postoperative chest physiotherapy to reduce the risk of postoperative pneumonia. Bulbar palsy, poor cough, and reduced gastric motility increase the risk of aspiration.
- Ventilation is sensitive to sedative drugs (barbiturates, benzodiazepines, propofol, volatile agents) and opioids and the central response to hypoxia and hypercarbia may be reduced. Central or obstructive sleep apnoea may occur.
- Cardiovascular involvement is common at all stages of the disease and does not correlate with the severity of muscle involvement. An ECG is required to look for conduction defects (atrial fibrillation, bradycardia, ectopic activity, heart block). An echocardiograph may be indicated to look for evidence of heart failure secondary to cardiomyopathy. Patients are sensitive to the myocardial depressant effects of volatile agents. There is a low threshold for invasive arterial pressure monitoring.
- Myotonia may be precipitated by cold, suxamethonium, anticholinesterases, shivering, surgical manipulation, and diathermy of muscle. The patient should be kept warm throughout the perioperative period. Direct infiltration of the muscle with LA may reduce myotonia during handling. Myotonia does not respond to non-depolarising muscle relaxants.

- Suxamethonium is contraindicated. It may cause in masseter spasm, difficulties with intubation and ventilation, difficulties with the surgical procedure and potassium release. Intubation can be achieved using non-depolarizing muscle relaxants, volatile agents or an induction agent and a short acting opioid.
- Non-depolarizing muscle relaxants can be used safely. Myotonic patients are more sensitive to their effects and may not require them to facilitate intubation or surgery. Neuromuscular monitoring should be used. Anticholinesterase drugs should be titrated cautiously as their effects are not always predictable and they can provoke muscle contraction. The use of a short acting neuromuscular blocker may make their use unnecessary.
- Regional techniques can be used but muscle relaxation does not always occur. Postoperative regional analgesia avoids the need for opioids.
- A weak link between malignant hyperthermia and myotonia may exist. Volatile agents have been used in many cases without problems. Temperature and end tidal CO_2 should be monitored.
- These patients should be cared for in a HDU after all but the most minor of procedures due to the high incidence of postoperative cardiorespiratory complications.

Mucopolysaccharidoses

- The mucopolysaccharidoses are a group of inherited disorders of metabolism resulting from a deficiency of the lysosomal enzymes that breakdown complex carbohydrates known as glycosaminoglycans (GAGS).
- The resultant accumulation of these partially degraded GAGS in cells of the connective tissue throughout the body impairs cell function and leads to the clinical manifestations of the diseases. The clinical effects and disease progression depends on the enzyme that is deficient and the sites of deposition. Deposition continues throughout life and clinical features worsen with age, except in Sanfilippo syndrome.
- Life expectancy and quality of life are reduced.
- Inheritance of these disorders is autosomal recessive except for Hunter's syndrome which is an X-linked disorder.
- These patients tend to present to anaesthetists on lists that reflect their clinical problems—ENT, orthopaedic, neuroimaging, neurosurgery, ophthalmology, and general surgery for hernia repair.
- Classification of the disorders is based on the specific enzyme deficiency rather than on clinical features.

Clinical features

MPS I (iduronidase deficiency) has three variants. **Hurler's syndrome** (MPS I H: gargoylism), **Scheie's syndrome** (MPS I S) and **Hurler/Scheie's syndrome** (MPS I HS). Hurler's is the most severe variant and Scheie's the mildest.

- *Hurler's syndrome (*incidence 1:100000 live births) characterized by dysmorphic features—coarse features, short stature, short neck, frontal bossing, hypertelorism, depressed nasal bridge, macroglossia, gum hypertrophy.
  - Airway problems (see below).
  - ENT: obstructive sleep apnoea, deafness.
  - Cardiac disease is very common—cardiomyopathy, thickening of the ventricular septum, mitral and aortic valves, and coronary artery disease.
  - CNS: progressive mental retardation, hydrocephalus, corneal clouding.
  - Hepatosplenomegaly with a protuberant abdomen and a high incidence of inguinal and umbilical herniae.
  - Death usually occurs in the first decade of life secondary to cardiorespiratory failure.
- *Scheie's syndrome* (incidence 1:600000 live births) is a much milder variant.
  - Characterized by joint stiffness, corneal clouding, and no mental retardation.
  - Features may be coarse with excessive body hair, macroglossia, glaucoma, and mitral and/or aortic incompetence in older patients.
  - Patients tend to present with orthopaedic complications—carpal tunnel, joint stiffness, back pain, spondylolisthesis.
  - Patients have a normal life expectancy.
- *Hurler-Scheie's syndrome* is extremely rare and intermediate in severity. Patients can live into adulthood.

MPS II: Hunter's syndrome
- Rare, sex-linked recessive (X-chromosome), incidence 1:140000 male births, mainly Caucasians.
- Mild and severe forms. Severe form shares many features of Hurler's syndrome in a milder form and less severe skeletal involvement. Progressive neuro-degeneration results in a vegetative state and death in teenage years.
- Mildly affected patients are at risk of cervical cord compression secondary to thickening of the dura and ligamentum flavum. MRI at the craniocervical junction is useful to assess compression and stability before any airway manipulation under anaesthesia to reduce the risk of quadriplegia.

MPS III: Sanfilippo's syndrome (types A, B, C, and D)
- This is the commonest variant of MPS in the UK.
- Mild dysmorphism.
- Affected children have severe mental retardation with difficult aggressive hyperactive behavioural disturbances.
- Death occurs in the teenage years.

MPS IV: Morquio's syndrome (A and B)
- Rare.
- Normal intelligence.
- Aortic incompetence in adults.
- Severe bone dysplasia—dwarfism, kyphosis (restrictive lung disease), pigeon chest.
- High risk cervical of cord compression from minimal trauma secondary to a hypoplastic, poorly ossified dens with and poor ligamentous support. Often require frequent MRIs and prophylactic occipitocervical fusions. Instability may also occur in the lower spine.
- Life expectancy depends on neurological complications and cardiorespiratory disease secondary to restrictive lung disease.

MPS VI: Maroteaux–Lamy syndrome
- Rare.
- Normal intelligence.
- Coarse features.
- Difficult intubation.
- Cardiomyopathy and atlanto-axial instability reported.
- Progressive airway narrowing leading to cor pulmonale and death in the early twenties.

MPS VII: beta-glucuronidase deficiency
- Extremely rare.

Anaesthetic problems and management
- Airway: most common major problem of MPS during anaesthesia.
  - Hurler's, Hunter's, and Maroteaux–Lamy syndromes commonly present with airways which are difficult to maintain and intubate.
  - This worsens with age. Fibreoptic endotracheal intubation is frequently necessary (□ Chapter 5).

- The features are of a short neck, small high larynx, limited atlanto-axial mobility, thickened tissues (mouth, tongue, and pharynx), worsening airway obstruction, difficult laryngoscopy, small hypopharynx, large fairly fixed epiglottis and excessive secretions.
- Previous anaesthetic records are useful if recent and occasionally imaging of the airway may be available.
- Unscheduled tracheostomy should be discussed as an option for airway management.
- Guedel airways can worsen the airway achieved and nasal may be better.
- Respiratory:
  - Obstructive sleep apnoea may initially respond to adenotonsillectomy.
  - Recurrent upper and lower respiratory infections.
  - Excessive secretions.
  - Progressive narrowing of distal airways.
- CVS:
  - Valve, septum, or coronary artery deposition of GAGs may be difficult to detect due to poor patient mobility and communication.
  - May present with heart failure, dysrhythmias, ischaemia, sudden death.
- Atlanto-axial instability in Morquio syndrome.

This difficult group of patients are best managed in a specialist centre by a multidisciplinary team familiar with the management of the many problems encountered.

Osteogenesis imperfecta

- Osteogenesis imperfecta is a connective tissue disorder caused by an abnormality of type I collagen resulting from mutations in the pro-collagen genes in chromosomes 7 and 17.
- Bone fragility is the hallmark feature.
- There is extra skeletal involvement affecting skin, fasciae, ligaments, tendons, sclera, and the inner ear.
- Four groups are currently classified although other variations of these groups are thought to exist:
  - Types I and IV inheritance are autosomal dominant and they are less severe.
  - Types II and III inheritance are autosomal recessive and they are fatal or progressive.

Clinical features

Type I

- Most common (80%).
- Usually presents as pathological fractures in toddlers or older children, especially in the lower limb. These are sometimes mistaken for non-accidental injuries.
- Spinal deformity can occur due to vertebral collapse from osteoporosis. Fractures may be less common after puberty.
- Other manifestations include blue sclera, hypotonia, hypermobile joints (may dislocate), hernias and thin atrophic skin. Early onset deafness is common due to otosclerosis (50% of adults). Aortic regurgitation and mitral valve prolapse can occur. Teeth may be affected with a bluish, yellow or translucent discolouration (dentinogenesis imperfecta). Stature is often normal.

Type II

- Severe form of skeletal abnormalities resulting in intrauterine or neonatal death.

Type III

- Progressive severe skeletal abnormalities. Fractures occur at birth and through infancy.
- Chest deformity with kyphoscoliosis and a prominent sternum increases susceptibility to recurrent bronchopneumonia.
- Sclera are often normal. Short stature. Macrocephalic.
- Left untreated, death usually results from cardiorespiratory failure in third or fourth decade. Pamidronate therapy in severely affected patients (age <3 years) has been found to ↑ bone mass density, improve symptoms of pain and poor mobility, as well as reduce the incidence of fractures.

Type IV

- Similar to type I.
- Fractures are present at birth in about 25% of cases and are common in childhood. At puberty, the frequency of fracture tends to reduce. Fractures often heal with a bowing deformity. Long bone deformity and kyphoscoliosis are more severe than type 1.

- Patients have short stature, pointed mandible and mid face hypoplasia. The sclera are normal and deafness is not a feature. Skull deformity can occur leading to basilar compression.

Anaesthetic problems and management

Patients tend to present for reduction of fractures, scoliosis surgery, neurosurgery, middle ear surgery, and dental surgery.

- Careful handling and positioning of the patients with appropriate padding is important to minimize the risk of further fractures. Large abnormally shaped heads will require careful positioning often with a pillow under the chest.
- Airway manipulation should be gentle due to the risk of mandible fractures, vertebral fractures from excessive neck extension, and damage to fragile teeth. Midface hypoplasia and micrognathia may make the choice face mask important.
- Severe kyphoscoliosis may result in a restrictive lung defect and awkward positioning.
- Cardiac lesions occur and may require antibiotic prophylaxis.
- During anaesthesia patients can become mildly hyperthermic, sweaty, and acidotic reflecting an increased metabolic state. It is wise to delay surgery if the patient is pyrexial. Intraoperative pyrexia, acidosis, and hypercarbia in this group of patients have been reported and is thought to be unrelated to malignant hyperthermia. It generally responds to active cooling alone. Temperature should be monitored.
- Fasciculations caused by suxamethonium may result in fractures.
- Platelet dysfunction has been reported despite a normal platelet count. A history of easy bruising requires further investigations before major surgery or a central regional anaesthetic technique.

Prematurity

- Premature birth is defined by the World Health Organization as a gestational age of <37 weeks or 259 days irrespective of birth weight. It is divided into moderate prematurity (31–36 weeks gestation) and severe prematurity (24–30 weeks gestation).
- The incidence of prematurity is 6–11 % of live births.
- Prematurity is associated with an increased neonatal and infant morbidity. It accounts for 85% of early neonatal deaths not caused by congenital conditions in Great Britain. Premature neonates have a higher risk of respiratory distress syndrome and subsequent chronic lung disease, sepsis, intraventricular haemorrhage, neurodevelopmental disorders, necrotizing enterocolitis, retinopathy of prematurity and anaemia.
- The risks are greater for low birth weight newborns (< 2500 g) and more so again for very low birth weight newborns (< 1500 g).

Clinical features

Respiratory

- The respiratory system in preterm infants is immature. The diaphragm is the main muscle of respiration and fatigues easily due to a low content of type I muscle fibres. Chest wall compliance is high, accessory inspiratory muscles are inefficient, airway resistance is increased (narrow airways), and the work of breathing to maintain their tidal volume may cause respiratory distress or apnoea. FRC is low.
- Premature babies may require ventilatory support for respiratory distress syndrome. Prolonged ventilation may result in pneumonia, barotrauma, hyaline membrane disease, and residual lung damage. The acute lung injury can lead to areas of emphysema, collapse, fibrosis, and thickening of pulmonary arterioles. This bronchopulmonary dysplasia (BPD) results in CXR changes (areas of hyperinflation, cystic pulmonary infiltrates, reticular pattern giving rise to a honeycomb lung appearance) and prolonged (>28 days) dependence on oxygen therapy and occasionally IPPV/CPAP. Treatment is with steroids, diuretics, bronchodilators, and often home oxygen.
- Infants presenting for surgery with BPD require higher peak ventilation pressures and F_iO_2 to achieve an acceptable S_pO_2. Postoperatively nasal CPAP or IPPV may be necessary. Regional techniques for some procedures e.g. inguinal herniotomy are sometimes used.
- Apnoeic episodes in preterm infants are common (up to 30%) and may be associated with bradycardia. Even after 56 weeks postconceptual age (PCA) the incidence can still be 1%. Risk factors for this include
  - Low gestational age <45 weeks.
  - Preterm infant born <34 weeks.
  - A history of apnoeas.
  - Anaemia (haematocrit <30%).
  - Chronic lung disease.
  - General anaesthesia can increase the risk of apnoea for 12–24 hours postoperatively.

- Recommendations to reduce the incidence of postoperative apnoea and aid its detection include:
  - Patients <60 weeks PCA are monitored for 12–24 hours postoperatively following general or regional anaesthesia with an apnoea monitor and pulse oximeter.
  - Theophylline (8 mg/kg IV) or caffeine citrate (10 mg/kg IV) can be given post-induction to high-risk groups.
  - Clonidine should not be used as an additive in caudal epidural blocks in this patient group. There are case reports describing an increased incidence of respiratory depression.

Cardiovascular

- Blood pressure is lower while cardiac output and heart rate are higher than in full term infants. Cardiac output is mainly rate dependent.
- The sympathetic system is immature and the heart is influenced mainly by the parasympathetic system.
- Hypoxia rapidly results in bradycardia and decreased cardiac output.
- There is decreased responsiveness to vasoconstrictor or vasodilator agents.
- There is poor autoregulatory control of cerebral blood flow and so fluctuations in blood pressure may increase the risk of intraventricular haemorrhage.
- IV access in preterm infants can be very difficult after prolonged stays in SCBU.

Neurological

- Preterm babies have a higher risk of intraventricular haemorrhage (IVH) with subsequent long term neurological deficits. Up to 40% of newborns <34 weeks PCA may have an IVH.
- The risk of IVH is increased with increasing prematurity, low birth weight, respiratory distress syndrome, coagulopathy, hypoxia, and acidosis. Fluctuations in blood pressure, over transfusion, and anaemia are avoided as far as possible.
- Retinopathy of prematurity (retrolental fibroplasia) is related to gestational age and duration of oxygen therapy. These patients may require anaesthesia for laser therapy. In order to avoid an unnecessarily high F_IO_2 in this group an $S_pO_2 > 90\%$ is accepted rather than striving for a value near 100%.

Thermoregulation

- Preterm infants have a larger body surface area to body weight ratio than term infants leading to an increase in heat losses.
- They have less subcutaneous fat and rely on reduced stores of brown fat for non-shivering thermogenesis to generate heat in response to cold.
- Volatile agents inhibit non-shivering thermogenesis.

- Various measures are taken to keep the infant warm during the perioperative period. The operating theatre temperature is raised (26–28°C), the baby lies on a warming mattress and is covered by a warm air blanket. An overhead heater may be necessary during exposure for induction and IV access, limbs are wrapped in gamgee, the head is covered with a bonnet or gamgee, and anaesthetic gases are humidified and warmed. IV and cleaning fluids are also warmed.
- Temperature is monitored during surgery.

Fluid and electrolyte balance

- Total body water in the preterm infant can be over 75% body weight with an estimated circulating blood volume of 90–100 mL/kg.
- Maintenance fluids increase over the first few days of life.

Day	1	2	3	4	5
mL/kg/24 hours	60	80	100	120	150

- Care should be taken not to over transfuse fluids in this group. Drug dilutions are kept to a minimum, syringe pumps used to administer fluids or for invasive monitoring lines and accurate fluid balance charts kept.

Glycaemic control

- The risk of hypoglycaemia in newborns and especially preterm infants is high.
- Glucose loading with resultant hyperglycaemia is tolerated poorly.
- Regular blood glucose measurements are required to guide therapy.

Haematological

- Preterm infants are commonly anaemic due to poor red blood cell production from an immature marrow. Transfusion is considered if the haemoglobin is <8 g/dL.
- Values for coagulation parameters (especially APTT) are different in preterm babies compared to term babies and adults. Local reference values should be consulted.
- Preterm babies may be thrombocytopenic and neonatal advice should be sought to exclude sepsis as a cause.
- All newborns should have received vitamin K at delivery. If major surgery is urgent and this has not been given, a coagulation screen is done. FFP may be needed.

Sepsis

- Reduced cellular and tissue immunity increases the incidence of sepsis.
- Aseptic techniques should be used for invasive procedures.

Gastrointestinal

Necrotizing enterocolitis is a disease of low birth weight premature infants. Gut ischaemia results in mucosal injury, perforation, peritonitis, fluid and electrolyte abnormalities, sepsis, and shock. Patients require fluid resuscitation and correction of coagulopathies before surgery. Intra-operative fluid and blood losses can be large (📖 Chapter 12).

Renal failure

- Renal failure is a decline in the ability of the kidneys to excrete their normal solute load. It is associated with the accumulation of nitrogenous waste, fluid retention, and electrolyte abnormalities.
- It may be acute in onset often presenting with oliguria (< 300mL/m^2/ 24 hours or < 0.5 mL/kg/hour in infants) reflecting a reduction in renal perfusion and glomerular filtration rate (GFR).
- The aetiology of acute renal failure (ARF) is divided into three categories (Table 15.2).

Table 15.2 Aetiology of acute renal failure in children

Prerenal (most common)	Renal	Post renal
Hypovolaemia secondary to: • Gastroenteritis • Burns • Blood loss • Ileus	Haemolytic uraemic syndrome	Posterior urethral valves
Birth asphyxia	Acute glomerulonephritis e.g. Henoch–Schönlein purpura, post-streptococcal	Obstructive uropathy at: • Pelviureteric junction • Vesicoureteric junction
Post cardiac surgery	Myoglobinuria	Neuropathic bladder
Renal artery or vein occlusion	Haemoglobinuria	Renal calculi
	Renal vein thrombosis	Trauma
	Arterial occlusion	Blocked catheter
	Nephrotoxins	
	Interstitial nephritis	
	Vasculitis	

- Aetiology varies with the age of presentation of the child.
  - The commonest cause of renal failure in neonates is perinatal asphyxia.
  - Haemolytic uraemic syndrome is the commonest cause in infants and older children in developed countries while gastroenteritis is the commonest in developing countries.
- Urinalysis will help differentiate between prerenal and renal causes.
  - In prerenal ARF urine osmolality is >500 mosmol/L and urinary Na is <20 mmol/L.
  - In ARF of renal origin the osmolality is <350 mosmol/L and urinary Na is >40 mmol/L.
- ARF is characterized by oliguria, oedema, hypertension, vomiting, lethargy, electrolyte abnormalities, and a metabolic acidosis.

- Renal failure that occurs over several months or years is termed chronic renal failure (CRF). Common causes include:
  - Chronic glomerulonephritis
  - Pyelonephritis
  - Malformations of the renal tract
  - Hereditary renal diseases (Alport syndrome, polycystic disease)
  - Haemolytic uraemic syndrome.
- Presentation is usually non-specific with lethargy, fatigue, headache, anorexia, vomiting, growth failure, peripheral oedema, polyuria or enuresis.

Clinical features

Renal failure results in pathophysiological changes that affect most organ systems. These changes often influence the conduct of anaesthesia.

Fluid, electrolyte, and acid–base balance

- Sodium levels may be high, low, or normal depending on the underlying aetiology of renal failure.
- Glomerulonephritis is associated with salt and water retention, peripheral oedema, hypertension, and a tendency to cardiac failure. Salt restriction is required.
- Congenital renal disease and obstructive uropathies are more commonly associated with being unable to concentrate the solute load leading to polyuria, salt loss, and the risk of hypovolaemia. Salt supplements and extra fluid are required.
- Hyperkalaemia is a medical emergency affecting cardiac conduction with the potential for precipitating a cardiac arrest. ECG changes include peaked T waves, reduced R wave amplitude, a prolonged QRS interval, and small or absent P waves. A–V block, ventricular tachycardias and cardiac arrest may follow.
- Acidosis exacerbates hyperkalaemia as intracellular potassium is exchanged for extracellular hydrogen.
- Drugs that may cause hyperkalaemia include angiotensin converting enzyme inhibitors, potassium sparing diuretics, NSAIDs, β-blockers, aminoglycosides, and some anti-neoplastic drugs (ciclosporin).
- Potassium intake from diet, parenteral nutrition, and IV fluids should be closely monitored.
- In chronic renal failure hydrogen ion clearance is impaired and the body is reliant on bicarbonate, phosphate from bone salts, and the protein buffer system to maintain a normal pH. As these buffers are used the patient develops a metabolic acidosis.
- Other electrolyte abnormalities include ↓ *ionized* calcium, ↑ phosphate and ↑ magnesium.

Haematological

- Reduced erythropoeitin synthesis and ↓ red cell survival (secondary to uraemia) give rise to a normochromic normocytic anaemia. Chronic upper gastrointestinal losses, ↑ bleeding tendency, and dietary deficiencies of iron and folate add to this.
- The haemoglobin may stay around about 8 g/dL and may be allowed to fall to 6 g/dL if patients are not symptomatic.

- Patients who are symptomatic may be treated with recombinant human erythropoietin therapy. Blood transfusions are avoided if possible as they may precipitate volume overload, hypertension, and cardiac failure.
- Platelet aggregation and adhesiveness is impaired in chronic renal failure. This may be detected by a prolonged bleeding time preoperatively or by excessive bleeding perioperatively. Desmopressin 300 nanograms/kg or pooled cryoprecipitate may be given for excessive intraoperative bleeding. Other coagulation parameters tend to be normal.

Cardiovascular

- Systemic hypertension is common in CRF usually as a result of salt and water retention with volume overload or an abnormal renin–angiotensin–aldosterone axis as the cause.
- Hypervolaemia, hypertension, and anaemia may all precipitate congestive heart failure.
- Many patients with CRF undergo regular haemodialysis facilitated by an A–V fistula in their upper limb. This limb should be padded and wrapped in gamgee to protect the fistula and highlight its presence. Venous or arterial access should be avoided in the limb. Any pressure from blood pressure cuffs or lying on the limb must also be avoided. It is also sensible to use veins in the legs or back of the hands, saving the veins in the antecubital fossae for any future fistulae. Previous central venous access for haemodialysis lines may make future access in these sites difficult.

Gastrointestinal

- Uraemia results in anorexia, nausea, and vomiting.
- There is reduced gastric emptying and increased acidity with a higher prevalence of gastric ulceration. Gastro-oesophageal reflux occurs in up to 70% of cases.
- Acute renal failure is a hypercatabolic condition. Nutritional management must ensure adequate calorie intake, electrolyte, and fluid provision. Calories are given mostly as combinations of carbohydrates and fats (intralipid). Dietary proteins are not restricted in children and intake can be increased in patients on dialysis.

Immunity

- May be reduced secondary to uraemia and immunosuppressive therapy and strict asepsis for procedures is necessary.

CNS

- Altered conscious level or convulsions can be precipitated by uraemia, abnormal electrolytes (hyponatraemia), or hypertension.

Management of renal failure

- Conservative management of fluid and electrolyte abnormalities using nutritional manipulation and drugs.
- Renal replacement therapy:
  - Peritoneal dialysis: continuous ambulatory peritoneal dialysis (CAPD) or continuous cycling peritoneal dialysis (CCPD). This is the most common form of dialysis. It can be carried out at home. The main complication is peritonitis.
  - Haemodialysis: an indwelling venous catheter is required with the risk of catheter infection. Therapy is more complex, expensive, and disruptive to life with regular hospital visits.
- Renal transplantation. This is the best mode of renal replacement with better survival rates than in dialysis patients. Immunosuppressive regimens (ciclosporin, steroids, and azathioprine) have improved graft survival rates—1-year survival of cadaveric renal transplant of 80% versus 90% for live donor transplantation.

Anaesthetic problems and management

- Fluid and electrolyte balance are optimized by the renal physicians. This may involve the timing of dialysis before and after surgery. Urea and electrolytes, FBC, and coagulation values post-dialysis should be checked before surgery. Potassium levels should be <5.0 mmol/L even for urgent procedures. Patients may be hypovolaemic following dialysis.
- Perioperative fluid management requires knowledge of the daily fluid allowances and care in matching fluid losses associated with surgery. Central venous monitoring may be necessary where large fluid shifts are predicted. Fluid replacement is generally with saline, avoiding potassium-containing solutions.
- Patients with hypertension and at risk of cardiac failure should have an ECG and CXR preoperatively.
- Patients are often on multiple medications. Antihypertensive and anti-failure therapy should not be stopped preoperatively. Steroid therapy should also be continued and may require perioperative supplementation. Diuretics may affect electrolyte balance.
- A–V shunts and central venous lines should be protected. Haemodialysis lines should not be routinely used for infusions and care must be taken to site IV access away from current and potential future sites for A-V shunts. Non-invasive blood pressure cuffs should not be used on the same limb as a shunt.
- Pre-emptive 'top-up' transfusions are not required. Haemoglobin as low as 6 g/dL may be acceptable for surgery associated with minimal blood loss. Blood should be available and given if necessary.
- Suxamethonium results in a transient rise in extracellular potassium of 0.5–1 mmol/L. Its use in patients with renal failure is safe if plasma potassium is within normal limits (<5.5 mmol/L). It is generally only used for emergency surgery on unfasted patients or in cases with gastro-oesophageal reflux.

- Drug pharmacokinetics and pharmacodynamics are altered in renal failure.
  - Induction agents. Thiopental is a highly protein bound drug (75–80% bound to plasma albumin). In CRF, hypoalbuminaemia and acidosis increase availability of free active drug. This combined with an increased sensitivity in uraemic patients means that a reduced dose should be given. The dose of propofol should also be reduced.
  - Non-depolarizing muscle relaxants. Renal elimination is significant in the clearance of pancuronium, gallamine, and tubocurarine. Atracurium clearance is unaffected by renal failure due to Hoffman elimination making it an ideal choice. Vecuronium and rocuronium can also be used safely.
  - The elimination of anticholinesterases is prolonged in parallel with non-depolarizing muscle relaxants and so recurarization is unlikely to occur.
  - Volatile agents. The metabolism of enflurane and sevoflurane produce fluoride and there is a theoretical risk of nephrotoxicity. Prolonged used of these agents is usually avoided. In practice, this is not a clinical issue.
  - Analgesics. Renal clearance plays a large part in the clearance of opioid analgesics and their metabolites. Morphine and pethidine are both metabolized by the liver to active metabolites (morphine-6-glucuronide and norpethidine) that may accumulate and cause side effects (e.g. norpethidine and seizures). PCA lockout periods are usually increased (up to 15 min) and patients are monitored for respiratory depression. Fentanyl, alfentanil, and sufentanil are more benign from the point of view of accumulation and active metabolites.
  - LA. The duration of action may be reduced in CRF. Reduced protein binding may increase the risk of toxicity.
  - The risks and benefits of central neuraxial blocks are weighed carefully in this group of patients who may have platelet dysfunction. NSAIDs should not be prescribed for postoperative analgesia in patients with known renal failure.
- Postoperative management involves regular input from the renal team particularly on fluid balance, electrolyte management, and the need for dialysis.

Table 15.3 Emergency treatment of hyperkalaemia

Drug	Dose	Onset	Duration	Side effects
8.4% NaHCO$_3$	1–2 mmol/kg IV over 30 min	30 min	1–2 hours	Hypernatraemia Fluid overload Alkalosis
10% Ca gluconate	0.5–1 ml/kg IV over 20 min	Instant	Min	Hypercalcaemia Bradycardia
10% dextrose	500 mg/kg as a rapid bolus Can then infuse 500 mg/kg/hour if necessary	30 min	1–2 hours	Hyperglycaemia. If plasma glucose >10 mmol/L add insulin 0.05 IU/kg/hour
Salbutamol	1.25–10 mg nebulized	30 min	2 hours	Tachycardia Hypertension
Calcium resonium	125–250 mg/kg oral or rectal (not nasogastric tube)	60 min	4–6 hours	Constipation
Dialysis		Min	Hours	Hypotension

Calcium gluconate is the treatment of choice if there are ECG changes.

Sickle cell disease

- Sickle cell disease is a haemoglobinopathy with autosomal dominant inheritance affecting synthesis of the β-chain of the globin molecule. There is a substitution of valine for a glutamic acid residue at the sixth amino acid position in the β-chain resulting from a genetic mutation on chromosome 11.
- Sickle cell anaemia (HbSS) is the more severe homozygous expression of the disease and gives rise to a chronic haemolytic anaemia, episodes of acute pain, respiratory compromise, end organ damage, and usually premature death.
- Sickle cell trait is the more benign heterozygous form (HbAS) often with no anaemia, no clinical signs and symptoms, sickling only under severe hypoxic conditions, and it confers some protection against Falciparum malaria.
- Tropical Africa and Madagascar have the highest incidence of the disease affecting up to 40% of the population. It is also relatively common in Turkey, Greece, other Mediterranean countries, and North Africa. In the UK, HbSS affects about 0.25% of the black population while HbAS affects up to 10%.

Clinical features

- Sickle cell disease is characterized by abnormally shaped red blood cells. Red blood cells containing deoxygenated HbS become sickle shaped when exposed to hypoxia, acidosis, low temperatures, or cellular dehydration.
- The deoxygenated HbS polymerises into long crystals that stack together and distort the shape of the red cell membrane.
- The sickle cells are less compliant and more adhesive than normal red cells, increasing the viscosity of the blood and reducing flow in the microcirculation.
- Microvascular thrombosis may result with occlusion of vessels potentially worsening local hypoxia and creating a cycle of sickling with further vascular compromise to tissues such as spleen and bones. Initially this cycle is reversible but with repeat sickling it becomes irreversible and these cells have a reduced lifespan of about 20 days.
- Sickle cell disease presents after the age of 6 months as the concentration of HbF decreases.
- The presence of fetal haemoglobin is protective against sickling and increased levels are associated with milder disease. HbF levels are between 5–15% (HbS 85–95%) in sickle cell disease.
- In areas where the incidence of sickle cell disease is high, pregnant women and neonates are screened.
- In those with the disease, mortality is high in the first 5 years of life from infection (pneumococcus, haemophilus, and salmonella), sequestration crisis (sickling within organs with blood pooling) and aplastic crisis (a sudden fall in haemoglobin usually following parvovirus infection).

- Preventative measures include vaccinating children against pneumococcus and H. influenzae, prophylactic penicillin from 4 months of age, folate supplements, and educating parents to recognize the signs of an acute sequestration crisis.

Anaesthetic problems and management

- Patients at risk are screened using the *Sickledex* test. This exposes red cells to sodium metabisulphite (an antioxidant which deoxygenates the sample) and causes sickling in the presence of HbS. It does not differentiate between HbSS, HbAS, and HbSC. If the test is positive and there is time, haemoglobin electrophoresis is performed.
- Avoidance of sickling.
  - The primary goal is to maintain adequate oxygenation during the perioperative period. Sickling becomes irreversible at an arterial oxygen tension below 5.5 kPa and all the red cells are sickled at a S_aO_2 <50% in patients with HbSS. Patients may have impaired oxygen delivery resulting from chronic anaemia, chronic lung damage, and a damaged vascular supply so may have a limited reserve during hypoxic episodes. Postoperatively there should be a low threshold for giving supplemental oxygen. Local hypoxia during the use of tourniquets may be a contraindication to their use.
  - Avoid acidosis.
  - Avoid hypothermia. Temperature is monitored and warming blankets etc used to maintain normothermia. Postoperative hypothermia and shivering may increase the risk of sickling.
  - There is little evidence to support the practice of fluid loading.
  - If there is evidence of active infection, elective surgery should be postponed.
- Dilution of sickle cells.
  - This is controversial and not without risk. Theoretically, reducing the percentage of HbSS by the prophylactic transfusion of normal HbA should prevent complications of sickle cell disease. This is achieved by exchange transfusion or by simple transfusion.
  - Studies comparing exchange transfusion and simple transfusion do not show any significant difference in the incidence of sickling but report a higher incidence of iatrogenic complications from exchange transfusion.
  - Preoperative prophylactic transfusion is recommended for homozygous patients undergoing major surgery. This can be performed 1–2 days before elective surgery with a transfusion goal of reducing the HbSS to 30% and achieving a haematocrit of 30%. Fresh blood is preferred for intra-operative transfusion.
  - There is a high incidence of alloimmunization in this group (antibodies to Rhesus, Kell, and Lewis blood groups) and extended phenotype matching to detect other antigen groups is required.
- Renal and respiratory end organ damage from chronic disease should be assessed.
- Hydroxyurea can benefit some patients with sickle cell disease by increasing the production of fetal haemoglobin. This reduces the tendency to sickle, in turn reducing the severity and frequency of crises.

- These patients have a much higher morbidity and mortality associated with surgery than normal and there is a lower threshold for referral to HDU or ITU postoperatively.
- The high incidence of sickling in cell savers prevents their use in sickle cell disease.
- Management of sickle cell crises:
  - Pain: acute recurrent episodes can occur. Affects long bones, ribs, vertebrae or abdomen (a surgical cause should be excluded). Analgesic requirements are often complex with opioid tolerance from previous admissions. A multimodal approach led by the pain team and guided by any previous effective analgesic recipes for individual patients is useful. These patients are kept warm and well hydrated.
  - Acute chest syndrome: pyrexia, respiratory distress, pulmonary infiltrates on CXR, and chest pain. This may result from infection (e.g. viral, mycoplasma) or postoperatively secondary to diaphragmatic splinting and atelectasis. Preventative measures are important—physiotherapy, adequate analgesia, early mobilization, and attention to any worsening of respiratory function. Treatment requires oxygen supplementation and, in severe cases, ventilatory support. Bronchodilators, dexamethasone, and broadspectrum antibiotics (if a postoperative pneumonia is suspected) may all be of benefit. In anaemic patients with acute chest syndrome blood transfusion may improve arterial oxygenation and outcome if there is hypoxia.
  - Sequestration crisis: this is the second leading cause of death in children with sickle cell disease. The main problem is pooling of blood in the spleen with acute hypovolaemia. Treatment is with transfusion of whole blood for volume replacement.
  - Aplastic crises (sudden fall in haemoglobin and reticulocytes) or haemolytic crisis (often accompanies painful crisis) require blood transfusion and analgesia.
  - For management of acute severe pain 🕮 see Chapter 6.

Sedation for diagnostic and therapeutic procedures

Anthony Moores

Overview

- For various reasons, all children who require therapeutic and diagnostic procedures are not anaesthetized. Sedation of children outside the operating theatre is an important area of paediatric medicine.
- It is required by many specialties (radiology, dentistry, accident and emergency, medical paediatrics), is often administered by non-anaesthetists and may take place outside hospital.
- Sedation is defined by the American Society of Anaesthesiologists as a drug-induced depression of consciousness during which patients may respond to verbal commands or light tactile stimulation.
- Depths of sedation are defined as:
  - **Minimal sedation** (anxiolysis): patient responds normally to verbal commands. Respiratory and cardiovascular functions are unaffected.
  - **Moderate sedation/analgesia** (conscious sedation): patient responds purposefully to verbal commands and/or light tactile stimulation. The airway is patent, ventilation is adequate, and cardiovascular function usually unaffected.
  - **Deep sedation/analgesia**: patient cannot be easily roused, responds purposefully to repeated or painful stimulation. Airway obstruction and respiratory depression may occur. Cardiovascular function is usually unaffected.
- As the depth of sedation increases, protective reflexes may be lost, ventilatory function impaired, and safety compromised if administered by someone without current advanced airway management skills.
- The most common complications of paediatric sedation are respiratory:
  - Upper airway obstruction
  - Respiratory depression
  - Hypoxia
  - Hypercarbia.
- These tend to occur with deeper levels of sedation.
- Sedation with a single agent is usually safer than the use of two or more agents. The use of a sedative and a local anaesthetic technique, if possible, is preferable to combining a sedative and an opioid.
- The drugs and techniques should carry a margin of safety wide enough to render unintended loss of consciousness unlikely.
- Sedation for a given procedure in a child should be as safe as general anaesthesia under the same circumstances. If it is not, then a general anaesthetic is preferable although it may be difficult to arrange.
- The Royal Colleges of Radiologists and Anaesthetists advise that sedation practice by non-anaesthetists be limited to conscious sedation where the child responds purposefully to verbal commands and/or light tactile stimulation.
- Procedures requiring sedation may be associated with pain. Attempting to use sedative drugs to provide analgesia is an underlying reason for many complications of sedation. Where possible the pre-emptive use of local anaesthetics and systemic analgesics or other measures (nitrous oxide) should be used to reduce pain perception.

- Safety in sedation requires properly trained staff, appropriate patient selection (and exclusion), patient preparation, protocols, facilities and equipment, adequate post sedation care, and ongoing audit of results and complications. Multidisciplinary sedation teams in paediatric hospitals demonstrate high success rates and good safety records.
- In certain settings general anaesthesia may be safer, more efficient, cost effective and reliable than sedation (MRI, cardiac catheterization). Procedures associated with pain or that require the patient to lie still for long periods (oesophagogastroscopy, interventional radiology, cardiac catheterisation) are often better carried out under general anaesthesia.

Management of sedation

Selection criteria

- Patients should undergo a preoperative assessment to classify their ASA status and identify any problems or contraindications for techniques carried out under sedation.
- ASA I and II children are appropriate for sedation as outpatients.
- ASA III and IV should be sedated on an in-patient basis, involving an anaesthetist trained in paediatric sedation and anaesthesia in an appropriate setting.
- Infants up to the age of 1 year are particularly sensitive to sedative drugs and are upgraded by two ASA classes. Children aged 1–5 years are upgraded by one class, except if sedated with nitrous oxide alone.

Contraindications

- Abnormal airway
- Raised intracranial pressure
- Depressed conscious level
- History of sleep apnoea
- Respiratory failure
- Cardiac failure
- Neuromuscular disease
- Bowel obstruction
- Active respiratory tract infection
- Known allergy or adverse reaction to sedative(s)
- Child too distressed despite adequate preparation
- Older child with severe behavioural problems
- Consent refusal by parent or patient

- Patients who become disinhibited or unmanageable during sedation should be rescheduled for a general anaesthetic.

Consent

Written informed consent from parent/guardian or patient is required as for procedures under general anaesthesia.

Parents

Parents usually wish to stay with the sedated child. This is usually appropriate and helpful although in some cases parental anxiety unsettles the child.

Facilities

- The environment should be 'child-friendly'.
- Equipment and drugs to minimize complications and manage those that do occur are required.
  - Oxygen source and the equipment to deliver high concentrations
  - Airway equipment—facemask, airways, LMAs, ETTs
  - Suction
  - Tipping trolley
  - Resuscitation equipment

- Monitoring equipment
  - Oximeter
  - ECG
  - NIBP
  - Capnography
  - Temperature measurement
  - Antagonists to benzodiazepines and opioids
- Recovery facilities.

Requirements are less rigorous in some settings e.g. community dentistry where only nitrous oxide is used. Specialty association guidelines give the relevant advice.

Personnel

- Have a number of roles:
  - Assess patient and obtain consent before sedation and procedure.
  - Prescribe and administer sedation.
  - Monitor child during procedure.
  - Perform procedure.
  - Observe and care for child after procedure until recovered and fit for discharge.
- Roles of operator and sedationist/monitor should be separate.
- The sedated child must be monitored continuously.
- Training and competency are required in the role and management of complications plus ongoing maintenance of skills e.g. ALS updates.

Fasting

- Fasting for sedation should be the same as for a general anaesthetic:
  - Clear fluids: 2 hours.
  - Breast milk: 4 hours.
  - Formula milk: 6 hours.
  - Food: 6 hours.
- The only exception to this is if nitrous oxide (up to 50%) alone is being used.

Non-pharmacological techniques

- May reduce the need for sedative drugs.
- Expertise with children, good communication, and a sympathetic approach is important.
- Behavioural techniques such as distraction, play therapy, relaxation, and hypnosis, carried out by experienced staff, play specialists, and nurses may be used for non-painful procedures.
- The presence of a calm reassuring parent can also have a sedative sparing effect on the child.
- Infants up to the age of 4 months may undergo imaging in the radiology department when asleep, post feeding in a warm environment with no sedation.
- Sedation is not an appropriate technique for an uncooperative child.
- Forcible restraint by staff or parents is no longer considered to be acceptable.

Analgesia

- For painful procedures local anaesthetic creams (EMLA or amethocaine gel) can be applied for cannulation, lumbar puncture, and prior to infiltration of local anaesthetic solutions in the relevant area.
- Pre-emptive oral analgesics (paracetamol, NSAIDs, or codeine phosphate or morphine) may be given.

Monitoring

- Regular and documented assessment of:
  - Level of sedation
  - Respiratory rate
  - Arterial oxygen saturation
  - Heart rate.
- NIBP, temperature, capnography, and pain assessment are appropriate under some circumstances.

Recovery

- Dedicated area.
- One to one observation and care.
- Monitoring as during the procedure until recovered.

Discharge criteria

- Awake or easily rouseable.
- Unobstructed airway.
- Normal ventilation: S_pO_2 > 95% in air.
- Haemodynamically stable.
- Pain free.
- No vomiting.
- Appropriate behaviour and responsiveness for age and development.

Drugs used for sedation

Benzodiazepines

Midazolam

Oral, IV, or intranasal administration.

- Oral:
  - Dose 0.5–0.75 mg/kg (up to 20 mg).
  - Onset time 30 min.
  - Duration 60–90 min.
  - May produce amnesia.
  - Provided as a commercial preparation intended for oral administration. The IV preparation is often used for oral administration. This has a bitter taste and is best mixed with a small volume of diluting juice.
- IV:
  - Dose 0.05–0.2 mg/kg.
  - Onset is rapid (2–3 min).
  - Duration 45–60 min.
  - Has a variable effect. Some children may display paradoxical excitement.
- Intranasal:
  - Dose 100–150 mcg/kg.
  - Onset time 10–15 min.
  - Duration up to 60 min.

Caution is required if simultaneous administration with opioids. Apnoea and/or prolonged sedation may occur. Doses should be reduced.

Diazepam

- Usually given IV.
- Dose 0.05–0.1 mg/kg up to 0.25 mg/kg.
- Onset is slower than midazolam (4–5 min).
- Duration is longer (60–120 min).
- Reduce dose with opioids.

Temazepam

- Oral tablets or solution of 10 mg/5 ml.
- Dose 0.5–1.0 mg/kg.
- May be combined with droperidol.

Flumazenil

- Benzodiazepine antagonist.
- Used to treat over sedation or reverse sedation with benzodiazepines Should be available where benzodiazepines are used.
- Dose 20–30 mcg/kg IV. The dose can be repeated every minute up to a maximum of 1 mg.
- Duration of action is 30–60 min and *resedation* should be anticipated.

Opioids

Morphine

Oral or IV administration.

- Oral:
  - 200–300 mcg/kg.
  - Onset 15–30 min.
  - Duration up to 2 hours.
  - Some sedation but usually combined with a sedative drug.
- IV:
  - 100–200 mcg/kg IV.
  - Onset time 5–10 min.
  - May be titrated to effect (starting with 100 mcg/kg with further increments of 50 mcg IV up to 200 mcg/kg) for painful procedures in combination with another sedative drug.
  - When given with a benzodiazepine there is a high incidence of side effects (over sedation and respiratory depression) and so the dose must be reduced.

Fentanyl

Fentanyl, alfentanil and remifentanil are potent IV opioids with a rapid onset that should only be used by staff with training and current experience in paediatric airway management and ventilation. If the pain associated with the procedure requires these potent drugs then a general anaesthetic may be a safer option.

Anaesthetic agents

Thiopental and propofol

- Potent IV anaesthetic agents licensed for use only by staff with training in paediatric anaesthesia and current relevant skills. They produce a high incidence of apnoea, airway obstruction, and hypoxia.
- Target controlled infusion programmes for propofol are being developed for children for use by anaesthetists.

Ketamine

- A potent 'dissociative' anaesthetic agent used for sedation, anaesthesia, and analgesia.
- Oral, IM, and IV administration.
- Since airway obstruction, respiratory depression and apnoea are less likely than with other anaesthetic agents ketamine has become popular worldwide for non-anaesthetists to administer for painful procedures requiring sedation and cooperation.
- However, it does produce adverse effects—copious airway secretions and occasional laryngospasm and apnoea. Safe use as a sedative requires administration in accordance with an appropriate protocol and the ability to manage the occasional airway complications that occur.
- An antisialogogue is often administered simultaneously to reduce airway secretions.
- Emergence delirium is believed to be less common in children than in adults but this may be a reflection of difficulty in assessment.

- Oral 5 mg/kg (often with midazolam).
- Intramuscularly 4–5 mg/kg.
- IV 1–2 mg/kg.

Nitrous oxide

- Inhalational anaesthetic agent.
- Onset is rapid (30–60 sec).
- Produces anxiolysis, analgesia and sedation.
- Patients must be cooperative.
- Concentrations of 30–70% are used.
- When used in accordance with an appropriate protocol and without other sedatives or analgesics nitrous oxide is extremely safe and practically devoid of respiratory and cardiovascular side effects.
- Nitrous oxide is a highly diffusible gas causing expansion of air pockets.
- Contraindications:
  - Bowel obstruction
  - Pneumothorax
  - Pnemoperitoneum
  - Intracranial air (after skull fracture or surgery)
  - Pulmonary cysts or bullae.
- Adequate scavenging is required to protect staff from the potential effects of long-term exposure.

Others

Chloral hydrate

- Dose 25–100 mg/kg oral.
- Onset time 45–60 min.
- Duration of action 60–120 min.
- Dose can be repeated after 30 min 25–50 mg/kg to a maximum total of 2 g or 100 mg/kg (whichever is less).
- It has an unpleasant taste and can cause gastric irritation.

Triclofos

- Dose 30–50 mg/kg oral.
- Prodrug of trichloroethanol.
- Weaker than chloral hydrate (1 g triclofos = 600 mg chloral hydrate).
- Less gastric irritation.

Melatonin

- Induces natural sleep for MRI or EEG investigations.
- Variable dose 2–10 mg oral.

Antihistamines and phenothiazines

Such as trimeprazine, promethazine and chlorpromazine are rarely used. They act on several receptors, have unpredictable effects, and a long duration of action. If given with opioids, hypotension and apnoea may occur.

Key references and further reading

Chapters 2 and 8

Litz, RJ, Popp M, Stehr SN, et al. Successful resuscitation of a patient with ropivacaine-induced asystole after axillary plexus block using lipid infusion. Anaesthesia 2006; **61**: 800–1.

Rosenblatt MA, M Abel, GW Fischer et al.. Successful use of a 20% lipid emulsion to resuscitate a patient after presumed bupivacaine-related cardiac arrest. Anesthesiology 2006; **105**: 217–18.

Weinberg G, Hertz P, and Newman J. Lipid, not propofol, treats bupivacaine overdose. Anesthesia and Analgesia 2004; **99**:1875–1876.

Weinberg G. Lipid infusion resuscitation for local anesthetic toxicity: proof of clinical efficacy. Anesthesiology 2006; **105**: 7–8.

Chapter 3

Forsyth I, Bergesio R, and Chambers NA. Attention-deficit hyperactivity disorder and anaesthesia. Pediatric Anesthesia 2006; **16**: 371–3.

Chapter 4

Arafat M and Mattoo TK. Measurement of blood pressure in children: recommendations and perceptions on cuff selection. Pediatrics 1999; **104**: 30–4.

Fine GF and Borland LM. The future of the cuffed endotracheal tube. Paediatric Anaesthesia 2004; **14**: 38–42.

Chapter 6

Baker C and Wong D. QUESTT: a process of pain assessment in children. Orthopaedic Nursing 1987; **6**: 11–21.

Chapter 7

Dalens B, Vanneuville G, and Tanguy A. Comparison of the fascia iliaca compartment block with the 3-in-1 block in children. Anesthesia & Analgesia 1989; **69**: 705–13.

Marhofer P, Greher M, and Kapral S. Ultrasound guidance in regional anaesthesia. British Journal of Anaesthesia 2005; **94**: 7–17.

Retzl G, Kapral S, Greher M, et al. Ultrasonographic findings of the axillary part of the brachial plexus. Anesthesia & Analgesia 2001; **92**: 1271–5.

Schwemmer U, Markus CK, Greim CA, et al. Sonographic imaging of the sciatic nerve and its division in the popliteal fossa in children. Paediatric Anaesthesia 2004; **14**: 1005–8.

Van Schoor AN, Boon JM, Bosenberg AT, et al. Anatomical considerations of the pediatric ilioinguinal/iliohypogastric nerve block. Pediatric Anesthesia 2005; **15**: 371–7.

Willschke H, Marhofer P, Bosenberg A, et al. Ultrasonography for ilioinguinal/iliohypogastric nerve blocks in children. British Journal of Anaesthesia 2005; **95**: 226–30.

Willschke H, Bösenberg A, Marhofer P, et al. Ultrasonography-guided rectus sheath block in paediatric anaesthesia – a new approach to an old technique. British Journal of Anaesthesia 2006; **97**: 244–9.

Chapter 10

Corbett IP, Ramacciato JC, Groppo FC, et al. Local anaesthetic use among GDPs. British Dental Journal 2005; **199:** 784–7.

Pawar DK and Marraro GA. One lung ventilation in infants and children: experience with Marraro double lumen tube. Pediatric Anesthesia 2005; **15:** 204–208.

Scottish Executive. An Action Plan for Dental Services in Scotland 2000.

Chapter 14

Rowney DA. Interhospital transfer of critically ill children. CPD Anaesthesia 2005; **7(2):** 69–76.

Chapter 15

Allt JE and Howell CJ. Down's syndrome. BJA CEPD reviews 2003; **3(3):** 83–6.

Ames WA, Mayou BJ, and Williams K. Anaesthetic management of epidermolysis bullosa. British Journal of Anaesthesia 1999; **82(5):** 746–51.

Cardwell M and Walker RWM. Management of the difficult paediatric airway. BJA CEPD reviews 2003; **3(6):** 167–70.

Dixon M. Treacher Collins syndrome. Journal of Medical Genetics 1995; **32(10):** 806–8.

Fernanda F and Cimaz R. Juvenile rheumatoid arthritis. Current Opinion in Rheumatology 2000; **12:** 415–19.

Firth PG. Anaesthesia for peculiar cells – a century of sickle cell disease. British Journal of Anaesthesia 2005; **95(3):** 287–99.

Gormley S and Crean P. Basic principles of anaesthesia for neonates and infants. British Journal of Anaesthesia 2001; **1(5):** 130–3.

Gratix AP and Enright SM. Epilepsy in anaesthesia and intensive care. BJA CEPD reviews 2005; **5(4):** 118–21.

Green DW and Ashley EMC. The choice of inhalational anaesthetic for major abdominal surgery in children with liver disease. Paediatric Anaesthesia 2002; **12(8):** 665–73.

Hata T and Michael M. Cervical spine considerations when anesthetizing patients with Down syndrome. Anesthesiology 2005; **102(3):** 680–5.

Kumar RJ. Anaesthetic considerations in patients with hepatic failure. International Anesthesiology Clinics 2005; **43(4):** 45–63.

Laguna P and Klukowska A. Management of oral bleedings with recombinant factor VIIa in children with haemophilia A and inhibitor. Haemophilia 2005; **11(1):** 2–4.

Lethagen S, Flordal P, Van Aken H, et al. The UK guidelines for the use of desmopressin in patients with von Willebrand's disease. European Journal of Anaesthesiology 1997; **14(14):** 19–22.

McAnulty GR, Robertshaw HJ, and Hall GM. Anaesthetic management of patients with diabetes mellitus. *British Journal of Anaesthesia* 2000; **85(1):** 80–90.

Manucci PM. Drug therapy: Treatment of von Willebrand's disease. *New England Journal of Medicine* 2004; **351(7):** 683–94.

Martin S and Tobias JD. Perioperative care of the child with arthrogryposis. *Pediatric Anesthesia* 2006; **16(1):** 31–7.

Moores C, Rogers JG, McKenzie IM, *et al.* Anaesthesia for children with mucopolysaccharidoses. *Anaesthesia and Intensive Care* 1996; **24(4):** 459–63.

Morgan KA, Rehman MA, and Schwartz RE. Morquio's syndrome and its anaesthetic considerations. *Paediatric Anaesthesia* 2002; **12(7):** 641–4.

Muraika L, Heyman JS, and Shevchenko Y. Fiberoptic tracheal intubation through a laryngeal mask airway in a child with Treacher Collins syndrome. *Anesthesia & Analgesia* 2003; **97(5):** 1298–9.

Schwartz D, Schwartz T, Cooper E, *et al.* Anaesthesia and the child with HIV infection. *Canadian Journal of Anaesthesia* 1991; **38(5):** 626–33.

Tracy MR, Dormans JP, and Kusumi K. Klippel–Feil syndrome: clinical features and current understanding of etiology. *Clinical Orthopaedics & Related Research* 2004; **424:** 183–90.

Tubridy N, Fontaine B, and Eymard B. Congenital myopathies and congenital muscular dystrophies. *Current Opinion in Neurology* 2001; **14(5):** 575–82.

White MC and Stoddart PA. Anesthesia for thymectomy in children with myasthenia gravis. *Pediatric Anesthesia* 2004; **14(8):** 625–35.

Wraith JE. The mucopolysaccharidoses: a clinical review and guide to management. *Archives of Disease in Childhood* 1995; **72(3):** 263–7.

Wongprasartsuk P and Stevens J. Cerebral palsy and anaesthesia. *Paediatric Anaesthesia* 2002; **12:** 296–303.

Chapter 16

Krauss B, Green SM. Procedural sedation in children. *Lancet* 2006; **367:** 766–80.

SIGN. Safe Sedation of Children Undergoing Diagnostic and Therapeutic Procedures. A national clinical guideline. Scottish Intercollegiate Guidelines Network 58, May 2004. Available at: www.sign.ac.uk/guidelines/published/index.html

Sury MRJ, Harker H, and Begent J, *et al.*. The management of infants and children for painless imaging. *Clinical Radiology* 2005; **60:** 731–41.

Index